The Doctors Book® of

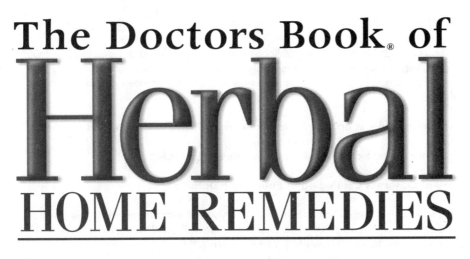

Herbal
HOME REMEDIES

Cure yourself with nature's most powerful healing agents

ADVICE FROM **200** EXPERTS ON MORE THAN **140** CONDITIONS

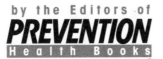

by the Editors of
PREVENTION
Health Books®

Foreword by VARRO E. TYLER, Ph.D., Sc.D.

RODALE

Library of Congress Cataloging-in-Publication Data

The doctors book of herbal home remedies : cure yourself with nature's most powerful healing agents : advice from 200 experts on more than 140 conditions / by the editors of Prevention Health Books ; foreword by Varro E. Tyler.
     p.   cm.
   title: Herbal home remedies.
   Includes index.
   ISBN 1–57954–096–1 hardcover
    1. Herbs—Therapeutic use. 2. Traditional medicine. I. Title: Herbal home remedies.
II. Prevention Health Books.
RM666.H33 D625 1999
615'.321—dc21
                                             99–050051

Distributed to the book trade by St. Martin's Press

2 4 6 8 10 9 7 5 3 1 hardcover

Visit us on the Web at www.rodaleremedies.com, or call us toll-free at (800) 848-4735.

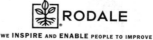

RODALE
WE INSPIRE AND ENABLE PEOPLE TO IMPROVE
THEIR LIVES AND THE WORLD AROUND THEM

About *Prevention* Health Books

The editors of *Prevention* Health Books are dedicated to providing you with authoritative, trustworthy, and innovative advice for a healthy, active lifestyle. In all of our books, our goal is to keep you thoroughly informed about the latest breakthroughs in natural healing, medical research, alternative health, herbs, nutrition, fitness, and weight loss. We cut through the confusion of today's conflicting health reports to deliver clear, concise, and definitive health information that you can trust. And we explain in practical terms what each new breakthrough means to you so that you can take immediate, practical steps to improve your health and well-being.

Every recommendation in *Prevention* Health Books is based upon interviews with highly qualified health authorities, including medical doctors and practitioners of alternative medicine. In addition, we consult with the *Prevention* Health Books Board of Advisors to ensure that all of the health information is safe, practical, and up-to-date. *Prevention* Health Books are thoroughly factchecked for accuracy, and we make every effort to verify recommendations, dosages, and cautions.

The advice in this book will help keep you well-informed about your personal choices in health care—to help you lead a happier, healthier, and longer life.

Notice

This book is intended as a reference volume only, not as a medical manual. The information given here is designed to help adults make informed decisions about their health. It is not intended as a substitute for any treatment that may have been prescribed by your doctor. You should consult your physician or a physician with expertise in herbs before treating yourself with herbs or combining them with any medications. Women who are pregnant or are considering becoming pregnant should not use herbs or other medications without seeking the approval of their doctors. If you suspect that you have a medical problem, we urge you to seek competent medical help.

The Doctors Book of Herbal Home Remedies Staff

EDITOR: Stephen C. George

WRITERS: Kelly Garrett, Doug Hill, Joely Johnson, Larry Keller, Diane Gardiner Kozak, Christian Millman, Julia VanTine, Judith West

CONTRIBUTING WRITERS: Barbara Loecher, Jordan Matus, Melinda Rizzo

ART DIRECTOR: Darlene Schneck

COVER AND BOOK DESIGNER: Lynn N. Gano

BOOK PROJECT RESEARCHER: Carol J. Gilmore

EDITORIAL RESEARCHERS: Elizabeth A. Brown, Adrien Drozdowski, Jan Eickmeier, Staci Hadeed-Sander, Grete Haentjens, Lois Guarino Hazel, Karen Jacob, Jennifer Bright Kaas, Terry Sutton Kravitz, Mary S. Mesaros, Deborah Pedron, Elizabeth B. Price, Paula Rasich, Elizabeth Shimer, Lucille Uhlman, Nancy Zelko, Shea Zukowski

SENIOR COPY EDITOR: Jane Sherman

LAYOUT DESIGNER: Donna G. Rossi

ASSOCIATE STUDIO MANAGER: Thomas P. Aczel

MANUFACTURING COORDINATORS: Brenda Miller, Jodi Schaffer, Patrick Smith

Rodale Healthy Living Books

VICE PRESIDENT AND PUBLISHER: Brian Carnahan

EDITORIAL DIRECTOR: Michael Ward

VICE PRESIDENT AND MARKETING DIRECTOR: Karen Arbegast

PRODUCT MARKETING DIRECTOR: Denyse Corelli

BOOK MANUFACTURING DIRECTOR: Helen Clogston

MANUFACTURING MANAGERS: Eileen Bauder, Mark Krahforst

RESEARCH MANAGER: Ann Gossy Yermish

COPY MANAGER: Lisa D. Andruscavage

PRODUCTION MANAGER: Robert V. Anderson Jr.

OFFICE MANAGER: Jacqueline Dornblaser

OFFICE STAFF: Julie Kehs, Mary Lou Stephen, Catherine E. Strouse

Prevention Health Books Board of Advisors

Jeffrey R. Lisse, M.D.
Professor of medicine and director of the division of rheumatology at the University of Texas Medical Branch at Galveston

Susan Olson, Ph.D.
Clinical psychologist, transition therapist, and weight-management consultant in Seattle

David P. Rose, M.D., Ph.D., D.Sc.
Chief of the division of nutrition and endocrinology at Naylor Dana Institute, part of the American Health Foundation, in Valhalla, New York, and an expert on nutrition and cancer for the National Cancer Institute and the American Cancer Society

Maria A. Fiatarone Singh, M.D.
Scientist I in the nutrition, exercise physiology, and sarcopenia laboratory at the Jean Mayer USDA Human Nutrition Research Center on Aging at Tufts University in Boston, associate professor at Tufts University School of Nutrition Science and Policy in Medford, Massachusetts, and professor of exercise and sports science and medicine at the School of Health Sciences at the University of Sydney in Australia

Yvonne S. Thornton, M.D.
Associate clinical professor of obstetrics and gynecology at Columbia University College of Physicians and Surgeons in New York City and director of the perinatal diagnostic testing center at Morristown Memorial Hospital in New Jersey

Lila Amdurska Wallis, M.D., M.A.C.P.
Clinical professor of medicine at Weill Medical College of Cornell University in New York City, past president of the American Medical Women's Association, founding president of the National Council on Women's Health, director of continuing medical education programs for physicians, and Master and Laureate of the American College of Physicians

Andrew T. Weil, M.D.
Director of the program in integrative medicine and clinical professor of internal medicine at the University of Arizona College of Medicine in Tucson

Douglas Whitehead, M.D.
Associate clinical professor of urology at Albert Einstein College of Medicine in the Bronx, associate attending physician in urology at Beth Israel Medical Center and co-founder and director of the Association for Male Sexual Dysfunction, both in New York City

Richard J. Wood, Ph.D.
Laboratory chief of the mineral bioavailability laboratory at the Jean Mayer USDA Human Nutrition Research Center on Aging at Tufts University in Boston and associate professor at the Tufts University School of Nutrition Science and Policy in Medford, Massachusetts

FOREWORD

HERBAL KNOWLEDGE YOU CAN TRUST

*S*ome readers will surely ask, "Why?" Why bother to make such a comprehensive collection of herbal folk remedies recommended by doctors for conditions ranging from aches and pains to yeast infections and everything in between? Aren't conventional remedies enough? If these things really worked, wouldn't they be part of mainstream medicine by now?

All of these are good questions that require answers.

History tells us that when observers first encounter any kind of culture different from their own, the natural reaction is to discard or discredit everything unfamiliar. People are distrustful of anything beyond their previous experience. New ideas are hard to sell. Early European settlers in the New World discounted the medicinal remedies of Native Americans because they involved unfamiliar plants. In doing so, much of the value of these healing remedies was neglected or lost. Dr. Albert Schweitzer said it very well: "In the hope of reaching the moon, men fail to see the flowers that blossom at their feet."

Indeed, it was only after many years that herbs found their way back into common use. Echinacea, goldenseal, saw palmetto, valerian, and garlic are good examples, and their use is now based on scientific and clinical studies. In several advanced nations—the United States is an exception—these and scores of other herbs are actually approved as drugs. There are numerous other herbs that work, too. We know that they work, thanks to decades of experience and anecdotal evidence.

That said, it must be readily admitted that while some herbal remedies are effective, others are not. Even the staunchest herbal advocates probably do not believe that carrying a buckeye or horse chestnut around in your pocket will ward off rheumatism or arthritis. Many such folk cures rely more on magic than on medicine.

These and other totally off-the-wall cures are not detailed in this book. That's because its 200 contributors were required to have some kind of training in herbal medicine in order to be consulted. They possess a wide variety of qualifications and degrees (M.D., N.D., Ph.D., Pharm D., and so forth) that provide the critical reader with some reassurance of the validity of the information presented. Many compilations of home remedies exist, but *The Doctors Book of Herbal Home Remedies* is unique because of the qualifications of the contributors. It's truly an herbal practitioners' book.

In the pages that follow, however, you will find much more than a compilation of herbal remedies from herbal experts. There is a chapter dealing with buying and using herbs, a list of reputable suppliers, and information on proper use of herbs. A brief summary of essential information about each of the specific health problems covered is also included for the busy reader. In short, the volume is easy to read and to understand. It is definitely user-friendly.

There is another value to a book of this sort, although it is one that is frequently overlooked. Much of the information on the home use of herbal remedies is fast disappearing from the American scene. The local drugstore is simply too convenient, and people are subjected to a continual barrage of propaganda in the various media that promotes numerous synthetic drugs. So instead of using an oatmeal bath to soothe itching skin, we buy a tube of antihistamine cream. It's easier to take an aspirin for a headache than to prepare a four-ingredient herbal tea. *The Doctors Book of Herbal Home Remedies* thus becomes an interesting repository of information, but it's my hope that this "home doctor book" will also serve as a basic sourcebook for physicians and scientists seeking new and effective cures for various diseases and conditions. In that way, some of the home remedies that you'll read about here may one day become a true part of mainstream medical practice.

I dislike long forewords to good books because they delay me from getting to the significant information that follows. Go ahead and read the rest of the book. The contents speak for themselves.

Varro E. Tyler

Varro E. Tyler, Ph.D., Sc.D.
Distinguished professor emeritus of pharmacognosy
Purdue University, West Lafayette, Indiana

CONTENTS

Part 1

USING HERBS AT HOME

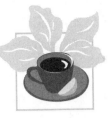

THE EVIDENCE
FOR HERBS

*Y*ou feel a cold coming on, so you take generous amounts of the herb echinacea—and feel well on your way to recovery.

You rub some liquid from an aloe plant on that nasty little burn your kitchen stove inflicted upon you—and lo and behold, it heals faster than anything you've experienced since childhood.

Too much anxiety is keeping you awake at night, so you swallow a 150-milligram capsule of powdered valerian twice a day—and soon find yourself calm and rested, without feeling groggy.

Those are just a humble handful of an uncountable number of natural remedies from the plant kingdom that are yours for the healing. "For a majority of your medical problems, there is a reasonably effective and safe medicine somewhere in the herbal world that you can apply yourself at home," says David Field, N.D., a naturopathic physician, licensed acupuncturist, and president of the California Association of Naturopathic Physicians in Santa Rosa. "That's good news."

As we all know, good news travels fast. Herbs have become the medicines of choice for so many people in recent years that the coinage "herbal renaissance" has taken its place right alongside "information age" as a defining description of our times. You are not alone in your interest in the healing power of herbs.

The best guess is that you're sharing that interest with about 60 million Americans. That's how many people—about one-third of the

U.S. adult population—use herbs medicinally, according to a national survey commissioned by *Prevention* magazine. And they use them for lots of common ailments, from allergies to premenstrual syndrome, from diarrhea to depression.

What's more, the boom is just beginning. "In the next 10 years, you're going to see herbal medicine really explode," says William Warnock, N.D., director of the Champlain Center for Natural Medicine in Shelburne, Vermont. "We're still at the bottom part of a curve that's sloping up, and we have a long way to go before we reach the top."

If *renaissance* means "rebirth," then herbal renaissance is indeed an apt description of what's going on. "Herbs have always been part of human culture," says Mark Blumenthal, executive director of the American Botanical Council in Austin, Texas, and editor of *Herbal-Gram*, a peer-reviewed quarterly journal on medicinal plants. "We are reawakening basic human wisdom. We are re-understanding and re-accessing our heritage, which is the use of plants for medicine."

The phrase "plants for medicine" is pretty good shorthand for what herbal remedies are all about. It's true that etymological conservatives may still insist on defining "herb" as a nonwoody plant that withers to the ground after flowering, but in the real world, when we talk about herbs, we're talking about much more than that. "An herb is any plant that can be used for medicine or nutrition," says Mary Bove, N.D., a naturopathic physician at the Brattleboro Naturopathic Clinic in Vermont and a member of Britain's National Institute of Medical Herbalists. "And that can be anything from a mushroom to an apple tree."

To be considered medicinal (not nutritional or culinary), an herb must have health benefits that come from something more than normal food doses, says Connie Catellani, M.D., medical director of the Miro Center for Integrative Medicine in Evanston, Illinois. "Adding garlic to your food regularly may offer some herbal benefits, but you need a stronger dose if you hope to speed recovery from the flu or lower blood pressure levels," she says.

Of course, not all plants are therapeutic, but those that are number in the thousands. Medicinal value is not only found in all types of plants (flowering plants, seaweed, trees, fungi, shrubs, and so forth), it can also show up in all *parts* of a plant—the leaves, stem, roots, flowers, seeds, fruit, or rhizome (the underground part of the stem).

Furthermore, you have lots of options for getting those benefits out of the plant and into your body. You can make a tea from just about any plant part. You can swallow plant material in capsules, drink it as a tincture, apply it as a poultice or salve, inhale it as steam or essential oil, drink it as juice, or just eat it.

Even with all the sophisticated delivery systems, though, it's the plant, not the technology, that cures. The chamomile that you grow on your windowsill or buy fresh from your local health food store may serve your needs better than the most rigidly measured standardized herb extract coming out of a "phytomedicine" laboratory.

"That's because most herbs have a multitude of active ingredients that work synergistically to provide a balanced action," says Chanchal Cabrera, a member of Britain's National Institute of Medical Herbalists, a professional member of the American Herbalists Guild, and an herbalist in Vancouver. Some of these naturally occurring ingredients even help to protect against the overly powerful effects of others, thus providing a natural system of checks and balances, according to Cabrera.

"Herbs are the most democratic form of medicine there is. Anyone with a good plant identification book and access to unpolluted fields and woods can harvest their own herbs and make their own medicines," she says.

HERB APPEAL

The deduction is simple: Interest in herbal medicine is soaring worldwide because more and more people are becoming convinced of herbs' therapeutic value. The *Prevention* magazine poll found that a majority (53 percent) of herbal remedy consumers consider herbs to be just as effective as or more effective than conventional medicines.

"Results have contributed to the trend. What we do works," says David McLeod, an herbalist and acupuncturist who is president of the National Herbalists Association of Australia in Sydney.

Still, the fact remains that herbs themselves aren't much more effective today than they were a few decades ago or even a few millennia ago. If they have always worked, why are so many of us turning to herbal medicine now?

There are lots of answers.

Herbs are often safer. In fact, when compared with pharmaceutical drugs, there's no contest. "Looking at the weight of the evidence, conventional medicines are potentially much more harmful than herbs," says Robert Rufsvold, M.D., a family practitioner at the New England Center for Integrative Health in Lyme, New Hampshire.

That doesn't mean, though, that you can swallow any piece of flora without consequences. "Natural" does not always equal "harmless." In fact, some herbs have the potential for abuse. Others are downright toxic.

Herbs have fewer side effects. Most herbs are gentle and often have no side effects, herbal practitioners point out. That can seldom be said for pharmaceutical drugs. "A lot of people who perhaps should be treated with conventional medicine just can't tolerate it because of the side effects," says McLeod.

Herbs offer an option. For all of the wonders that it works, modern conventional medicine has disillusioned its share of people. If it's not the side effects, it's the expense, the impersonal approach, or the occasional ineffectiveness. "One reason for the growing popularity of herbal medicine is simply the health-care consumer's growing dissatisfaction with conventional medicine," says Shiva Barton, N.D., a licensed acupuncturist and lead naturopathic practitioner at Wellspace, a complementary health center in Cambridge, Massachusetts.

The desire for an option is not limited to patients. "Every time I write a prescription, I have to think if there is an alternative to a pharmaceutical drug," says Dr. Rufsvold. "Is there something else that might also work? Something that might not be as powerful or act as fast but might be safer?"

Herbs dig deeper. "There's more of a desire today to promote health rather than just manage disease," notes Maureen Williams, N.D., a naturopathic physician in Quechee, Vermont. Herbal medicine generally does just that, by working with the body to treat underlying conditions rather than simply covering up symptoms or killing germs (although herbs can do those things, too).

"Too often, we M.D.'s are apt to just jump in and try to fix things rather than working with the body's natural healing ability," Dr.

Rufsvold says. "Of course, sometimes that is necessary, depending upon the acuteness and severity of the illness or injury. But for many less severe or chronic conditions, a gentler, safer approach should be considered."

Herbs are natural. It's hard to imagine anything more natural than a plant, and more and more people want it that way. "If you're trying to live a more natural lifestyle, you want your medicine to somehow reflect that," says Amy Rothenberg, N.D., a naturopathic physician in Enfield, Connecticut. "Herbs fit that bill."

Herbs work at home. Naturopathic doctors and other qualified herbal practitioners can help you improve your health. Qualified herbal practitioners include medical doctors and pharmacists who have studied herbal medicine, naturopathic doctors, doctors of oriental medicine (O.M.D.'s) or people certified in Chinese herbology, and herbalists who are members of professional herbal organizations around the world, such as the American Herbalists Guild and Britain's National Institute of Medical Herbalists. But herbs also let you help yourself, in the privacy of your own home. "If you go to the health food store and get an herb, you're very likely to achieve some success," Dr. Warnock says. "Part of the appeal is being able to gain some control over your health destiny. "

That doesn't mean that all conditions are self-treatable or even herb-treatable, but, says Cabrera, "If you have a simple, self-limiting condition that you would normally be quite confident to self-medicate with a conventional over-the-counter product from the drugstore, that's a good and safe time to treat yourself with herbs."

How Herbs Work

Herbs work differently than drugs do, with a different goal. So it's a mistake—albeit a common one—to misjudge the efficiency of herbal medicine by comparing the results to what conventional medicine might have done in the same situation. "It isn't a question of substituting an herb for a pharmaceutical drug," says Dr. Catellani.

What's the difference? Mostly this: While conventional medicine attacks the disease, herbal medicine works with the body's natural

A Brief History
of Herbal Medicine

*M*ankind's love affair with herbs goes back a lot farther than the use of medicinal plants by neolithic types around 10,000 B.C. If you really want to start at the beginning, you have to go back to early evolutionary times, before humans were humans.

Plants may have jumped off to a big head start, but flora and fauna have been evolving together for hundreds of millions of years. It's that longest of long-term relationships, practitioners of natural medicine say, that makes plants a body's best friend.

Our metabolic systems evolved at the same time that plants began to synthesize a greater and more complex number of organic compounds, believes David Field, N.D., a naturopathic physician, licensed acupuncturist, and president of the California Association of Naturopathic Physicians in Santa Rosa. "Thus, we're used to plants and we know how to work with them. That's why herbal medicine exists."

Once mankind settled down, it didn't take long to discover this beneficial coexistence. Of all the very old civilizations that developed herbal medicine, those in China and India mean the most to us today, for the simple reason that we still use herbal remedies from their extremely sophisticated medical systems. Ginseng is a shining example.

Later, in classical times, when Greeks and Romans were laying the foundation for Western medicine, medicinal plants remained key. Hippocrates listed some 400 of them, many of which, such as garlic, hawthorn, and thyme, are still important today. Galen, often hailed as the father of modern medicine, connected plant

healing process. Hence, an antibiotic will kill off bacteria, but an herbal treatment such as echinacea will support your immune system in resisting the infection.

Isn't an antibiotic faster? Probably, "but that's like comparing ap-

qualities to the four bodily "humors"—choleric, phlegmatic, melancholic, and sanguine. The Greek botanist Dioscorides compiled a materia medica (a compendium of medicinal plants) in the first century A.D. that was considered authoritative in some circles until the middle of the nineteenth century.

Such herbals dominated European popular medicine throughout the Middle Ages, giving way to more learned pharmacopoeia when science started taking off in the seventeenth century. Meanwhile, in the Western Hemisphere, Native Americans on both continents developed a rich tradition of herbal medicine.

In the modern New World, herbal and other natural medicines vied with what would become "conventional" medicine until the quasi-official Flexner Report in 1910 canonized the latter and effectively suppressed the former. This was soon followed by a technological revolution so stunning in its medical advancements that herbal medicine was relegated to quaint folklore.

The suppression began to shift in the 1960s, as so many things did. "In the 1960s, people started questioning whether technology had all the answers," says William Warnock, N.D., director of the Champlain Center for Natural Medicine in Shelburne, Vermont. "Then it became a progression from questioning in the 1970s what technology was doing to the outer environment to questioning in the 1980s what it was doing to the inner environment—our bodies."

ples to oranges," Dr. Catellani says. "The echinacea may work more slowly, but you're building up antibodies, you're increasing immune system activity, and you're much less likely to get the next thing that comes around. "

In other words, an antibiotic may "defeat" a disease, but the herb makes you healthier.

None of this is to say, though, that herbs can't work in the same length of time as a conventional drug. Dr. Catellani cites the natural antidepressant St. John's wort as an example of an herb that acts at least as fast as its pharmaceutical cousin. And, although natural medicine as a rule addresses the underlying causes of an ailment rather than hiding the symptoms, lots of herbs make you feel better right away. This book includes many remedies that do just that.

Still, herbs work best if you adjust your mindset to the natural way of doing things. "Herbs stimulate the body to act optimally," Dr. Williams says. "They are generally used to move the body toward health, not to force change. If force is needed, such as in life-threatening situations, herbal medicine is not adequate."

That simple fact—that herbal medicine and conventional medicine each has its place—has created integrative medicine, which offers the best of both treatment worlds. This promising new marriage moves herbal medicine and other natural modalities away from the medical fringes and toward the mainstream.

"I refer people to M.D.'s, and they send people to me," says Dr. Field, "and there's nothing better than doing both systems when appropriate."

Because herbs work naturally and gently with few side effects, they're usually the right first choice, according to Dr. Field. "The best approach is to use the least invasive procedure first, such as herbs," he says. "But there are times when herbal medicine alone is not adequate."

THE CASE FOR HERBS

The increasing popularity of integrative medicine logically implies a growing acceptance of herbs by conventional physicians. Indeed, in European countries such as France, Italy, Austria, and Switzerland, natural remedies are regularly prescribed by M.D.'s. Germany has taken the global lead in modern scientific research on herbs.

Most of the evidence for medicinal herbs is still empirical (the result of practical observation) rather than scientific (based on con-

Herbs in the Bible

*I*t happens every Christmas. Some overcheered caroler insists on asking anyone who'll listen, "Just what *were* frankincense and myrrh, anyway?"

Well, you can tell the wag that they were—and are—medicinal plants. True, the Three Wise Men may have had the sweet-smelling incense properties of these gummy tree resins in mind when they took them as gifts to Bethlehem, but both were also used as antiseptics in biblical times. In fact, says Blair Montague-Drake, an herbalist in Kendall, Australia, and author of *A Biblical Herbal: The Greatest Herbal Story Ever Told*, the Israelites applied soothing solutions of myrrh to the fresh circumcisions of conquered enemies forced to convert to Judaism. That, too, was no doubt considered something of a gift at that most uncomfortable moment.

These are gifts that have kept on giving. Myrrh was a treatment for anemia in Elizabethan times, and it's still used today as a mild herbal stimulant, among other things. Frankincense, as *Boswellia serrata*, is an anti-inflammatory that's still helping people with asthma.

Good ol' frankincense and myrrh are just two of the scores of medicinal plants referred to in the Bible, proving that there's not much new under the sun, herbally speaking. A garden description in the Song of Solomon, for example, is herb-filled: ". . . Spikenard and saffron, calamus and cinnamon, with all trees of frankincense; myrrh and aloes . . ." Today, we benefit from all of those, although we may call spikenard (*Aralia nudicaulis*) wild sarsaparilla and calamus (*Acorus calamus*) sweet flag.

trolled experiments). For most M.D.'s—even those open to herbal alternatives—that's not good enough.

"The larger body of evidence for herbs is based on thousands of years of use, with a kind of empirical knowledge developing around that," Dr. Rufsvold says. "But from a purely scientific point of view, there's not as much research as many of us would like to see, and that includes natural practitioners as well as conventional physicians."

Nevertheless, herbs have a lot more research behind them than ever before. "Despite sorely limited funding, scientific research is increasingly verifying the safety and efficacy of herbal medicine," Dr. Williams says. "They are 'proving,' in effect, what was already known empirically."

Not surprisingly, some of the better-known medicinal plants are some of the most thoroughly studied. Examples include ginkgo, saw palmetto, garlic, black cohosh, and ginger. One 1997 ginkgo study on Alzheimer's patients, published in the *Journal of the American Medical Association*, provides some good insight into both the promise and the problem of still nascent scientific herbal research.

"Going by the standard cognitive measures, the patients taking the ginkgo extract seemed to do a little better compared to the placebo group," says Linda Hershey, M.D., Ph.D., professor of neurology at the State University of New York at Buffalo and chief of neurology at the Buffalo Veterans Affairs Medical Center. "What was most remarkable was that the relatives or caretakers—the ones who were actually with the patients more—saw a much more dramatic improvement with ginkgo than the doctors did." The journal report was accompanied by an editorial note hailing ginkgo as "an intriguing addition to the drugs thought to be helpful" for patients with Alzheimer's disease.

Still, Dr. Hershey cautions, more of this kind of research has to accumulate in order for ginkgo or any other herbal medicine to gain widespread medical acceptance. "This study alone didn't make doctors jump up and down," she says. "In general, there's not enough evidence to move doctors to begin prescribing herbs, but there's certainly enough to encourage further research."

Remember, Dr. Rufsvold says, that the purpose of such further research is to seek the truth and promote better health, not just to vindicate herbal medicine. "As we study herbals, hopefully we will gain an even larger body of evidence for their efficacy and safety," he says. "But I also suspect that in doing the studies, we may find that some of the herbs in common use today won't show the effectiveness we'd like to see. If so, they should be dropped."

So as the herbal renaissance blossoms, "don't go overboard" might qualify as good advice. There's a corollary piece of good advice, though: "Don't go underboard." Waiting for ironclad, proof-positive evidence for an otherwise safe herb that's been shown to work in the real world for centuries can be unnecessarily frustrating, says Dr. Rufsvold. "When you come right down to it, probably a majority of conventional medicines in our pharmacy today were not put to the standard of double-blind, placebo-controlled, randomized clinical trials," he explains, referring to the gold standard scientific test for a new drug. "So there's a tradition of empiricism in conventional medicine, too, and it's not necessarily a wrong one."

Or, as Dr. Barton puts it, "A lack of scientific proof is no reason for not using an herb that works. If it's safe and appears to be effective, why not?"

HOME HERBALISM 101

*H*erbal remedies have been around for a few thousand years or so, but it's never been easier to use them at home than it is right now.

Unlike your ancestors, you don't have to go traipsing through the woods for elusive flora or surrender your soul to some mysterious shaman. You don't have to change your religion, your politics, or your clothes. All you have to do is get to know some friendly medicinal herbs and make the decision to get involved with your own well-being.

"It's really just a question of taking control of your health again," says David Field, N.D., a naturopathic physician, licensed acupuncturist, and president of the California Association of Naturopathic Physicians in Santa Rosa.

AN EMBARRASSMENT OF HERBAL RICHES

The first thing that you've probably noticed about herbal medicine these days is that there are *lots* of options out there—lots of traditions (such as Western, Chinese, and Indian), lots of herbs themselves, and lots of ways to use them. It can seem bewildering.

But, truth be told, the sheer volume of choices makes it easier, not harder, to find the herbal remedy that's right for you. And since this book does most of the work for you by describing the best herbal remedies for whatever ails you, all you have to do is open your front door and let those herbs into your home.

In fact, you've probably already done it. "Look at your spice rack in the kitchen and realize that those are herbs and that some of those herbs have medicinal qualities," says Lorilee Schoenbeck, N.D., a naturopathic physician at the Champlain Center for Natural Medicine in Shelburne, Vermont. Then shift your gaze to the vegetable bin, where those garlic cloves, for example, have lots of medicinal uses. In fact, says Dr. Schoenbeck, "The most direct way to use herbs as medicine is actually to put them in your food. Think of herbs as concentrated foods, and the whole idea of herbal medicine is less intimidating." That's right, herbs are foods, and some foods—cranberry, oats, and others you'll find in this book—have herbal healing qualities.

Of course, the lion's share of herbal remedies aren't side dishes at dinner, so it helps to familiarize yourself with the most common ways to take your herbal medicine. Let's take a look.

TEAS: TAKING TIME TO HEAL

When you hear the word *extract* (as you often will in herbal medicine), remember that it's just a loose term for any method of getting the healing constituents out of a plant so that you can enjoy its benefits without eating it. And what's the easiest, most common, and often most pleasant way of extracting the good stuff from an herb? With hot water, of course.

That's right: The basic tea that you're so familiar with is one of the most oft-recommended herbal remedies you'll find. That very familiarity is one of its advantages. "The best herb form is the one you're most likely to use," says Amy Rothenberg, N.D., a naturopathic physician in Enfield, Connecticut.

Sure, making tea takes longer than popping a pill, but that's also a plus. "Sick people need to slow down," says Dr. Shoenbeck. "An additional therapeutic value of tea is that you have to pay attention to yourself at least long enough to make it and drink it." Also, you're more "involved" with the herb when you make tea—you see it, touch it, and taste it. "That's something you lose with pills," she says. "Actually tasting the herb can be an important part of the remedy. The taste activates something in you internally."

The problem is, teas sometimes activate your tastebuds when you'd rather they wouldn't. Certain medicinal teas taste great and others are neutral, but some are downright nasty. A lot, especially those from traditional Chinese medicine, even smell rank. "You start brewing up some of those Chinese herbs, and everyone else finds a good excuse to leave the house," says Robert Rufsvold, M.D., a family practitioner at the New England Center for Integrative Health in Lyme, New Hampshire. Fortunately, medical practitioners who prescribe herbs tend to take these things into account.

"When it comes to teas, I try to make them taste good," says Connie Catellani, M.D., medical director of the Miro Center for Integrative Medicine in Evanston, Illinois. "Taking a few drops of a bad-tasting medicine is one thing, but drinking two or three cups of it is something else."

TINCTURES: HEALING DROP BY DROP

Alcohol, as it happens, is nature's great extractor of an herb's healing properties. Thus, one of the best ways to take your herbal medicine is in an alcohol-based liquid extract called a tincture. Modern technology has improved the process considerably, but tinc-

Know Your Herbs By Name

*L*ike every other living thing on the planet, each herb has a botanical name in addition to its common name. So "*Silybum marianum*" and "milk thistle" refer to the same plant, kind of the way "John Wayne" and "The Duke" refer to the same man. The botanical name is always based on Latin and consists of two words. The first (*Silybum*) is capitalized and refers to the genus. The second (*marianum*) is lower case and narrows it down to the species. If there are several similar species in one genus, you'll see that indicated by "spp." If two species of the same genus are listed, you may see the genus abbreviated (*S. marianum*).

Now, that wasn't so hard, was it? The difficulty isn't mastering the botanical names; it's convincing yourself that they're worth bothering with. Our position is that your home herb preparation will be easier if you familiarize yourself with the botanical names of at least the herbs you'll be using. Here are some reasons.

To get the right herb. Sometimes, the same common name is used for two or more completely different herbs. Old man's beard is a common name for the lichen *Usnea spp.*,

tures are essentially the result of soaking an herb in alcohol for several weeks. They are widely available, easy to take, often recommended, and kind of nifty-looking in those smart little dark apothecary bottles capped with droppers.

Alcohol is such an efficient extractor that tinctures are usually more potent than teas. Virtually all of the properties of the plant itself are in the liquid, including the taste. Also, the absorption rate is swift, meaning that the healing constituents get into your bloodstream faster than with, say, pills.

Better yet, alcohol acts as a preservative as well as an extractor, so tinctures are long-lasting. The shelf life of herbs in other forms may

but it's also been used for other, totally unrelated plants, such as fringe-tree bark (*Chionanthus virginicus*). "You should know the botanical names so that when you go to the store, you get the right thing," says Rena Bloom, N.D., a naturopathic physician in Denver.

To use a mutual language. Many herbs have several common names. You may know a plant as bedstraw, your friends may call the same plant cleavers, and your grandmother may call it goose grass. All of you can call it *Galium aparine*.

To be specific. When you say "elder," you can be referring to several different species. *Sambucus canadensis* and *S. nigra* are both elder, but they have quite different effects and aren't used the same way in herbal medicine, according to Dr. Bloom. Without nailing down the precise species with the botanical name, you could end up taking the wrong medicine.

We've listed botanical names for all the herbs in this book in the chart on page 548. Whenever you need to familiarize yourself with the terminology for a specific herb, you can turn there for a quick reference.

be measured in months or even weeks, but some tinctures can sit in your medicine chest for several years and not lose a thing. Even non-alcohol, glycerin-based tinctures—often called glycerites—can last for several years when stored. So we're talking medical efficiency in the short run and cost efficiency in the long run.

Tincture doses are often given in drops, droppers, teaspoons, or milliliters. Most tinctures come in bottles with droppers that allow you to measure drops and sometimes milliliters. To ensure that you achieve the proper dosage when measuring in teaspoons, use a standard liquid measuring spoon, not a teaspoon from your silverware drawer, says Mark Stengler, N.D., a naturopathic physician in

Oceanside, California, and author of *The Natural Physician: Your Health Guide for Common Ailments*. Drugstores sell measuring spoons and dosing syringes marked with both teaspoons and milliliters. These may be easiest to find near the children's medicine section.

CAPSULES AND TABLETS: SWALLOWING HEALTH

One of the most convenient ways to get your herb dosage is with capsules or tablets. You know how to swallow a pill, it's easy to tell how much you're taking (just read the label), and these days, you can find herb capsules as easily as vitamins. With capsules or tablets, you make an end run around the bad-tasting herbs. You also avoid the alcohol that's in the majority of tinctures, which is an issue for some people.

A common capsule is simply filled with the dry powder of an herb that's been ground up. This isn't exactly the most effective herb form, though, since the process of grinding exposes more of the herb to air and makes it oxidize quickly. There's a good chance that it could lose most of its healing power by the time you buy it.

Technology has stepped in to build a better herb capsule. Processes such as freeze-drying yield a dry herbal extract that makes a more potent and stable capsule. "Freeze-dried extracts are far superior to air-dried whole herbs," says Andrew Weil, M.D., director of the program in integrative medicine at the University of Arizona College of Medicine in Tucson and author of *8 Weeks to Optimum Health*.

Hard-core herbalists usually prefer teas or tinctures to any kind of capsule or tablet. Aside from the problem of oxidation, herbs in capsules are harder for your body to absorb. You also sacrifice that helpful sensory connection with the herb itself, since you hardly taste, touch, or smell anything when you swallow a capsule. Still, in the real world, herb capsules are godsends. "Sure, an encapsulated product might have slightly less efficacy sometimes," Dr. Rothenberg says. "But if you take the right amount, it's going to be a lot more effective than not taking anything."

Oils and Water: They Do Mix

Herbal oils are sensual herbal remedies. While *oil* may refer to an herb that's been extracted into something like virgin olive oil, the version that you'll probably use most is the essential kind. Essential oil is distilled from an herb via a complicated evaporation and condensation process that yields an extremely concentrated liquid.

What about the sensual part? Well, a lot of home remedies using essential oils take the form of aromatherapy or hydrotherapy. As its name implies, aromatherapy taps into your sense of smell to soothe and promote healing. Since the essential oils of herbs are highly aromatic, you have a match made in olfactory heaven, whether the oil is diluted for massage or diffused for breathing.

One way of breathing in the herb is through steam inhalation, which melds aromatherapy and hydrotherapy. Hydrotherapy is a venerable natural healing technique that exploits the healing powers of water. It's also a great way to get herbs into your system. Steam treatments, hot baths, and foot soaks are just some of the ways to combine essential oils (or often the dried or fresh herb itself) with water for a pleasant herbal home remedy.

Other Herbal Options

If teas, tinctures, capsules, and essential oils are the Big Four, there are still plenty of other ways to use herbs. Here's a rundown of some that you can take advantage of.

Solid extract. A favorite with naturopaths, a solid extract is actually a gooey syrup that's a concentrated source of herbal medicine. Surprisingly, many solid extracts—of hawthorn berry or licorice root, for example—don't taste half-bad, says Dr. Catellani.

Juice. If you have access to generous amounts of fresh herbs and have a good, heavy-duty juicer, this is an excellent way to make your medicines, says Chanchal Cabrera, a member of Britain's National Institute of Medical Herbalists, a professional member of the American Herbalists Guild, and an herbalist in Vancouver. "It is about as simple and unprocessed as you can get and provides your body with a host of vitamins, minerals, and other trace elements along with the medicine," she says. Aloe is one herb that's often used in juice form. The problem is that aloe (and many others) taste pretty bad and don't keep long, says Cabrera.

Salve. It's often better to put herbs on your body than in it. Relief from muscle pain is a case in point. An herbal salve, usually prepared with olive oil and/or beeswax for good consistency and penetration, is a good way to do that. Salves also let you take advantage of herbs that are dangerous if taken internally, such as arnica. So do similar topical herbal products (those that are applied to the skin) such as ointments, balms, creams, and lotions.

Poultice. Herbal remedies can be pretty darn simple. A poultice is little more than mashed or ground herbs in the form of a soft, semi-liquid, pulplike mass that is usually spread over wounds, bites, or sores and held in place with a bandage or cloth.

Compress. Here's another simple concept that can work. All we're talking about here is a cloth or pad that you press to your skin. As an herbal remedy, you will probably soak the material in a tea or a water-diluted tincture and then hold it near the source of inflammation or muscle pain. If it's hot, it may be called a fomentation.

How to Buy Herbs

Unless you're ready to dedicate half your life to growing herbs in your garden and the other half to studying botany so that you can safely harvest them in the wild, you'll get most of your herbal medicines the new-fashioned way—by buying them.

Thanks to the herbal renaissance and the market it created, you can find just about any herb from alfalfa to yellow dock with no problem. If you live near a city of any size, using herbal remedies is as simple as a trip to any of the well-stocked health food stores and sometimes to one of the larger drugstores or grocery stores. If you live in an area that's not as well-supplied, mail-order companies will deliver herbs to you post-haste, as any glance at the Internet or health-oriented magazines will confirm.

"Ten years ago, I used to have to make the herbal remedies myself for my patients," says Willow Moore, N.D., D.C., a naturopathic physician and chiropractor at the Maryland Natural Medicine Center in Owings Mills. "Now they can buy them themselves."

That same herbal renaissance has also complicated herbal shopping, however. "Growing interest in herbal medicine has stimulated the proliferation of both high-quality herb suppliers and marginal ones," says Dr. Weil. That's the good doctor's polite way of saying that there's a lot of junk out there.

How do you avoid the junk? Mainly by being a wary shopper. If you need aspirin, you're probably not averse to simply running into any place that's open, grabbing a bottle of whatever says "aspirin" on the label, and trusting that the Food and Drug Administration has determined that it's perfectly good aspirin. Unfortunately, you can't take the same lackadaisical approach to the wide-open and still mostly unregulated herb market.

"You have to be very proactive," says Cabrera. To be a proactive procurer, heed the following tips.

Buy by reputation. "A basic ground rule is always to buy from a reputable herb supplier," Cabrera says. Check a store or mail-order company's reputation the way you'd check any reputation—by asking questions, talking to friends, reading up, and using common sense. "There's no set way to judge," she says, "but in the end, you should feel confident that you can trust the supplier."

Grill the store owner. "Talk to the health food store owner and ask a lot of questions," Cabrera says. "Where are they getting their herbs? How are they assuring quality? How do they keep track of how long the herbs have been in stock? The owner of a good store will know these things." And insist on answers before you buy. "If a shopkeeper doesn't have this information or won't provide it, that tells you something," she says.

Don't get hung up on size. There are big herb companies that have earned their reputation, but bigger doesn't necessarily mean better, Cabrera says. "There are a lot of really good, home-grown herb suppliers," she says. Also, it's worth noting that at the smaller stores, you're more likely to get the owner's personal attention and the information you need.

(continued on page 24)

Your Herbal Medicine Starter Kit

*S*o many herbs, so little shelf space . . .

If you're a beginning home herbalist, you'll find it easier to make sense out of the wide world of herbal remedies by first getting to know a limited number of them up close and personal. To help you on your way, we asked herbal experts to suggest the best herbs to stock in a modest herbal medicine chest. We used their answers to come up with a Top 10 list of safe and effective herbs that are easy to get, easy to keep, and easy to use.

Of course, specific conditions will call for herbs that may not be on this list, and you'll want to expand your repertoire as time goes on. But as a basic medicine chest for general health, the following herbs are a great starter kit.

1. Echinacea. The number one herbal remedy for colds, flu, sore throats, and other respiratory infections, echinacea is an immune system booster and antibiotic. Keep either a tincture or capsules of extract handy, because you need to start taking echinacea as soon as symptoms appear.

2. Garlic. This is a multipurpose natural wonder. How many herbs can lower blood pressure, reduce cholesterol, boost immunity, fight infection, *and* flavor your spaghetti sauce? Keep plenty of natural garlic around to use as a clove-a-day cardiovascular tonic, but also stock up on capsules to take for high blood pressure, infections, and other conditions.

3. Chamomile. You probably love chamomile as a pleasure tea, but you'll love it even more as a relaxing herbal remedy for a plethora of problems, from indigestion to insomnia to a stuffy nose. Buy dried chamomile flowers in bulk so that you can make medicinal teas stronger and more economically than most tea bags allow.

4. Hawthorn. With heart disease as America's top health enemy, you can use a friend like hawthorn. It's a proven improver of cardiovascular health that you can keep on hand as a tincture, capsules, or a solid extract. Use it as a tonic for your heart or medicinally when cardiovascular problems arise.

5. Aloe. Put aloe in the first-aid section of your herbal medicine chest, because it's a first-rate cut, bite, and burn healer. The juice also helps an upset stomach. A good way to have aloe handy is to keep a small live plant so that you can break open a leaf as needed to get at the healing liquid.

6. Valerian. This is nature's sleeping aid and anxiety alleviator, a safe sedative that you can take as tincture or capsules.

7. Ginkgo. Ginkgo is known as a memory enhancer, and that's reason enough to include it in your medicine chest. But it also improves circulation, which can bring many health benefits. Keep it for the long term as a tincture or capsules.

8. Eucalyptus. Nothing beats inhaling some good herbal steam when you're hit with a chest or head cold, cough, stuffy nose, sinusitis, and so on—and nothing beats the volatile oils from eucalyptus leaves to make that steam work. The oil can be released from the leaves themselves in water, or you can buy a little vial of the essential oil.

9. Oregon grape root. A frequent companion to echinacea as a remedy for respiratory infections, Oregon grape root has essentially the same healing berberines as goldenseal. It's also good to have the capsules around for intestinal problems such as diarrhea or an upset stomach.

10. Ginger. This much-loved warming herb acts as an anti-inflammatory, so it's a big help for arthritis and bursitis. You can also take it for chest congestion, nausea, and even motion sickness. It's available in lots of forms, including tinctures, syrups, and capsules, but be sure to have the cut or powdered root on hand for a deliciously healing ginger tea.

Buy what you need, not what they sell you. The commercial herb business tends to dream up a lot of whiz-bang herbal potpourris that have more to do with sales than with healing. It's not necessarily that they're bad, but they can distract you from your particular herbal remedy. Stick to your guns and buy exactly what you need, suggests Dr. Rothenberg. "The market pushes a lot of combinations that are probably not what many herbalists would recommend," she says.

GETTING LOOSE: BUYING HERBS IN BULK

There are two basic ways to buy herbs. One lets the suppliers do the preparing and packaging of the tinctures, capsules, oils, salves, and other herbal medicines. Your role is to check for quality, buy the product, take it home, take it, and feel better. The other way is to purchase the actual loose plant in bulk. You can buy it fresh or dried. You can buy the whole herb or certain parts, such as the leaves, root, bark, flowers, or fruit. You can buy it intact or cut up. However you buy it, you'll take it home and make it into medicine yourself.

You're surely going to be doing both kinds of shopping. The higher-tech products such as extracts in capsules and essential oils aren't the kinds of things that you're likely to whip up in your garage. On the other hand, you need the loose herb to make some teas as well as to prepare certain poultices, baths, compresses, and the like. You even have the option of extracting your own tinctures.

Even bulk herbs can be packaged so that you can buy fixed, weighed amounts, such as 1 ounce, 4 ounces, or even 1 pound, in some kind of sealed bag—a must if you're ordering by mail. Frequently, though, you'll help yourself to what you need, just like buying coffee beans at the co-op. "Herb stores will have big containers of herbs— leaves, roots, flowers, or whatever," Dr. Schoenbeck says. "Just measure out as many ounces as you want and put it in a bag to take home."

Such self-service shopping is cost-effective, since you buy only what you need (perhaps just the right amount to follow a remedy in this book) and there are no packaging costs. It's also kind of fun.

Again, though, you have to pay attention to what you're buying, or you can end up with a decidedly nonmedicinal pile of leaves. Here are some tips to make sure that you get what you pay for.

Trace the age. Once an herb has been unearthed, its flowers and leaves start to deteriorate, especially if they're finely chopped.

"A big chunk of dried root or bark might keep for a year or two, but if it's been cut and sifted, or if it's the leaves or flowers, it's good for 6 months, max," Cabrera says. "It has a finite life span." So ask the store owner or manager how long ago the herb was picked. "Track down not just how long it's been in the store but also how long it was in a warehouse or with brokers before it got to the store," she says.

Rate the display. Air and light are enemies of herb potency. A store that protects its herbs properly from those two things is more likely to be selling good ones. Make sure the herbs are in airtight containers that are either dark or stored out of the light. "If they're in those big clear plastic bins with flip-up lids, they're not protected," Cabrera says.

Check the color. A sign of age is fading color, Cabrera says. "Look for a nice bright color before you buy."

Sniff around. A stale-smelling herb is probably an impotent herb, so give it the sniff test before you buy. "Check for that really fresh, herby smell," Cabrera says. "Nothing musty or dusty."

Give your herbs a good home. Herbs are just as sensitive to light and oxygen after you buy them as they are in the store, so follow the same storage rules at home that you demand from the place where you got them. "Keep your herbs stored in a tightly covered glass container," Dr. Schoenbeck says, "and keep that container somewhere away from light exposure."

THE HERBAL STANDARD

You hear lots of laments about declining standards in the modern world, but not in herbal medicine. Indeed, standardization is a trusty aid in your herb quest. Why? Well, when you buy herbs in capsule or tincture form, it helps to know whether the product has a certain standard percentage of the herb's most important healing constituent (or constituents). A standardized extract has been tested and found to contain enough of the principal active constituent for the herb to do its healing.

For example, there are lots of capsules on the market for the popular immune-boosting herb echinacea. If the label indicates that the capsules contain an extract with at least 15 percent of the polysaccharides known as echinacasides, you can be fairly confident that this standardized product will have the desired effect. If not, you could be swallowing an ineffective substance.

Not everyone loves standardized extracts. Some natural practitioners consider standardization a contradiction of a widely adopted tenet in herbal medicine that *all* of the plant's chemicals work together to heal. Still, using a set amount of one constituent as a marker for overall plant potency is the closest thing to consumer protection that exists in herbal medicine. As Dr. Weil puts it, "Standardization is the best assurance that a product contains what it's supposed to contain in amounts sufficient to produce a desired effect."

It also depends on how sick you are. The more serious and pervasive the problem, the more you want to start looking at standardized preparations, says Robert Rountree, M.D., a holistic physician at the Helios Health Center in Boulder, Colorado. "But if you're at the lower end of the disease spectrum, where you're looking more to prevent than to treat, then increased potency as determined by standardization isn't as important as just being sure that you take the herb on a daily basis," he says.

Preparing and Using Herbs

Chances are that you're already an experienced home herbalist. If you've ever dropped a mint tea bag into hot water, you've converted bulk herbs (the stuff in the bag) to medicine (the mint tea itself), even if you never thought of it that way. In fact, the next time a friend asks you what you're doing, don't say, "Making mint tea." Say, "I'm preparing a liquid extract of *Mentha piperita* by infusing the dried leaves with hot water." She'll be impressed, and you'll be telling the truth.

The best thing about home herbal remedies (other than the fact that they work) is the way they let you get involved in your own healing. "There's a big difference between taking a drug and using an herbal remedy," Dr. Schoenbeck says. "You actually see the herb, smell it, interact with it. When you connect with the idea that a living plant is delivering healing properties, you open up a whole new dimension of healing."

In other words, preparing your own herbal medicine is part of the healing. Just knowing that should help you overcome your fear of herb preparation. Even more inspiring is the fact that using herbs at home ranges in difficulty from the very easy (making a tea) to the extremely easy (putting some drops of tincture in water and drinking it) to the embarrassingly easy (swallowing a capsule).

Making Herbal Teas

To be an expert herbal tea brewer, you need to know three things: one, how to boil water; two, the difference between a teaspoon (the littler one) and a tablespoon (the bigger one); and three, the difference between a root and a leaf.

Once privy to that inside info, you can make the two kinds of tea remedies most often called for in herbal medicine. If you're using the "soft" parts of a plant (the leaves or flowers), you steep the herb by pouring boiling water over it and letting it stand, or steep, for a set amount of time, usually between 5 and 20 minutes. That's called an infusion, and it's not any different from the method Earl Grey would use.

The plant's harder parts (the root, rhizome, or bark) yield their healing properties more reluctantly, so to use them, you have to decoct rather than infuse. With a decoction, you usually place the herb in the water before you bring it to a boil, then let the mixture simmer (rather than steep) for 10 to 30 minutes.

That's it. Strain out the dregs and drink up. Sure, there are lots of variations on these themes; those are explained with the individual remedies in this book. But knowing these two basic tea preparations puts all herbal tea remedies within easy reach. The following tricks of the trade will help, too.

Be strong. "Most Americans don't make their teas strong enough," says Dr. Catellani, "so they stop using them for medicine because they don't get results." Remember, medicinal teas usually aren't pleasure teas, and you have to adjust the herb-to-water ratio accordingly. A heaping teaspoon of the cut-up dried herb per cup of water is the low end of the scale. Medicinal strength is usually more like a tablespoon (which is about 3 teaspoons) per cup, or even more.

(continued on page 30)

FINDING DR. GOODHERB

*T*here are times when nothing but a pro will do—one who's well-versed in herbal remedies and can not only assist you in becoming a better home herbalist but also help you heal when home remedies aren't enough. Herb-savvy health-care practitioners can tailor herbal remedies to your special needs and can put together complex formulas for complex problems.

The professional that you seek can be an herbalist, a naturopathic physician (N.D.), a medical doctor (M.D.) or osteopathic doctor (D.O.) who uses herbs, or some other qualified healer such as a chiropractor, a licensed acupuncturist (L.Ac.), or a practitioner of Traditional Chinese Medicine. That's a lot of options, but even with the booming interest in herbal medicine, finding someone who's qualified to practice it is still no cinch. Here are some tips for a successful search.

Ask your doctor. Sometimes, you find what you're looking for where you least expect it. "The first thing to try is to ask your doctor if he'll work with herbal medicine," says Robert Rountree, M.D., a holistic physician at the Helios Health Center in Boulder, Colorado. "You may be surprised." Even if your doctor won't deal with herbs, he may be able to refer you to someone who does.

Go where the action is. "Ask the people at your local health food store if they're aware of any doctors who are sending their patients over," Dr. Rountree suggests. "That's a great way to find out." Don't forget to ask your fellow customers, too.

Contact the guild. Most herbalists aren't licensed to practice medicine, but the good ones are well-trained in herbal healing. The best way to find a qualified one is to contact the American Herbalists Guild (AHG) to find out if any of their professional members are located near you. "They keep a register of all the professional members—herbalists who have passed an extensive peer-review process," says Chanchal Cabrera, a professional member of the AHG, a member of Britain's National Institute of Medical Herbalists, and an herbalist in Vancouver. The address is American Herbalists Guild, P. O. Box 70, Roosevelt, UT 84066. The organization also includes a referral list of professional members on its Web site. If you have access to the Internet, use your Web search engine to find the guild's site.

Nab a naturopath. Naturopathic doctors with degrees from accredited natural medical schools such as Bastyr University in Kenmore, Washington, are often highly qualified physicians who practice a broad range of natural modalities, including herbal medicine. Their principal professional organization, the American Association of Naturopathic Physicians, offers a referral service that may put you in touch with an herbal practitioner near you. Write to 601 Valley Street, Suite 105, Seattle, WA 98109 or search for their Web site and physician database on the Internet.

Hunt for the holistic. Many medical doctors who use herbs in their practices consider themselves holistic physicians and may be affiliated with the American Holistic Medical Association. Their referral directory costs $5 and may help you pin down an herb-oriented holistic M.D. in your area. Write to the American Holistic Medical Association, 4101 Lake Boone Trail, Suite 201, Raleigh, NC 27607 for more information. You can also locate the organization's site on the World Wide Web.

Use more herb if it's fresh. Herb-to-water proportions usually assume that you'll be using dried herbs rather than fresh. If you're substituting fresh herbs for dried, you need to increase the amount because fresh herbs still have all that water in them. If a recipe calls for 2 tablespoons of dried herbs, count on needing about a handful of fresh herbs to end up with tea of the same strength.

Put a lid on it. If you're making just one cup of tea, you may be tempted to just steep the herb in the cup that you're going to use to drink the tea. Resist that temptation and use a covered pot or something else with a lid. That keeps volatile oils—oils in the herb that carry many of the healing ingredients—from evaporating, says Dr. Schoenbeck.

Blend the herb, not the tea. Lots of herbal remedies call for a tea made from several different herbs. Make the blend first with the dried herb, says Mary Bove, N.D., a naturopathic physician at the Brattleboro Naturopathic Clinic in Vermont and a member of Britain's National Institute of Medical Herbalists. For example, if a flu remedy calls for a cup of tea with equal parts of linden flowers, elder flowers, yarrow flowers, and peppermint leaves, don't make ¼ cup of each and pour the four teas together. Instead, mix the four dried herbs together in equal parts and then steep a full teaspoon (or whatever quantity is called for) of this blend in a cup of water.

Blend ahead. If you know that you're going to be drinking several cups of a blended tea in one day, Dr. Bove suggests that you mix enough of the dried herbs to make enough tea for that day. For that matter, go ahead and make enough of the blend for the entire winter, if you know you'll be using it. The dried herbs will keep just as well together as they would separately. All that matters is that you mix your blend with the same herb ratio as you would for a single cup.

Simmer first, then steep. Some tea remedies call for a blend of root or bark (which you simmer) with leaves or flowers (which you steep). What to do? The best approach, suggests Dr. Bove, is to do the simmering first, then use the resulting decoction to steep the dried leaves or flowers. The extra steeping won't hurt the decoction, but if you reverse the procedure, all that simmering will deplete the leaves or flowers of their healing properties.

Be sweet. A lot of herbal remedies will allow you a little honey to help those teas that are taste-challenged, but there are better ways, says Dr. Catellani.

She suggests a splash of a good-tasting tea such as licorice. Your best bet, though, may be natural juice, especially grape juice. "Grape juice will mask the flavor of just about anything," she says.

Using Tinctures

Unless you want to make them from scratch, using herbal tinctures is a snap. The hardest part may be mastering the measurements. A remedy's dosage—how much you take at a time—may be given in drops, by the dropper, by the teaspoon (or fraction thereof), or in milliliters. A typical dose might be a dropper, which is simply the amount it takes to fill the dropper that comes with your tincture bottle. That usually equals about ¼ teaspoon. Five milliliters fills a teaspoon.

Since good tinctures are readily available, most home herb users don't bother to make their own. If you have the urge to move up a level, there's a definite cost advantage to tincturing your own herbs. "A tincture of echinacea root might cost $10 an ounce," says Dr. Schoenbeck. "If you have an upper respiratory infection, you can go through that in a few days. But you can make that ounce of tincture yourself for about $2. That's an 80 percent saving."

Here are the basics of home tincturing from Dr. Schoenbeck. Put the finely cut herb and a 40 percent clear alcohol solution (vodka works fine) in a glass jar with a tight-fitting lid. You should use 1 part herb to 5 parts liquid, which roughly translates to putting in enough vodka to cover the herb with ¼ inch to spare. Store it in a dark place for 6 weeks, shaking the bottle once or twice a day. Then strain it, squeezing as much of the liquid from the herb as you can, and behold, you have a tincture.

As you may have guessed, it gets more detailed than that. For one thing, different herbs require different alcohol strengths, so vodka isn't always best. Each herb's specific requirements can be found in herbal compendiums, but Dr. Schoenbeck suggests another way to sharpen your tincturing skills. "Take a class that a lot of herb stores or herbalists offer," she says. "Having somebody show you how to do

ADVENTURES IN HERBALISM

ANCESTRAL HERBS

*H*ow old are herbal remedies?

"Older than man," says James A. Duke, Ph.D., an herbalist and ethnobotanist in Fulton, Maryland, and author of *The Green Pharmacy*. Zoologists have identified as many as eight species of primates that use plants for medicinal purposes, he says.

Evidence suggests that humans figured out herbal medicine pretty quickly, though. Scientists analyzing the grave of a Neanderthal man found in a cave in Iraq discovered that someone, presumably members of his family or tribe, had surrounded his body with clusters of flowers and branches. Of the eight species of plants identified, seven had medicinal properties. Among them were marshmallow root, now widely recognized as a tonic for sore throats and upset stomachs; yarrow, a common remedy for fevers and high blood pressure; and ephedra, which for thousands of years has been used to help fight colds, flu, and asthma.

Were the herbs planted there because they produce pretty flowers or because of their healing powers? No one can know for sure, but it seems that this was one Neanderthal who was well-prepared for his journey to another world.

it at least once will help you get comfortable. Then you can make tinctures forever, using books."

Whether your tinctures are bought or built, here are some hints for optimal use.

Test the measurement. Measuring in drops is far from an exact science, so you may want to test-drop to determine how many drops are in a dropper or how many droppers equal a teaspoon. "I suggest that you just count how many droppers it takes to fill a teaspoon the first time you use the bottle," says Dr. Schoenbeck.

Be sure it's alcohol. Sometimes, glycerin or even vinegar is used instead of alcohol in making tinctures. That's fine if you can't take the alcohol. Otherwise, though, double-check that the tincture uses alcohol. "Alcohol extracts are better," Dr. Rothenberg says. "Tinctures from alcohol are stronger and last longer."

Get a carry-on bottle. Tincture remedies often call for taking three doses a day, and that's not always easy to do. "Some people can do the morning and evening doses but can't get that third dose in because they don't want to drag the 1- or 2-ounce tincture bottle around with them during the day," says Dr. Rothenberg. The solution? She suggests measuring a dose into a very small glass vial with a tight cap and taking it with you in your pocket.

Evaporate the alcohol. One downside to tinctures is that some people don't care for their taste. Sweeter-tasting glycerin-based tinctures are one option, but glycerin doesn't extract as many medicinal qualities as alcohol can, says Dr. Stengler. If the taste of alcohol bothers you or you want to avoid alcohol, put one dose in a small amount of hot water and let it stand for a few minutes. The hot water will help the alcohol evaporate from the tincture but won't affect the strength of the herbal medicine. Add the alcohol-reduced tincture to a small amount of water, juice, or herb tea, or simply drink it by itself.

Make a grape juice cocktail. Tinctures can taste bad even when diluted. You can use grape juice to mask the taste just as you can with bitter teas, says Dr. Catellani. With tinctures, though, take it a step farther. "Use the frozen grape juice concentrate," she suggests. "Just scoop out about ¼ teaspoon and stir it into your tincture and water."

THE ART OF HOME HERB USE

This book offers specific herbal remedies for specific conditions, with clear instructions on how to prepare those remedies. But there's more to herbal medicine than just following instructions. "There's science in herbal medicine, but there's also an element of art," says Dr. Rothenberg.

"Besides the general guidelines, there are elements that you, the individual, bring into play. That's why so many people like herbs."

The things that you learn about herbs as you practice your home-herbalist skills expand your healing possibilities. The more you become personally involved with herbs, the healthier you can be. That's something to keep in mind as you consider these last tips for getting the maximum benefit out of your herbal home remedies.

Spread out the doses. When a remedy calls for three cups of tea a day or 1 teaspoon of tincture three times a day, that almost always means a morning-noon-night schedule, not a triple shot with breakfast. "Herbs work gently, so you don't need a whopping dose all at once," says Dr. Schoenbeck. "You'll absorb them better if you spread the doses out over the day."

Take most herbs between meals. "Almost all herbs like to be taken between meals so they don't have to compete for absorption with foods," Dr. Schoenbeck says. You'll find plenty of exceptions, of course, but between-meal dosing has another advantage. "Taking them at least 15 minutes before meals can aid your digestion, because they prime your digestive system for handling the food," she explains.

Make your own capsules. If you're taking capsules of whole powdered herb rather than extract, try making your own by buying the powdered herb in bulk along with a quantity of empty capsules, usually labeled "00." "You'll save money," Dr. Schoenbeck says.

Better yet, Cabrera suggests, you can make your own powdered dried herbs in a coffee grinder. "Turn it on and off so you don't overheat the herbs," she says. "If you grind enough to fill enough capsules for a week, they'll be fresher than what you buy at the store."

Refrigerate. "Capsules or any other kind of powdered herb should be kept in the fridge," Cabrera says. "That will prolong their shelf life a little bit."

Get a plan. Always remember that herbal remedies are just a part of natural healing. "Take your herbs in conjunction with vitamins, diet changes, and stress management," says Susan B. Kowalsky, N.D., a naturopathic physician in Norwich, Vermont. "Natural medicine isn't a matter of popping a different kind of pill. It's about lifestyle."

Part 2

HEALING
WITH HERBS

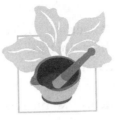

AN A-TO-Z GUIDE

*D*uring the first half of the twentieth century, the doctor-recommended remedy that people plucked from the shelf at the corner drugstore was likely to be an herbal remedy. Not until the discovery of antibiotics during World War II and the beginning of the modern "wonder drug" era did plant-based medicines fall out of favor in America. We eagerly embraced modern pharmaceuticals and left behind a way of healing that had served quite literally every culture on the planet for thousands of years.

Now, the poles have shifted again, and we want to know more about herbs. We're learning that with medicine, stronger and faster doesn't necessarily mean better. Herbs offer another way of healing, a more natural way to help the body help itself. With herbs, we can have medicines that are usually less invasive, easier on our bodies, and readily available.

Once again, drugstores (and grocery stores) are stocking their shelves with dozens of herbal products. Sandwiched between the vitamins and the aspirin, you'll find everything from aloe and black cohosh to witch hazel and valerian root. But what you won't find on all those packages is prescriptive advice. Because of federal regulations, manufacturers can allude to the possible usefulness of an herb, but they can't make direct claims about curing a specific disease or condition. This means that the job of figuring out exactly which herb to select is strictly up to you. That's a job that we can make a little bit easier.

In the following A-to-Z section, we've assembled the combined wisdom of nearly 200 medical doctors, naturopathic physicians, scientists, and professional herbalists to bring you the best, safest, most practical herbal remedies for common health conditions. Whether you're treating minor problems like blisters and bad breath or chronic conditions like arthritis and diabetes, you'll find advice in every chapter on which herbs to try, how to use them, specific dosages to take, and why the remedies work. You'll also find dozens of practical, easy-to-follow recipes for making your own herbal medicines.

Each chapter includes a "Fast Facts" feature to tell you at a glance the cause of the condition, some statistics on its incidence, and when it's time to call the doctor. You'll also get a taste of herbal adventure and folklore as you read the stories about the experiences of real-life herbalists that are sprinkled throughout.

Before you get started, though, a few caveats are in order.

- Never try to diagnose a medical condition yourself.

- Even if you've seen a doctor about a particular problem, don't substitute an herbal therapy for your prescribed treatment without discussing it with your doctor first. This is especially true if you have a chronic condition such as diabetes or high blood pressure.

- Don't try herbal medicines if you are pregnant or nursing.

- Don't give herbs to children without consulting a qualified health practitioner who can advise you about dosage and safety precautions that apply specifically to children. None of the advice in this book is intended for children under the age of 16.

- Use common sense when trying an herb for the first time. Although side effects are rare, if an herb causes any type of discomfort, stop using it and see your doctor immediately. Before you try the remedies in this book, check the safety guidelines for herbs and essential oils beginning on page 547.

ACHES AND PAINS

*P*ain is basically a signal—a warning that your body sends out when tissues are being damaged. When you overexert yourself, that damage comes in the form of tiny muscle tears. Doctors call it delayed-onset muscle soreness. It's a signal from your body to slow down and take a rest. It's just one explanation for aches and pains, though. Sometimes, the cause is a mystery.

Over-the-counter pain relievers like aspirin and acetaminophen offer one-dimensional relief—they mask the pain. Unlike herbal remedies, they won't relax tired, contracted muscles. These herbs will.

Bromelain

For pain brought on by overexertion, take 250 milligrams three or four times a day, 1 hour after meals. Any type of inflammation heals faster when you take bromelain, explains Jacob Schor, N.D., a naturopathic physician in Denver. It's safe to take this dose for long periods of time.

"When I've been skiing all day and know that I'm going to be sore from overexertion the next day, I take some bromelain before I go to bed," he says. "My muscles don't ache as much, and I recover faster."

An enzyme derived from the pineapple plant, bromelain helps you digest your food when you take it with meals. When taken on an empty stomach, bromelain promotes circulation and helps your body reabsorb all the by-products of inflammation. As a result, you heal faster. And in one study, patients who took bromelain also reported that they had less pain.

Bromelain strength is standardized in measurements called milk-clotting units (mcu) or gelatin-dissolving units (gdu), which indicate how much of the enzyme is needed to curdle milk or dissolve gelatin. Since 1,200 gdu equals roughly 2,000 mcu per gram, look for a product that lists a strength between 1,200 and 2,400 mcu or between

720 and 1,440 gdu, says Jacqueline Jacques, N.D., a naturopathic physician in Portland, Oregon, who specializes in pain management.

Ginger, Cloves, Orange, Lemon, and Cinnamon

Soak in a soothing herbal bath. A warm bath infused with these everyday pantry items stimulates sluggish circulation, relaxes stiff joints, and eases muscle pain, says Phoebe Reeve, a professional member of the American Herbalists Guild and an herbalist in Winchester, Virginia.

To prepare this infusion, fill a pan with about 1 pint of water. Add one sliced lemon, the peel of one orange, a cinnamon stick, an inch-long piece of fresh ginger cut into slices, and five whole cloves. Bring to a boil, cover, and simmer for about 20 minutes, then strain it into a tub of warm bathwater. It's safe to use this remedy whenever necessary.

Willow and Meadowsweet

For natural pain relief, take 10 drops of a combined tincture of these herbs four times a day. The aspirin-like substances in these herbs ease inflammation and pain in sore muscles and joints, says Reeve. This herb combination is easier on the stomach than aspirin. If your stomach is especially aspirin-sensitive, try rubbing 25 milliliters of the tincture directly on the sore muscle or joint. You can buy the tinctures already combined or mix equal parts of each. It's safe to take this remedy whenever it's needed.

Lavender, Peppermint, Rosemary, and Bergamot

Put 6 to 10 drops of any combination of these pain-soothing essential oils in your bath. When you ache all over, soak in a warm bath infused with anti-inflammatory essential oils to melt away the pain, says Reeve.

Fast FACTS

Cause: If you look up "aches and pains" in a medical book, you'll find that there are dozens of causes for this vague and general symptom. If accompanied by a fever, aches and pains can indicate an infection such as Lyme disease, chronic fatigue syndrome, hepatitis, toxic shock syndrome, or simply a cold or the flu. Without fever, the most likely cause of your aches and pains is an injury to a muscle, joint, or nerve.

Incidence: Pain is the universal human experience and the number one reason that people seek medical care.

When to see the doctor: If aches and pains worsen after 3 to 4 days or persist despite proper rest and other home remedies, consult your physician.

"The combination of warm water and essential oils stimulates circulation and allows the body to relax. If we can relax the muscle, blood and nutrients can flow to it," she explains. "This signals the body to start the healing process." To help your body absorb the oils, add ¼ cup of Epsom salts to the bathwater. It's safe to use this remedy whenever needed, but don't use more than three drops of peppermint oil.

Cramp Bark

To relax overcontracted muscles, take 5 milliliters of a 1:5 tincture three times a day. Just as its name implies, cramp bark is used primarily to relax tight, painful muscles. When muscles become rigid in response to pain, cramp bark can bring effective relief, says Keith Robertson, a member of Britain's National Institute of Medical Herbalists and director of education for the Scottish School of Medical Herbalism in Glasgow. You'll feel better as your muscles relax, blood flow improves, and the by-products of inflammation are reabsorbed. It's safe to use this remedy until symptoms subside.

Cramp Bark Cream

Although you can take it internally, cramp bark makes a wonderful topical cream to soothe aching muscles, says Keith Robertson, a member of Britain's National Institute of Medical Herbalists and director of education for the Scottish School of Medical Herbalism in Glasgow.

Try this basic recipe to make your own personal brand of relaxation. Rub a small amount of cream directly on achy muscles and joints up to three times a day. Unlike an ointment, cream blends with the skin and allows it to breathe. It's safe to use this until symptoms subside.

- **5 ounces emulsifying wax**
- **2½ ounces vegetable glycerin**
- **2½ ounces water**
- **1 ounce dried cramp bark**
- **20 drops tea tree essential oil (optional)**

Melt the wax in the top of a double boiler. Stir in the glycerin, water, and herb. Simmer slowly, stirring occasionally, for 3 hours. If you try to rush the emulsifying process, the oil and water will separate.

Strain the mixture through cheesecloth or a fine sieve. Stir slowly and continuously until it cools and sets. To discourage mold growth, you can stir in the tea tree oil before transferring the cream to a sterilized dark glass jar. Store it in the refrigerator for up to 3 months.

Guaiacum

When you have a lot of pain and inflammation, drink three cups of decoction daily. Chronic aches and pains should be treated with a cleansing herb like guaiacum, says Robertson. It stimulates blood flow to the affected area, which helps reabsorb the dead and damaged cells caused by inflammation. Put 1 teaspoon of guaiacum wood chips in 1 cup of water and bring to a boil. Simmer for 15 to 20 minutes, then strain and drink. It's safe to drink this until symptoms subside.

ACNE

$\mathcal{W}$hether you're 15 or 50, hormones seem to play a large part in whether you get acne. Not chocolate. Or greasy foods. Or even poor hygiene.

At puberty, hormones called androgens rev up the oil-producing sebaceous glands. They also stimulate excessive shedding of dead skin cells, which in turn contributes to clogged hair follicles or pores that become blackheads or whiteheads.

Other hormonal changes, like the fluctuations that occur during the menstrual cycle, can also cause breakouts.

It's not clear why this unwanted vestige of adolescence persists in some people even when gray hair starts to sprout, or why some develop acne as adults after breezing through their teens with barely a blemish. But just because your skin is behaving like a teenager's doesn't mean that you can treat it that way.

"Most adults cannot tolerate the teenage acne products. They're too harsh and drying. Some natural products can act as alternatives to treat mild acne," says Marcey Shapiro, M.D., a family doctor in Albany, California, who combines natural healing with conventional medicine.

Experts say that you can use the following herbal remedies topically to unclog pores, fight pimple-producing bacteria, and dry up existing blemishes. Ideally, though, you want to stop acne before it starts, says Dr. Shapiro. Natural products aren't substitutes for dermatologist-prescribed antibiotics and sebum-reducing drugs, but they can help in many cases of mild acne.

Tea Tree

Rub a drop of this antiseptic essential oil on blemishes three times a day to discourage infection and promote faster healing. Tea tree, a plant native to Australia, provides one of the most effective natural antiseptics for the skin. "It's a pretty good, mild bacterial agent—about as strong as deodorant soap," says Dr. Shapiro. "It's not as potent as prescription medicines that we have for acne, but it may have some benefit for mild acne." You should see results within a month.

An Australian study found that a 5 percent tea tree oil gel proved as effective against acne as a 5 percent benzoyl peroxide lotion. While the gel was slower to take effect, it was much less drying to the skin. The volatile oil from the leaves and small branches of the tree contain a compound called terpinen-4-ol, a well-tolerated skin antiseptic. It also contains small amounts of a skin irritant called cineol, which can cause a poison ivy–like rash. The percentage of cineol in tea tree oil can vary widely, from less than 5 percent in high-quality oil to up to 65 percent in poor-quality oil.

For your own homemade pimple cream, mix 5 drops of tea tree essential oil with 1 teaspoon of an oil-free, fragrance-free lotion and apply it three times a day, advises Christine Steward, a medical herbalist in Worcester, England, and past president of Britain's National Institute of Medical Herbalists.

Witch Hazel

Blot acne-prone areas twice a day. It's an old-fashioned remedy that Grandma probably used, but witch hazel is still a very good astringent, says Dr. Shapiro. Using witch hazel daily helps remove excess oil and kill bacteria on the skin.

Leaves and young twigs of the witch hazel tree are distilled to make the bottled astringent that you see on store shelves. The herbal solution contains large quantities of tannins, which have drying and astringent effects that cause the proteins of the skin surface to tighten.

Witch Hazel and Sage

For added antibacterial strength, drop five fresh sage leaves into a 4-ounce bottle of witch hazel. Let the leaves stand in the witch hazel for about a week, then use as an astringent on the skin after

Fast FACTS

Cause: Hormones stimulate oil glands in the skin to produce excess sebum, an oily substance that keeps hair and skin lubricated. These hormones also make the skin shed an excess number of cells, which mix with the sebum to form a plug that clogs a hair follicle or pore. The blockage can form into either a blackhead or a whitehead. Blemishes typically erupt where sebaceous glands are the most numerous and productive—on the face, chest, back, neck, and shoulders. Acne is not caused by dirt or diet. Washing too often may actually make your acne worse.

Incidence: Women are more likely than men to experience the hormone fluctuations that trigger acne in adulthood. The incidence of chronic, mild to moderate acne among women ages 20 to 50 is increasing and affects an estimated 40 to 50 percent of all adult women to varying degrees.

When to see the doctor: Severe acne can lead to serious and permanent scarring. Resist the temptation to pick or squeeze blemishes. It increases the danger of infection and scarring. If your acne is so unsightly that it bothers you, consult a dermatologist to determine the optimal way to treat it.

---

cleansing in the morning and evening, says Steward. Research shows that the volatile oil in sage contains a compound called thujone, a strong antiseptic. Mixed together, the two create a pleasant-smelling solution that Steward says makes a great aftershave, too.

Lavender

To help heal blemish scars, dab them with a drop of oil. Better-known for its sweet aroma, lavender essential oil has significant antiseptic and antibacterial actions that can help acne scars heal faster, says Mercedes Cameron, M.D., family practitioner at The Woman's Place at St. Mary's Hospital in Grand Junction, Colorado. Use a drop of lavender oil on old blemishes and look for results within a week or two. Or Dr. Cameron says that you can look for lotions and cleansers containing lavender oil at health food stores.

Chasteberry and Calendula

Drink one to two cups of this hormone-balancing tea daily. Claudia Wingo, R.N., a medical herbalist in College Park, Maryland, and a member of the National Herbalists Association of Australia, recommends drinking a tea made with chasteberry and calendula if you're prone to breakouts caused by the fluctuations in estrogen and progesterone that accompany your menstrual cycle.

Also called vitex, chasteberry traditionally was chewed by monks to reduce unwanted libido. Research has confirmed that it does have a hormone-regulating action.

Once you ovulate, start drinking one to two cups of tea a day and continue until your period begins. The herbs need time to regulate your system, so it may take two or three cycles before you notice an improvement in your acne outbreaks, says Wingo. Don't try to speed things along by drinking more of the tea, though. That could actually make your skin look worse.

AGE SPOTS

*D*o your hands give away your age? was the question asked in a 1970s advertisement for a skin cream that promised to erase the speckled evidence of your years.

Like most Madison Avenue messages, that slogan was a mixture of fact and fiction. While it's true that age spots usually start cropping up in middle age, they have little to do with how old you are.

Like a slice of TV nostalgia, age spots are a blast from the past. Your past. A jumbled reminder of the golden glow you got each summer. A dead giveaway of hours spent in the sun—without sunscreen.

When repeatedly exposed to the sun, the skin tries to protect itself by producing an overabundance of melanin, a protective pigment that causes skin to tan when you're young. Get too much sun, and over time, that excess melanin will start to congregate in irregular patches that show up—usually on the hands and face—when you get older.

The result? Flat, freckle-like spots that give your complexion an uneven tone.

"Your first step toward clearer skin is prevention of further sun damage," says Marcey Shapiro, M.D., a family doctor in Albany, California, who combines natural healing with conventional medicine. Start wearing sunscreen with a sun protection factor (SPF) of at least 15 on a daily basis, and be sure it's the type that blocks both UVA and UVB rays. Apply it to your face and the backs of your hands first thing in the morning, before you put on any makeup. Reapply it after you wash your hands. Unless you're willing to stick to a preventive regimen, there's really no point in fading the spots you have. Without sun protection, new spots will appear in a few months.

Although spots can be removed instantly with laser surgery, experts suggest trying a few of these natural skin lighteners for several months and seeing if your age spots begin to fade.

Kojic Acid

Use an over-the-counter bleaching cream containing this acid. Many of the conventional products used by dermatologists contain ingredients that come from plants. Kojic acid is one example. Derived from a Japanese mushroom, kojic acid can often make age spots look

50 percent lighter over time, says Dr. Shapiro. It's now an ingredient in many over-the-counter fading creams, and a fairly effective one, according to the latest research.

"With fading products, you don't want to get an overwhitened effect. It has to be strong enough to fade, yet weak enough to leave your normal pigmentation," says Dr. Shapiro. "And it has to work slowly enough so that you can control the end result, which makes creams containing kojic acid a wise choice."

Lemon

Rub dark patches with juice three times a day. Lemon juice acts as a natural bleaching agent. It lightens hair and freckles and may help make age spots fade, says Christine Steward, a medical herbalist and past president of Britain's National Institute of Medical Herbalists.

The citric acid in the lemon juice helps remove the top layer of dead skin cells, which helps even out variations in skin tone. She recommends rubbing fresh juice directly on the skin. It may take weeks or months to see results, but if it works for you, this remedy can be used until your age spots fade.

Aloe

Apply fresh gel liberally twice a day. Research has shown that the clear gel from the leaves of the aloe plant has a dramatic ability to heal wounds, ulcers, and burns. Its healing powers may also help clear away age spots, says Steward, although how it works it still a bit of a mystery. Aloe has been a beauty treatment since ancient times, and Cleopatra is said to have relied on it to keep her skin flawless.

Even if you don't have a green thumb, you can keep your own potted aloe plant in the house. To collect the gel, break off one of the

Cause: Technically known as lentigines, the flat, irregular brown spots are the result of excess pigment being deposited in the skin after years of sun exposure. They generally appear on chronically sun-exposed areas such as the face, hands, back, and feet.

Incidence: Virtually everyone gets age spots over the course of time.

When to see the doctor: Although most age spots are harmless blemishes, early stages of skin cancer can resemble them. If any spot enlarges, thickens, changes color, bleeds, or itches, have it checked by a doctor.

succulent leaves and split it open on a cutting board. With the edge of a dull knife, scrape the gel from the inner part of the leaf and place it in a small jar.

Comfrey

Rub infused oil into your skin three times a day. Although it's best-known as a wound healer, this herb has also been used with some success to heal scars on the skin. While age spots don't fall into the scar category, comfrey may still be worth a try, says Steward.

Make your own hot infused oil from dried comfrey leaves with this recipe, suggests Steward. In the top of a double boiler, mix 2 cups of dried leaves with 4 cups of olive, sunflower, or other good-quality vegetable oil so that the herbs are completely covered. Add water to the bottom of the double boiler and bring to a boil. Place the herb mixture over the boiling water and simmer gently for 1 to 2 hours on low heat. (Or you can use a slow cooker set on low.) Check the oil frequently and reduce the heat if it bubbles. If it begins to smoke, start over.

Remove the pan from the heat and let the mixture cool. The oil will be dark green when it's ready. Strain the mixture through cheese-cloth or a jelly bag, squeezing all of the oil from the pulp of the herb. Pour the infused oil into a sterilized, dark glass bottle and label it. Infused oils can last up to a year.

ALLERGIES

*A*llergies are mistakes. They're false alarms from your immune system, which responds to otherwise harmless substances as though they were invaders bent on harm. The results are well-known to allergy sufferers: sneezing and wheezing, coughing and itching, and all kinds of other discomforts that come from inflammation in the lungs, nose, eyes, and even the digestive tract. "The sneezing and wheezing, coughing and itching, and diarrhea are all efforts of the body to expel this foreign invader," says Connie Catellani, M.D., medical director of the Miro Center for Integrative Medicine in Evanston, Illinois.

Since so many of these misinterpreted substances hail from the plant world (pollen, trees, and grasses, for example), it seems only fair that medicine from the plant world should improve things. Indeed, there are lots of herbal remedies that can either help ease allergy attacks, reduce your long-term susceptibility, or both.

Herbs are a big part of the natural approach to alleviating allergies—but not all of it. "You're going to have to deal with allergies on more than just the herbal front," says Beverly Yates, N.D., a naturopathic physician at the Natural Health Care Group in Portland, Oregon, and Seattle. It's a good idea to use your herbal remedies in the context of an overall natural healing and prevention approach. One of the principal strategies involves avoiding those foods or substances that trigger your allergic reactions, which means that first, you have to identify them.

Practitioners of natural medicine may also recommend that you cut down on the animal protein in your diet, especially from cow's milk and chicken eggs, says Dr. Catellani.

Some of the following home herbal remedies may relieve symptoms right away. Others are long-term solutions. "The key thing is to try to normalize and balance the immune system before it goes bonkers and decides to start attacking the body's tissues," Dr. Yates says.

Wild Cherry

Drink one cup of tea a day for 2 months. A tea from the bark of the wild cherry plant will soothe and calm the upper respiratory tract, where lots of allergy symptoms show up on a year-round basis.

"Cherry bark is great for the throat and on up," Dr. Yates says, "especially if coughing is your predominant allergy symptom." Buy the bark in dried powder form. Use 1 tablespoon of herb per cup of water and steep it for 10 minutes. Use it daily for 2 months, then evaluate your symptoms. "If you feel relief, that's great. Stop taking the herb," says Dr. Yates.

You can also take your wild cherry in easy-to-find lozenges. "They will help provide relief and soothe your cough on an as-needed basis," Dr. Yates says.

Eyebright

Take 20 to 25 drops of tincture three times a day. This herb is for symptom relief, especially for the itchy or watery eyes, runny nose, and sneezing very common in all kinds of allergies. Eyebright helps normalize blood flow to the nose and eyes, says Dr. Yates.

Put the eyebright tincture into some water to dilute the taste and take it with or without food. "Take this when eye and nose symptoms are driving you crazy," Dr. Yates says.

Fast FACTS

Cause: Scientists think that the predisposition to allergic reactions may be inherited. The allergens that actually trigger the reaction can include pollen, mold, animal dander, house dust, food, drugs, insect stings, trees and grasses, and feathers or down.

Incidence: Including hay fever, asthma, and everything in between, allergies affect 40 to 50 million Americans.

When to see the doctor: If allergies are limiting your normal activities and affecting work or school attendance, it's time to see a doctor to find out what's going on inside your body and, if possible, what's causing the allergic reaction. Frequent bouts of other illnesses related to allergies, such as asthma, recurrent bronchitis and sinusitis, and eczema, also warrant a medical evaluation.

Nettle

Take 500 milligrams of freeze-dried leaf three times a day in capsule form. If hay fever is your problem, a medicinal preparation of this well-known herb may be your best friend. "Stinging nettle is the primary herb for hay fever," says Michael Traub, N.D., a naturopathic doctor in Kailua Kona, Hawaii. "It works like a natural antihistamine for hay fever symptoms."

Unlike pharmaceutical antihistamines that can cause drowsiness, nettle usually doesn't have any side effects, Dr. Traub notes, although symptoms may worsen initially for the first few days of use. Capsules of the freeze-dried leaf are available in health food stores. If you have severe symptoms, you can go higher than the recommended 500-milligram dose, he says.

Quercetin

Take 200 to 500 milligrams in capsule form three times a day. Quercetin is a bioflavonoid, a pigment found in foods such as grapes,

Home Run Allergy Relief

This formula is called a "home run" tincture because it touches all the bases, according to Beverly Yates, N.D., a naturopathic physician at the Natural Health Care Group in Portland, Oregon, and Seattle. It stabilizes the immune system, eases histamine symptoms, reduces eye and nose irritation, quells excess mucus production, corrects blood flow to the nose and eyes, and generally calms things down. All of the ingredients for the formula are available in health food stores or by mail order.

For allergy relief, put about 30 drops into an ounce or two of water and drink it down. Use the remedy three times a day for no more than a week at a time. Then slap yourself five for hitting a home run.

1	**ounce echinacea tincture**
1	**ounce goldenseal tincture**
1	**ounce licorice tincture**
½	**ounce eyebright tincture**
3 to 4	**drops horseradish tincture**

Blend the echinacea, goldenseal, licorice, eyebright, and horse-radish in a dark glass bottle.

green tea, tomatoes, and onions. It is highly regarded for reducing inflammation and providing relief from allergies.

"A lot of people who use quercetin regularly get good results," says Kathi Head, N.D., a Sandpoint, Idaho, naturopathic physician and an editor of *Alternative Medicine Review*. You can start with the lower dose and increase to the higher dose after a few weeks if you don't see a benefit, she says. If after 6 weeks, you still don't see results, quercetin may not be effective for you, but if you find that it helps, it's safe to take it daily on an ongoing basis.

Quercetin is especially helpful for hay fever, says Dr. Catellani, and you can take it at the first sign of hay fever season or even a week before. The season can begin as early as January in the southern United States but generally lasts from February or March through October.

Anal Fissures

*H*ere's a homework assignment for you. Let's say your feet are size 10. Go out and buy size 4 socks, then go home and try to put one on. No copping out or complaining that it's too small. Grunt, strain, and sweat, but do what you have to do to force that sock onto your foot.

What happens to the sock? It becomes stretched and worn. If you keep forcing your foot into it, it will eventually develop tears.

Now you know what your anus goes through on its way to forming anal fissures.

Anal fissures are small tears in the lining of your anus. Small though they are, the distress that comes with them is not. "Fissures are quite literally a pain in the butt," says Brenda Snowman, M.D., a physician in Cleveland, Tennessee. Although they may ache throughout the day, they hurt most when you have a bowel movement, and they can cause bright red blood to appear in your stool.

You have them because you eat too little fiber and drink too little water, which leaves your stool hard, dry, and exceptionally difficult to pass. Your anus wasn't designed to handle that kind of material.

The first thing you want to do, says Dr. Snowman, is start tossing back some extra water. People with anal fissures are generally in a state of chronic dehydration. Their bodies absorb all the moisture they can from food to meet their internal needs, leaving stools dry.

You've likely heard that the ideal amount is six to eight 8-ounce glasses of water a day. Now you need to practice drinking at least that amount faithfully if you want to give your fissures a chance to heal. Plus, some of the herbal remedies that follow depend on drinking enough water for them to work.

Witch Hazel

Apply as needed. Witch hazel extract is available on pretty much any drugstore shelf, says Dr. Snowman. Its cooling, astringent action

Fast Facts

Cause: Anal fissures come about from eating low-fiber foods and drinking too little water. The result is hard, dry stools that tear open the sensitive tissues in your anus.

Incidence: Most people who live with chronic constipation will develop anal fissures. They are more common among women because women tend to be constipated more often due to higher progesterone levels and lower intakes of dietary fiber.

When to see the doctor: If you have rectal bleeding that doesn't resolve within 2 weeks, has no pain associated with it, or is recurrent, you need to consult a physician. The same applies if you notice blood in your stool or on the toilet paper after a painful bowel movement. While bleeding is common with anal fissures, you need to rule out the possibility of a more serious condition, such as colon cancer.

Once you have a diagnosis, you can usually self-treat fissures successfully. Check with your doctor, though, if they don't go away within a few months.

---

can go a long way toward soothing the torn tissue in your anus. The herb also acts as a mild analgesic, or pain reliever, when applied topically. As a bonus, it's an antiseptic that can keep the tears from becoming infected.

Although you can apply it as your discomfort dictates, a good time to use witch hazel is when you're wiping after a bowel movement. Simply dampen a wad of toilet paper with the extract and use it to clean yourself. Not only does the homemade wet-wipe make for a gentler experience, it also gives you the healing properties of witch hazel.

Psyllium

Take according to the label instructions. It only makes sense that since constipation and hard stools got you into this predicament, the reverse can get you out. Psyllium, available in products like Metamucil, is a high-fiber plant. Fiber prevents constipation and softens stools. Since psyllium products vary, check the label for the correct dose.

Here's an important note from Dr. Snowman: Don't use psyllium if you're unprepared to increase your water intake. Adding bulk to your diet without adding water will make you more constipated than before. In the worst cases, it can also cause a dangerous bowel obstruction. Again, you need a minimum of six to eight 8-ounce glasses of water a day.

Aloe

Apply gel twice a day. Aloe vera has a rich tradition of speeding healing, says Miles Greenberg, N.D., a naturopathic physician in Kapaa, Hawaii, and president of the Hawaii Society of Naturopathic Physicians. In its pure gel form, it can help do the same for fissures. Wash your hands and brush under your fingernails with antibacterial soap before applying the gel to the outside of the anus with your clean finger. Slide some up into the torn area as well.

"It's soothing and has mild antibiotic properties as well," explains Dr. Greenberg, which is good for keeping the area clean and helping to avoid infections in the tears.

Goldenseal

Apply balm once a day. Goldenseal is one of the most versatile plants in the herbal medicine cabinet, says Dr. Greenberg. It's a strong antibiotic, so it can reduce inflammation if your fissures are infected and extremely tender.

To make the balm, use about a tablespoon of the powdered herb and add a small amount of olive oil or beeswax. Mix until it forms a sticky paste. As with aloe, clean your hands and apply the balm to the outside of the anus as well as to the inner tears. Leave it on until your next shower.

ANGINA

$\mathcal{S}$ome people describe the chest pains of angina pectoris as so intense that they feel as if elephants are standing on their chests. Which leads to the following riddle: How much can herbs (measured in milligrams) move elephants (measured in tons)? Answer: Plenty, but not by themselves.

Angina is serious stuff, the result of insufficient blood flow (and hence an insufficient oxygen supply) to the heart. Its severe chest pains usually go away in a matter of minutes, but the danger doesn't.

"Angina is a big red flag, a possible prelude to a heart attack," says Robert Rountree, M.D., a holistic physician at the Helios Health Center in Boulder, Colorado. "Any flag that big and that red calls for a thorough evaluation by a medical doctor. I only recommend herbs or other natural medicine as something to do in addition to whatever conventional medicine your doctor prescribes."

That conventional medicine often takes the form of nitroglycerin, which helps get blood and oxygen to the heart, thereby easing angina pain and helping prevent further attacks. Longer-term treatment may also include drugs such as beta blockers or calcium channel blockers, which are prescribed for many heart conditions.

Conventional and natural medicine experts agree that a healthier lifestyle is also essential for controlling angina. Managing stress is high on the list.

"Stress is an important contributing factor to heart disease," says George Milowe, M.D., a holistic physician in Saratoga Springs, New York, "so relaxation techniques such as yoga or meditation can be very helpful." Exercising to strengthen your cardiovascular system can also be beneficial, Dr. Milowe says, although people who have angina obviously should exercise only as prescribed by their doctors.

In addition, of course, the health of your diet dictates the health of your heart. "But it's not just a question of what you shouldn't eat, such as saturated fats," Dr. Rountree says. "Also look for beneficial foods that you can eat. Intensely colored fruits and vegetables confer protection to your heart. Blueberries, raspberries, tomatoes, sweet potatoes, and certain winter squashes all have these rich pigments that make them exceptionally good heart foods."

Dr. Rountree also points out that it's a short step from heart-healthy foods to heart-healthy herbs. "The idea that what you eat will have a beneficial effect segues neatly into using herbs," he says. "They're right on the cusp between the nutritional and the medicinal."

Hawthorn

Take 1 teaspoon of tincture or ¼ teaspoon of solid extract two to four times a day, or take two 500-milligram capsules two or three times a day. "The way to treat angina is with anything that increases blood flow to the heart," says Ian Bier, N.D., Ph.D., a naturopathic physician, licensed acupuncturist, and natural medicine researcher in Portsmouth, New Hampshire. "Hawthorn is a very powerful one for that."

Hawthorn helps with angina in several ways. For one, it has a strengthening effect on the heart itself. What's more, the berries of this common shrubby tree help improve the cardiovascular conditions that lead to angina, such as clogged arteries, high cholesterol, and high blood pressure. It is easy to find in a variety of forms.

Motherwort

Drink three cups of tea a day or take 1 to 2 milliliters of tincture three times a day. Motherwort is another good heart herb. Not only is it a healthy tonic for the heart muscle itself, it also helps lower blood pressure and has a general calming effect on the cardiovascular system. "Motherwort's particularly good for people with a kind of 'nervous' heart condition," Dr. Rountree says.

Motherwort is widely available in health food stores in many forms. You can make a tea by steeping 1 teaspoon of the dried leaves and flowering tops in 1 cup of hot water. Strain the tea before drinking. Since it's no taste treat, Dr. Bier suggests using a little bit of honey as a sweetener.

You'll taste it less in tincture form. For angina, Dr. Bier suggests putting a dropper (about a milliliter) or two in some water. It's safe to take this dose long-term as a cardiac tonic.

Garlic

Take capsules providing 8,000 micrograms of allicin potential daily. Good old garlic helps control several cardiovascular conditions that can lead to angina or aggravate it. It helps lower cholesterol and blood pressure levels. It reduces the risk of blood clotting. And it fights atherosclerosis (clogged arteries).

Nobody's claiming that garlic is going to cure your angina, but natural medicine experts agree that any plant that does so much for your cardiovascular system should be a regular part of your diet. "Try to eat a clove a day with your food at least five times a week," Dr. Bier suggests.

If you have angina—or any other heart condition, for that matter—you'll need more garlic in a more concentrated form, says Dr. Rountree. That's where garlic capsules come in. There are plenty of them out there in health food stores and drugstores. He suggests that you bypass the popular but less potent "aged garlic" and instead look for capsules containing allicin potential (allicin is the main active constituent that is responsible for the good things that garlic does for your heart). You can take it for several months.

Ginkgo

Take one 40-milligram capsule three times a day. Ginkgo is a popular herb that's good for a lot of things, including heart con-

Fast FACTS

Cause: Physical exertion, a heavy meal, or exposure to cold can trigger an angina attack, which is caused by a low blood supply to the heart. Risk factors such as high cholesterol, high blood pressure, a high triglyceride count, stress, diabetes, and genetic factors all can lead to angina.

Incidence: Angina pectoris, along with heart attack and other forms of coronary heart disease, affects more than 13 million Americans.

When to see the doctor: Seek prompt medical care the first time you experience an angina attack and during any subsequent episode that differs from your usual pattern or duration.

ditions such as angina. Like garlic, it helps with cardiovascular problems associated with angina, especially high blood pressure. The active ingredient in ginkgo appears to help get the blood flowing to the heart by opening up the blood vessels, and that's just what you need if you have angina. It is generally safe to take this herb for long periods.

Valerian, Skullcap, Hawthorn, and Ginger

Take 1 teaspoon of this tincture formula three times a day. According to Ralph T. Golan, M.D., a holistic general practitioner in Seattle and author of *Optimal Wellness: Where Mainstream and Alternative Medicine Meet*, it makes a lot of sense to take advantage of calming herbs such as skullcap and valerian to help deal with the stress that's so often a factor in heart conditions such as angina. It also makes sense to combine those herbs with the overall heart benefits of hawthorn and with circulation-stimulating ginger.

You can get all of these things by whipping up a simple liquid formula with herbal tinctures that are easily found in good health food stores, then making that formula part of your daily routine. Mix 2 parts each hawthorn and skullcap, 1 part valerian root, and ½ part ginger. "Take this for at least a year, while you're cleaning up your lifestyle," Dr. Golan says.

ANXIETY

*P*art fear, part apprehension, and part plain old worry, anxiety is a familiar companion to many people, but not a very personable one. Too much anxiety can keep you up at night, bring on tension headaches, and leave you feeling restless, irritable, and downright exhausted.

If that companion is knocking at your door more often than you'd like, herbal remedies can help you bid it a calm farewell, says George Milowe, M.D., a holistic physician in Saratoga Springs, New York.

While the remedies in this chapter are generally considered to be safe for regular use, you should try to identify what has you so anxious and address the underlying cause, Dr. Milowe suggests. Cut back on coffee, tea, and other sources of caffeine, since caffeine is a notorious stimulant that can make you feel even more jittery. Try to get some anxiety-relieving exercise and take time to relax.

You might also try taking 500 to 1,000 milligrams of magnesium, says Dr. Milowe, who calls the mineral nature's tranquilizer. Supplemental magnesium may cause diarrhea in some people, and if you have heart or kidney problems, check with your doctor before taking it.

While you're at it, ease up with these herbs.

Anxiety-Free Tea

When anxiety creeps into your mind, sometimes you just want fast relief. In that case, you'll want this quick calm-down blend of herbal tea, courtesy of Candis Cantin-Packard, a professional member of the American Herbalists Guild and director of the Evergreen Herb Garden and Learning Center in Placerville, California. To make the tea, scoop out 1 teaspoon of the blend and steep in hot water for 10 minutes, then strain. Drink one to three cups a day as needed.

- **I ounce dried Siberian ginseng**
- **I ounce dried licorice**
- **I ounce dried skullcap**
- **½ ounce dried marshmallow**
- **½ ounce dried valerian**

Combine the ginseng, licorice, skullcap, marshmallow, and valerian in a wide-mouth jar.

Kava Kava

Take capsules that provide 60 milligrams of kavalactones three times a day. Kavalactones are the active anxiety-fighting ingredients in the herb kava, says Dr. Milowe.

Compared with drugs commonly prescribed for anxiety, kava has shown similar results without the side effects, says Susan B. Kowalsky, N.D., a naturopathic physician in Norwich, Vermont. When you buy capsules, look for a brand that is standardized to 30 percent kavalactones.

Valerian

Take a 150-milligram capsule twice a day. A popular anxiety remedy throughout Europe, valerian can calm your nerves and help

Fast FACTS

Cause: High-stakes, high-stress situations—or worrying about being in these situations—can cause anxiety. Persistent anxiety may be a symptom of a physical problem, such as a thyroid disorder. Some research suggests that changes in the production of certain brain chemicals, or neurotransmitters, may contribute to severe anxiety.

Incidence: Everyone feels anxious in certain situations, such as driving during a snowstorm or awaiting a medical diagnosis, for instance. About 5 percent of Americans have what's called generalized anxiety disorder (GAD), which means that they're chronically anxious about a variety of different things. GAD is twice as common in women as in men.

When to see the doctor: If anxiety is interfering with your work or relationships or is so severe that you find yourself unable to speak or often even think straight, see a doctor or licensed therapist.

---

you sleep better, which in turn can take the edge off edginess. Research suggests that certain ingredients in valerian—compounds called valepotriates and valeric acid—bind to the same brain receptors as the anti-anxiety drug diazepam (Valium). But valerian doesn't appear to cause the same side effects as diazepam; there's no grogginess or dependency.

Chamomile

Drink one cup of tea three times daily. Research has found that an active ingredient in chamomile, apigenin, has a significant anti-anxiety effect. Serve yourself a soothing cup three times a day, drinking the last one just before bedtime if your jitters are keeping you awake at night, says Anne Cowper, a medical herbalist in Morisset, Australia, and a member of the National Herbalists Association of Australia.

To brew yourself a perfect cup, put 2 teaspoons of dried chamomile flowers in a mug, pour in 8 ounces of boiling water, cover, steep for 15 minutes, and strain. If the chamomile you buy is ground to a fine powder (some shops sell it this way), add just 1 teaspoon to an 8-ounce cup, says Cowper. Chamomile is mild but effective, and it can be used long-term without concern.

Dried chamomile doesn't have a long shelf life, so check for freshness. The chamomile flowers you use for tea should be yellow and white. If they're straw-colored, they're too old. Whole flowers last longer than ground ones. Store yours in dark glass jars away from light and heat to prolong their healing properties.

Passionflower

Take 40 drops of tincture in water before or with meals, or drink one cup of tea three times daily. Another popular European anti-anxiety remedy, passionflower is available as a tincture and dried for tea. Most tinctures are alcohol-based, so diluting them with water makes them easier on your stomach, Cowper explains.

You can also brew some passionflower tea. Put 1 teaspoon of dried passionflowers in a cup, pour in 8 ounces of boiling water, cover, steep for 15 minutes, and strain the tea before you drink it. Passionflower is safe to take regularly, but it is best taken as a medicinal tea in times of stress rather than as an everyday tea, she says.

Kava Kava, Ginkgo, and Gotu Kola

Take 20 to 40 drops of a mixture of these tinctures in water before or with meals three times daily. This mixture is especially good for the kind of anxiety that can accompany a big event such as a job interview or an exam, Cowper says. You should be able to find tinctures of kava, ginkgo, and gotu kola at health food stores. Mix equal quantities of the three tinctures and store the blend in a small bottle or other container. You should notice results within a day or two, but this remedy is best if taken regularly around stressful times, says Cowper.

ARTHRITIS

*A*mong the more than 100 diseases that we call arthritis, there's one common thread—joint pain and inflammation. Actually, there are two common threads, because in all cases of arthritis, there's no cure.

The two types that you've heard the most about—osteoarthritis and rheumatoid arthritis—have very different causes, explains Jeffrey R. Lisse, M.D., professor of medicine and director of the division of rheumatology at the University of Texas Medical Branch at Galveston. Osteoarthritis occurs when you wear down the cushiony material between your joints. When that material is worn to a nub, the bones start to rub together, causing pain, stiffness, and even swelling in the joints.

Rheumatoid arthritis is caused by an overactive immune system. The way that it does its dirty work isn't entirely clear, but the result is painful, swollen, hot joints.

Treatment usually zeros in on relieving the day-to-day aches and stiffness with a combination of medication, rest, exercise, and the use of heat and cold. Research on newer, better arthritis drugs is ongoing and incredibly promising. For now, though, it's standard practice for doctors to prescribe one of the many nonsteroidal anti-inflammatory drugs (NSAIDs) to ease the pain and inflammation of rheumatoid arthritis, says Dr. Lisse. For osteoarthritis, they start with acetaminophen to relieve pain, but if that doesn't work, they go on to NSAIDs.

The problem is that while NSAIDs may mask the pain, they can and do cause intestinal bleeding that lands thousands of people in the hospital each year. Test-tube research suggests that long-term use of these drugs may even damage joint tissue. Caught in a proverbial Catch-22, you're faced with two choices—live with the pain or run the risk of developing nasty side effects.

Sometimes, if NSAIDs aren't powerful enough to treat arthritis, doctors prescribe steroids. "Treating inflammation with steroids is like cutting down a tree to get rid of a hornet's nest high up in the branches. The pain is gone, but the side effects are costly," says C. Leigh Broadhurst, Ph.D., a nutrition consultant and herbal researcher based in Clovery, Maryland. "Herbal medicine may hold the key to reducing pain and inflammation without the undesirable side effects."

Herbal remedies aren't as effective if you eat a poor diet or have an unhealthy lifestyle. Holistic practitioners start by recommending a diet of whole grains, vegetables, and fruits, with very little meat, dairy, or refined carbohydrates, for their arthritis patients, says Ruth Bar-Shalom, N.D., a naturopathic physician in Fairbanks, Alaska. A daily multivitamin and antioxidant supplement is crucial, she says. Research suggests that it can help preserve joint tissue.

While some plants offer simple pain relief, the general aim of herbal treatment is to improve the cleansing of the congested tissues around the joint. Herbs that stimulate blood flow, digestion, and elimination encourage the body to eliminate toxins that cause inflammation.

Boswellia

To ease chronic pain, take 450 milligrams in capsule form four times a day. An extract from the frankincense tree may hold the key to relieving pain from arthritis without undesirable side effects, says Dr. Broadhurst.

Inside the fragrant tree are chemicals called boswellic acids. Research suggests that these acids interrupt inflammation early on by preventing the production of biochemicals in our bodies that start the pain process. In other words, instead of trying to stop the train when it's barreling down the track at 100 miles an hour, boswellia cuts the engines while it's still pulling out of the station.

The bark of this tree, which is grown on the dry hills of India, is cut to collect the aromatic gum resin that's used to make a standardized extract. The extract has been shown to improve blood supply to the joints and prevent the breakdown of tissues affected

An Essential Arthritis Rub

When pain is localized in one joint, try this recipe for a pain-relieving rub developed by Douglas Schar, a medical herbalist in London, editor of the British Journal of Phytotherapy, *and author of* Backyard Medicine Chest. *"A medicated rub made with pure essential oils can ease inflammation and joint pain,"* he says. Apply a dab to the sore joint four times a day.

20 drops lemon essential oil
20 drops sandalwood essential oil
1 small jar petroleum jelly, minus 1 tablespoon

Mix the lemon and sandalwood oils well into the petroleum jelly.

by all types of arthritis. It's safe to take boswellia for arthritis indefinitely.

Turmeric

To relieve chronic pain and inflammation, take one or two 400- to 500-milligram capsules of extract three times a day. Curcumin, the powerful anti-inflammatory substance in turmeric, isn't a drug, but it can act like one, says Dr. Broadhurst.

"If my fate were such that I could have only one medicinal plant, it would be turmeric," Dr. Broadhurst says. Although it has been used for thousands of years in India for cooking, dyeing, and medicinal uses, turmeric was largely overlooked in North America until the 1970s. When modern science finally took a closer look, the results were impressive.

When compared to the popular anti-inflammatory drug phenylbutazone (Butazolidin) in a clinical study, curcumin was found to be equally effective at treating arthritis. It's okay to take curcumin for arthritis indefinitely.

Ginger

For pain relief without side effects, eat some type of ginger every day. Unlike many arthritis medications that may wreak havoc with your digestive system, ginger is a stomach soother. Long used as a treatment for nausea, research now suggests that it may help ease the aches and pains of arthritis, says Dr. Broadhurst.

In a study from Denmark, three-quarters of the people with arthritis who took a daily dose of ginger reported some relief from pain and swelling without any side effects.

For the best medicinal benefits, look for fresh, organically grown rhizome, sometimes mistakenly referred to as a root. If it is old, shriveled, moldy, or chemically treated, it will not yield the same amount of active substances. To keep a steady supply on hand, peel the ginger and cut it into thick slices. Place them in a clean jar, pour in enough vodka (as a preservative) to cover, and put a lid on the jar. You can store it in the refrigerator indefinitely. You should eat about 1 teaspoon of grated ginger every day.

Cayenne

Rub some hot-pepper cream on the sore joint three or four times a day. Creams and ointments containing capsaicin—the hot stuff in hot pepper—stimulate the release of your body's own painkillers, says Jacqueline Jacques, N.D., a naturopathic physician in Portland, Oregon, who specializes in pain management. These creams are commonly available in drugstores.

Scientists believe that capsaicin also interferes with the action of your body's pain messenger, which is called simply substance P. When cayenne is applied to the skin, it also stimulates blood flow in the joint, which will help promote healing. Use a standardized ointment containing 0.075 or 0.025 percent capsaicin.

It's safe to use cayenne long-term, but if your pain persists for more than 3 to 4 weeks, consult a doctor. And here's a word to the wise: Be sure to wash your hands after you use the cream to avoid "burning" other parts of your body, and never put the cream on a rash or open wound.

Fast FACTS

Cause: No one knows what causes most forms of arthritis, but a lifetime of using and abusing your joints can contribute to deterioration, swelling, and pain.

Incidence: Arthritis is the number one chronic health problem, afflicting nearly one in six Americans. That's 43 million people, and nearly two-thirds of them are women. The most common form of the disease, osteoarthritis, affects 20.7 million Americans. It is sometimes called wear-and-tear arthritis, and the chances of developing it increase after age 45. Rheumatoid arthritis affects about 2 million people in the United States.

When to see the doctor: If you develop pain, stiffness, or swelling in a joint that persists for more than 2 weeks, contact your doctor. Many things can be done to reduce the impact of arthritis on everyday life. The key is early diagnosis.

Juniper

Massage diluted essential oil into the sore joint three or four times a day. To stimulate blood flow and help cleanse the aching joint, Keith Robertson, a member of Britain's National Institute of Medical Herbalists and director of education for the Scottish School of Herbal Medicine in Glasgow, recommends a gentle massage with juniper oil. Made from the berries of the juniper tree, this versatile oil will also ease pain and tension.

Mix a few drops of the woody-scented essential oil with 1 cup of vegetable oil and apply to the painful joint. Don't use the oil for more than 2 weeks.

Guaiacum

When you have a lot of pain and inflammation, drink three cups of decoction daily. Guaiacum is a specific herb for the pain and swelling caused by rheumatoid arthritis, says Robertson. It stimulates blood flow to the affected area and flushes away the dead and damaged cells caused by inflammation.

To make the decoction, put 1 teaspoon of guaiacum wood chips in 1 cup of water and bring to a boil. Simmer for 15 to 20 minutes, then strain.

Asthma

*P*anic.

It's sometimes part of a severe asthma attack, and for a very good reason. The wheezing and tight-chested feeling during an attack can have you quite literally fighting for your very breath. What's not to feel panicked about?

An asthma attack occurs when an irritant—it could be stress, severe cold, a wisp of smoke, or something you're allergic to—causes spasms in the bronchi, passageways that carry air into the lungs. When you have bronchial spasms, the passageways constrict, forcing you to gasp for air.

That's no time to be debating the relative merits of natural and conventional medicine. During an attack, airway-opening drugs known as bronchodilators are used to provide quick relief, usually in the form of inhalers. Inhaled steroids may be used for slower-acting, anti-inflammatory relief.

Even though steroids have side effects, few practitioners in the natural healing community would quarrel with their use in such situations. "When asthma symptoms are severe, there's a time and place for conventional medicine," says Connie Catellani, M.D., medical director of the Miro Center for Integrative Medicine in Evanston, Illinois.

Herbal medicine has its place, too, and it can be of great help to people with asthma, says Dr. Catellani. For one thing, not all asthma cases approach panic-land. "Most people have mild to moderate, intermittent asthma," she says. "They can usually use their home herbal medications on an as-needed basis."

Moreover, asthma attacks don't just happen. They are the periodic consequences of a chronic disorder that is marked by airway inflammation. Fortunately, herbs deal with that broad picture as well. "You need more than bronchodilation," Dr. Catellani says. "There's an inflammatory aspect to asthma, and you want to reduce that, too."

So herbs will help, but they'll be more helpful if they're used as part of a lifestyle plan. As with any allergic condition, you need to find out what's provoking the attacks and avoid that trigger. For some people, that means trying to dodge notorious allergens like pollen or dust.

"Chronic food allergies or sensitivities also put people at risk for asthma," says Dr. Catellani. For others, asthma might be associated with hard exercise or emotional stress. You could also have a low-level infection that's causing asthma, and you'll need antibiotics to get that infection cleared up. While you're chasing after the cause, however, you can turn to these herbal home remedies for help.

Grindelia

Take 20 to 30 drops of tincture two or three times a day. You can help prevent bronchial spasms with tincture derived from the dried buds of the grindelia plant, says Feather Jones, a professional member of the American Herbalists Guild and director of the Rocky Mountain Center for Botanical Studies in Boulder, Colorado.

"Grindelia is very good as an antispasmodic, which means that it helps relax smooth muscles like those found in the airways," she says. "Because of this ability, it works nicely to prevent the bronchial tubes from constricting. It's also a bronchodilator, so it opens bronchi that are already constricted." The tincture is available in health food stores.

ADVENTURES IN HERBALISM

HOREHOUND FOR HACKING

*B*ecause of her asthma, Tierney Salter had been plagued by a chronic cough since birth. She never made it through an 8-hour snooze without having to endure at least one bout of coughing. By the time she was 18, she had seen specialists all over her state and had a medicine cabinet brimming with prescription-strength asthma cough medicines. Nothing worked.

When she was a freshman at the University of California at Santa Barbara, one of her roommates suggested that she try some white horehound for her cough. Horehound, an unassuming mintlike plant that frequently grows on roadsides and in waste areas, is used in herbal medicine to treat chest colds, bronchitis, and whooping cough.

Since her roommates had to put up with her nocturnal coughing, Salter felt that she owed it to them to try the remedy. "I went to a little health food store near campus and bought 25 cents worth of horehound," says Salter. She took it home and made a cup of tea before going to bed that

Boswellia

Take two or three 150-milligram capsules twice a day for 6 months or more. Boswellia comes from a gummy tree whose resins contain acids that act as anti-inflammatories, among other things. That makes boswellia an effective partner with its fellow Ayurvedic herb *T. asthmatica* for treating chronic asthma.

"Boswellia acts like an army call against your immune system's inappropriate and inflammatory response," Dr. Yates says. "It calms, soothes, and helps keep all that thickness and congestion from building up in the respiratory tree, which is part of what makes it so hard to breathe with asthma."

night. "It was horrible-tasting stuff. I called it horrible hore-hound."

For the first time in years, she slept through the night without coughing.

The experience sparked an interest in herbal medicine. Salter decided to major in cultural anthropology so that she could study herbal traditions in other cultures. After graduation, she studied herbology at the College of Natural Medicine in Santa Fe, New Mexico. There, she learned the nuts and bolts of botanical medicine and regularly ventured into the fields of the Southwest to learn how to collect wild herbs and prepare them for medicinal uses.

When she graduated in 1982, Salter realized that there was a shortage of quality herbal products on the market. To fill the niche, she started The Herbalist, a Seattle business specializing in the manufacture of herbal formulas.

Although she now can manage her asthma with other herbal remedies, Salter still downs a cup of that horrible horehound tea when she has a stubborn cough.

The dose for boswellia is similar to that for *T. asthmatica*. Look for a product with 60 percent boswellic acids. "If you can get both of them, take them together," Dr. Yates says. "If not, taking just one of them will be just fine. You're not going to go wrong with either *T. asthmatica* or boswellia."

Ginkgo

Take 40 milligrams in capsule form two or three times a day. "Ginkgo is a very good herb for asthma," says Shiva Barton, N.D., a licensed acupuncturist and lead naturopathic practitioner at Well-

Fast FACTS

Cause: There's a long list of potential triggers that cause the airway spasms that are the hallmark of an asthma attack. They include allergens such as food, pollen, dander, and dust; infections such as sinusitis; certain drugs; and even exercise.

Incidence: Asthma cases are actually increasing. It affects all age groups, although about a third of the approximately 15 million people with asthma in the United States are under age 18.

When to see the doctor: Asthma is serious business—a potential killer. You should seek medical help if you experience episodes of wheezing, shortness of breath, or unexplained persistent cough.

---

space, a complementary health center in Cambridge, Massachusetts. "It works by relaxing the smooth muscle in the lungs and decreasing inflammation there."

Take one capsule two or three times a day and see if there's some improvement in a month or two, Dr. Barton suggests. If you experience positive results, reduce the dosage to the lowest amount that you need to feel well, she says.

Green Tea

Drink a cup a day. The same green tea that you enjoy so much with sushi or other Japanese food is also a good anti-inflammatory that helps calm mucus secretion in asthma. You can drink it semi-regularly over the long haul and daily when asthma symptoms are particularly bad.

You can find green tea as supplements, but drinking tea made from the unfermented dried leaves makes more sense. You can find them loose or in tea bags in Japanese or Asian food stores, and they're becoming more available in health food stores and grocery stores.

The key is to make a medicinal-strength tea. "If you use a tea bag, steep it for a good 10 minutes," says Emily Kane, N.D,. a naturopathic doctor and licensed acupuncturist in Juneau, Alaska. "You should definitely get that little backbite from the tannins. That's how you know it's strong enough."

Green tea is a healthy substitute for coffee in general, but it does contain caffeine, so keep your consumption at a moderate level. It contains roughly half the amount of caffeine that's found in coffee.

Cayenne

Add ⅛ teaspoon to your tea. Red pepper can also help during mild asthma attacks. It appears to improve circulation and enhance dilation of the bronchial passages, according to Kathi Head, N.D., a Sandpoint, Idaho, naturopathic physician and an editor of *Alternative Medicine Review*.

Cayenne works as a tea itself, but few natural practitioners are sadistic enough to recommend a strong medicinal tea made with hot pepper. Instead, during acute phases, get the cayenne from your spice rack and sprinkle ⅛ teaspoon into your green tea or chamomile tea, suggests Dr. Head. For these, she recommends steeping a tea bag or ½ teaspoon of loose tea in hot water for 5 to 10 minutes.

Red Raspberry and Alfalfa

Women, drink one to two cups of tea a day before and during menstruation. Many women with asthma find that their symptoms worsen during the estrogen peaks preceding menstruation, according to Dr. Yates. If you experience this, try a strong tea made by steeping 1 tablespoon each of dried alfalfa and red raspberry leaves in 1 cup of hot water for 10 minutes. "It's a pretty good-tasting tea," Dr. Yates says, "and it can really help."

ATHLETE'S FOOT

*I*f you have athlete's foot, don't blame it on the locker room. Scientists have tried. In studies conducted by the American Academy of Dermatology, researchers attempted to infect healthy skin with athlete's foot—and failed. What's more, one family member can have it without infecting others living in the same house. Why some people get athlete's foot and others don't is one of the unsolved mysteries of modern science.

What is known is that athlete's foot is a fungus. Like most fungal critters, it feels at home in moist, damp conditions such as inside shoes and socks, especially socks that haven't been washed. That's where the association between athlete's foot and stinky locker rooms started.

To avoid developing athlete's foot in the first place, wash your socks regularly and rotate the shoes you wear (athletic and otherwise) so that each pair has a chance to dry and air out. If you already have athlete's foot, here are some herbal remedies that can help you commit fungicide.

Tea Tree

Apply diluted oil twice a day. Researchers discovered early in this century that the tea tree of Australia possesses a variety of potent medicinal properties, with fighting fungus among them.

Beverly Yates, N.D., a naturopathic physician with the Natural Health Care Group in Portland, Oregon, and Seattle, suggests mixing tea tree oil with an equal amount of olive oil and rubbing it into the infected area.

Athlete's foot can toughen the skin, she says, which creates a barrier against medication. The olive oil helps to tenderize the skin so that the healing power of the tea tree oil can be better absorbed.

Victoria's Aromatic Foot Powder

The fungi that cause athlete's foot thrive where it's damp, which means that you can create an inhospitable environment for them by sprinkling a drying powder on your feet before you put on your shoes. Any drying powder that you use to combat athlete's foot should not contain cornstarch. Cornstarch is essentially a sugar and will feed the fungus, says Beverly Yates, N.D., a naturopathic physician with the Natural Health Care Group in Portland, Oregon, and Seattle.

Here's a recipe for an aromatic, cornstarch-free foot powder from aromatherapist Victoria Edwards, owner of Leydet Aromatics in Fair Oaks, California. After a shower, dry your feet, then sprinkle the powder on.

- 1 **cup bentonite or kaolin clay**
- 1 **tablespoon baking soda**
- 2 **drops thyme essential oil**
- 5 **drops rosemary essential oil**
- 2 **drops tagetes essential oil**

Place the clay, baking soda, and thyme, rosemary, and tagetes oils in a glass jar and shake.

Aloe and Tea Tree

Use a mixture of these two herbs to fight fungus. Aloe makes the skin tender, plus it promotes healing of injured tissues, says John E. Hahn, N.D., D.P.M., a naturopathic doctor and podiatrist in Bend, Oregon. Adding those properties to the antifungal powers of tea tree oil makes for a potent one-two punch. Dr. Hahn recommends mixing 3 parts tea tree oil and 1 part aloe gel. Twice a day, rub this mixture into the infected area until it's absorbed. You should apply the mixture for a minimum of 6 to 8 weeks for best results.

Fast Facts

Cause: Athlete's foot is caused by several types of fungi (the official name is *Tinea pedis*) that flourish in dark, moist environments.

Incidence: It is extremely common, and not limited to athletes. The American Podiatric Medical Association estimates that about 5 percent of the American population has foot infections, including athlete's foot, each year.

When to see the doctor: The rate of skin turnover on the human foot is 21 days, so give home remedies at least that much time to produce results. If you have a severe case, however, you should see a podiatrist or dermatologist sooner than that to determine if a different type of fungal or bacterial infection is responsible. Also see a doctor if you experience redness, swelling, and pain or see red streaks coming from the affected area.

Myrrh

Soak in a foot bath to relieve itching and dry up athlete's foot sores. Myrrh is an anti-inflammatory herb that's particularly effective on wet or "weeping" athlete's foot, Dr. Hahn says. Its astringent properties help dry up the wetness.

To prepare a myrrh foot bath, mix 1 tablespoon of extract in 1 quart of warm water. Soak your feet for 10 to 15 minutes once a day, Dr. Hahn says. If you have a particularly weepy case, use the soak twice a day for at least 7 days, or until the weeping stops.

Garlic

Take enough capsules to equal 7,500 micrograms of allicin in three divided doses a day. Allicin is the active ingredient in garlic, and it has potent antifungal properties. Be forewarned, however, that the amount of allicin in store-bought garlic capsules varies widely.

Kathleen Janel, N.D., a naturopathic physician with the Brattleboro Naturopathic Clinic in Vermont, recommends making sure that you get what you need by reading the label and gauging the appropriate daily dose by the amount of allicin you see listed there.

Lavender

Rub essential oil onto your feet once a day. Lavender is another herb that can help soothe and heal outbreaks of athlete's foot, says Michael Traub, N.D., a naturopathic doctor in Kailua Kona, Hawaii. Massage a thin coat of the oil directly into the infected area, he says. "It's antifungal, and it smells good," he says. "Also, people like rubbing it on their feet at night because it's calming."

BACK PAIN

Ever since our cave-dwelling ancestors decided to climb the evolutionary ladder and walk upright, our backs have been plagued by pain brought on by spastic muscles, pinched nerves, and slipped disks.

Each of us has about 25 bones in and around our backs, stacked on a column of fluid-filled, shock-absorbing disks. They're all held together by ligaments and muscles and controlled by a network of nerves. Even an array of high-tech diagnostic equipment can't always sort out this complex arrangement, so the exact cause of individual back problems is seldom known.

Despite this element of mystery, most run-of-the-mill backaches usually resolve on their own in about 4 to 6 weeks, says Scott

Haldeman, M.D., D.C., Ph.D., clinical professor in the department of neurology at the University of California, Irvine, and adjunct professor at Los Angeles Chiropractic College.

For the most part, conventional and herbal medicine approach treatment in much the same way. The goal is to control pain and inflammation and relax tense muscles during this healing interim, says Gayle Eversole, Ph.D., a certified nurse practitioner and professional member of the American Herbalists Guild in Everett, Washington. To achieve complete recovery, you'll probably need to do special exercises that are designed to strengthen your back and abdominal muscles.

When the pain hits, you might be tempted to hit the sack—and stay there—but doctors say to limit a period of rest to one day, then resume quiet activity. Moving around will help tone muscles and pump fluid back into the disks, says Dr. Haldeman.

Doctors usually recommend an anti-inflammatory drug like ibuprofen to ease pain and inflammation, or they may prescribe muscle relaxants. The trouble with these prescription drugs is that they can cause side effects like dizziness, clumsiness, fever, and irregular heartbeat.

Herbs offer gentler yet more effective relief, says Dr. Eversole. And unlike simple over-the-counter pain relievers, most herbal remedies for pain have a second benefit: They help you heal faster.

Valerian

Take two 250-milligram capsules four times a day or 20 drops of tincture every 2 hours. Although valerian is best-known as a mild sedative to treat insomnia, its soothing qualities can provide pain relief for a backache triggered by overworked, spastic muscles, says Jacqueline Jacques, N.D., a naturopathic physician in Portland, Oregon, who specializes in pain management.

Muscles in pain tend to tense up. An animal study showed that compounds in valerian relaxed smooth muscle cells, and relaxed muscles tend to heal faster, says Dr. Eversole.

"It also quiets the part of the nervous system that causes the sensation of pain," says Dr. Jacques.

The sedative effects of valerian also come in handy, since back pain tends to keep you tossing and turning at night. Unlike over-the-counter sleep aids, it won't leave you with a hangover effect the next morning.

One big problem with valerian, though, is that it reeks. The yellowish green oil from this relaxing root contains the same aromatic properties as human sweat. Unless you can endure a fragrance and flavor that have been compared to well-ripened gym socks, you'll probably want to take a capsule of valerian rather than a tincture, says Jacob Schor, N.D., a naturopathic physician in Denver. "If my patients opt for the tincture, I just tell them to pinch their noses and swallow," he says. It's okay to take valerian for back pain until your symptoms subside.

Turmeric

Take 400 milligrams of extract in capsule form three times a day. A dash of this ancient Indian herb can spice up a curry dish—or you can use it to help relieve a variety of aches and pains, says Dr. Schor. Locked in the orange yellow turmeric root is a powerful anti-inflammatory substance called curcumin, which has demonstrated an anti-inflammatory effect similar to that of ibuprofen and cortisone.

If you're trying to get rid of a nagging backache, don't reach for the spice bottle. It's best to take the concentrated extract of curcumin in capsule form, says Dr. Schor. You would need to eat about ¼ cup of turmeric to get the pain-relief power of two capsules of standardized extract.

Cayenne

Rub the sore area with red-pepper ointment three or four times a day. Creams and ointments containing red pepper stimulate the release of your body's own painkillers, says Dr. Jacques. Scientists believe that the active substance, capsaicin, also inter-

Pain-Pacifying Compress

For quick relief from lower-back pain, apply a compress soaked in a blend of pain-relieving essential oils and water, says Jacqueline Jacques, N.D., a naturopathic physician in Portland, Oregon, who specializes in pain management. This recipe combines the healing powers of peppermint, bergamot, and lavender to stop muscle spasms and quiet pain and inflammation. Adding Epsom salts to the water helps promote absorption of the essential oils through the skin. The magnesium in Epsom salts also acts as a muscle relaxant.

To make the compress, dip a small kitchen towel or a washcloth into the solution and wring it out. Apply it directly to the painful area for 15 to 20 minutes two or three times a day.

Use cold water for treatments for the first 24 hours after the onset of pain. Later, you can use warm water to make the solution or reheat leftover solution before using it. For added relief, lie on your back with your feet elevated while the compress is in place to help relieve the pressure on your lower back, says Dr. Jacques.

- **1 tablespoon Epsom salts**
- **1 gallon cold water**
- **3 drops peppermint essential oil**
- **3 drops bergamot essential oil**
- **4 drops lavender essential oil**

Mix the Epsom salts into the water, then add the peppermint, bergamot, and lavender oils and stir gently. Store extra solution in a dark glass container away from heat and light.

feres with the action of your body's pain messenger, called substance P.

Use a standardized ointment containing 0.075 or 0.025 percent capsaicin. "You won't get relief with the first application," says Dr. Jacques. It takes a few slatherings to wear out those pain messengers.

After you use the cream, be sure to wash your hands with soap to avoid a very uncomfortable burning sensation if you happen to touch other parts of your body. Also, never put the cream on a rash or open

Fast Facts

Cause: Most back pain is the result of overused muscles, ruptured disks, sprained ligaments, or irritated joints. In approximately 1 percent of cases, back pain is associated with tumors. Sometimes, no cause can be found.

Incidence: Lower-back pain is one of the most common medical problems. At some point in their lives, four out of five people experience it.

When to see the doctor: If you experience fever, pain that is considerably worse when you're lying down, or recent unexplained weight loss, or if pain persists for more than a week, call your physician.

wound. It's safe to use this remedy for long periods of time, but if pain persists for more than 3 to 4 weeks, see a doctor.

Willow

Take one or two capsules or 1 to 2 milliliters of tincture three times a day. Hippocrates recommended chewing the leaves of the willow tree for pain relief more than 2,400 years ago. In ancient Rome, the bark of the poplar tree (a member of the willow family) was prescribed for sciatic pain. This is a good, old-fashioned remedy for back pain, says Dr. Schor.

Today, herbalists still use the bark to treat pain and inflammation. Its active ingredient, salicin, is the chemical that was isolated in the 1800s to manufacture aspirin. So why not just pop an aspirin? Because willow doesn't cause stomach upset as aspirin can, explains Dr. Schor.

Because of the low salicin content of most commercial willow bark, you would need to drink $1\frac{1}{2}$ to 5 quarts of willow tea to get a dose equivalent to one aspirin. "Capsules are generally the easiest way to stomach willow. The herb has a horrid flavor," says Dr. Schor.

Peppermint, Lavender, and Rosemary

Blend four drops of each oil with ½ ounce of safflower oil to make a pain-relieving massage oil and use as needed. "Warm the oil to improve absorption and rub it directly on the painful area of your back two or three times a day," says Dr. Jacques. Essential oils provide pain relief when you inhale their aroma and when they are absorbed through your skin, she explains.

Peppermint, lavender, and rosemary all help to decrease pain, relieve inflammation, and keep muscles from going into spasms. Since stress is often a factor in back pain, their soothing psychological effect can also help, says Dr. Jacques.

BAD BREATH

$\mathcal{R}$ecords of bad breath date back to the earliest written medical texts, when, in 1550 B.C., Hippocrates suggested a mouth rinse made from herbs and wine. Roman dramatist Maccius Plautus, who lived about 200 B.C., decided that his wife's bad breath was just cause for infidelity.

It may seem that halitosis has chosen you, and only you, to grace with its signature smell, but rest assured, many others have dealt with it all along. "It's been a problem forever," says Anne Bosy, a researcher in oral malodor and founder of the Fresh Breath Clinic in Toronto.

The first thing you want to determine is whether you actually have bad breath. F. Michael Eggert, D.D.S., Ph.D., professor of dentistry at the University of Alberta in Edmonton, suggests this method: "Scrape the back of your tongue with a spoon and have a sniff of the stuff that comes off it." Pay attention to the type of smell.

Breath-Busting Mouthwash

Sure, you can head down to the drugstore and pick up a bottle of electric blue or red mouthwash, but why bother when it's so easy and cheap to make at home? Plus, this recipe from Flora Parsa Stay, D.D.S., a dentist in Oxnard, California, and author of The Complete Book of Dental Remedies, *doesn't contain the mouth-burning alcohol that's in most commercial preparations. Rinse and gargle with the mouthwash as needed, generally up to three times a day.*

- 1 cup warm water
- 1 teaspoon baking soda
- ¼ cup aloe juice
- ½ cup fresh parsley

Place the water in a small saucepan, add the baking soda, and stir until dissolved. Add the aloe. (The mixture will be cloudy.) Add the parsley and simmer on low heat for 30 minutes. Remove the parsley and let cool. Any leftover mouthwash can be refrigerated for up to a week.

A sour smell is normal and doesn't necessarily mean that you have bad breath. If it's a sulfuric smell similar to that of old eggs or an odor like bad meat, you need to take action. If you're not sure, ask a family member or close friend to help by smelling your breath, says Dr. Eggert. Then try these home halitosis helpers.

Parsley

Chew a sprig as needed. The ancient Romans munched on sprigs of parsley to freshen their breath. You'll see this custom echoed in the sprig of parsley on the side of your plate at a restaurant. Rome may have fallen, but at least the parsley cure for bad breath didn't go with it.

Parsley, says Bosy, contains chlorophyll, the same stuff used in some commercial breath fresheners. Fresh parsley costs much less, and you can use what's left over for cooking. Pick up a bunch of the herb at any grocery store, cut off a few sprigs, and chew them slowly, a sprig at a time. The longer it's in your mouth, the better. "Parsley doesn't just mask the smell, it actually deodorizes your mouth," she says.

Cloves

Chew as needed. For thousands of years, says Mel Rosenberg, Ph.D., a professor of microbiology at Tel Aviv University School of Dentistry in Israel who researches bad breath, the Iraqi people have used cloves to combat bad breath. And there's good reason for this tradition—cloves are rich in eugenol, an oily substance that is both antibacterial and highly aromatic. This oil is often used in toothpastes and mouthwashes. You don't have to spend the extra money to get fresh-breath benefits, though, since cloves are as close as your spice rack.

The cloves you need are the dried, round seed pods labeled "whole cloves." Simply take one clove, pop it in your mouth, and gently bruise it with your teeth. The aromatic oils can burn a little on sensitive tissue, so you'll have to keep them moving around, says Dr. Rosenberg. Keep at it for a few minutes or until you feel the essence permeating your mouth, then spit it out.

There are a couple of cautions, though. The seeds are small, so be careful you don't suck one down the wrong pipe. Also, don't use clove oil or powdered cloves, as they are both strong and can burn the tissues in your mouth.

Peppermint

Chew some leaves as needed. Is there anything as synonymous with fresh breath as mint? Peppermint is a rich source of menthol, another aromatic oil that is widely used in candy, toothpaste, chewing gum, and mouthwash. The best thing about fresh peppermint as a breath aid, says Dr. Eggert, is that it attacks on multiple fronts.

Fast FACTS

Cause: The causes of bad breath are many and include smoking, strong foods such as onions and garlic, and improper oral hygiene that allows festering bacteria to build up in your mouth. Even the mucus that drips from your sinuses onto the back of your tongue can create a powerful stench.

Incidence: Virtually everyone has bad breath at some time. About one-quarter of the population has halitosis on a regular basis.

When to see the doctor: If home remedies don't work for you, it's time to see a dentist. There are also specialists in oral malodor, who usually are affiliated with clinics associated with dental schools or major hospitals. You should also see a doctor if your breath has a fruity, sweet smell; a fishy odor; or a strong, cheesy smell, all of which may indicate medical problems.

Have you ever eaten garlic or onions and felt not only that your breath was bad but also that you were sweating out the odor? Well, you were. Some powerfully pungent foods are absorbed into the bloodstream, Dr. Eggert explains, and the smell comes out through your pores and through your lungs to your breath. Peppermint's volatile oils do the same thing. Not only do they help kill stinky bacteria in your mouth, but the oils also travel to your bloodstream and come out through the same avenues as the onions and garlic.

Fresh peppermint is available at some produce stands and supermarkets. Just break off a few leaves, chew them slowly, and swallow. Repeat as often as necessary, recommends Dr. Eggert. If you prefer a warm alternative, buy any of the commercially available peppermint teas and follow the package instructions.

Myrrh

Drink two cups of tea as needed. In the Christmas carol, myrrh "breathes a life of gathering gloom," but there's nothing gloomy about what it can do for your breath, says Flora Parsa Stay, D.D.S., a dentist in Oxnard, California, and author of *The Complete Book of Dental Remedies*. The aromatic nature of myrrh has been known since biblical times.

Add $\frac{1}{2}$ teaspoon of powdered myrrh, which is available in health food stores, to 2 cups of water and simmer for 30 minutes. Sip the tea and let the antiseptic fluid run over your tongue. Myrrh has a bitter taste, so be prepared for it.

Alternatively, you can dip your toothbrush into a tiny dab (not more than $\frac{1}{8}$ teaspoon), of powdered myrrh and get some of the same breath-freshening benefits by brushing with it after using your regular toothpaste. Be sure to brush your tongue, too. Then rinse well.

BLACK EYES

*I*t used to be that the first thing you thought of putting on a black eye was a thick steak. Times have definitely changed.

Some people get black eyes because of vitamin deficiencies that weaken the tiny blood vessels that run close to the surface of the skin there. Usually, though, they're simply bruises, the result of sudden and painful contact with hard objects. "Bruises around the eyes can be dramatic because the tissues there are extremely soft, like tissue paper," says Robert Abel Jr., M.D., clinical professor of ophthalmology at Thomas Jefferson University in Philadelphia. "In fact, the tissues around the eyes are so sensitive that bruises there often spread spontaneously from one eye to the other."

If you sustain a substantial knock to the eyeball, have it checked out by a doctor or an ophthalmologist, Dr. Abel says, to make sure that the eye hasn't been damaged by pressing against the bony structures around it. Most blows, though, bounce off those same bony structures and can cause bruising. (That's what they're there for, after all—to protect the eye.) In that case, what you need is a little TLC and some herbal first-aid.

Parsley

Apply parsley-laced ice cubes directly to the black eye. The first step to take in treating virtually any bruise, including a black eye, is to apply ice, says Dr. Abel. Cold constricts the blood vessels, thereby reducing inflammation and swelling.

Dr. Abel suggests a novel herbal twist on that old standby: ice cubes filled with parsley. Toss a handful of washed parsley and about $\frac{1}{4}$ cup of water into a blender or food processor and process until it looks like slush, he says. Then fill ice cube trays half full and put them in the freezer. Wrap a frozen cube in gauze and apply it to your closed eye as needed. Be careful not to get the water from the ice into your eye. It could contain bacteria from the parsley, which in turn could be transmitted to your eye.

Bromelain

Take three 500-milligram capsules four times a day until your black eye goes away. Bromelain is an enzyme derived from the pineapple plant that has anti-inflammatory properties. It's been tested on those who need it most: boxers. Researchers gave bromelain to 74 bruised boxers, while 72 injured boxers in another group were given a pill with no active ingredients (placebo). The result: More than 75 percent of the bromelain group healed in 4 days, compared to 14 percent of the placebo group.

"Bromelain works for any bruise resulting from injury, including black eyes," says C. Leigh Broadhurst, Ph.D., a nutrition consultant and herbalist based in Clovery, Maryland. "It helps digest some of the clotted blood that accumulates in a wound, which helps reduce inflammation, and basically cleans up the degraded tissues."

Fast FACTS

Comfrey

Soak the black eye with a compress. Comfrey contains allantoin, a chemical that promotes skin repair, and it's an anti-inflammatory. Both properties make it perfect for soothing the bruised tissues of a black eye.

Dr. Broadhurst recommends making a comfrey infusion by putting 10 to 12 drops of comfrey extract in 2 ounces of cold water. Dilute the mixture with 1 or 2 more ounces of water if this infusion stings. It won't hurt to refrigerate the mixture to make it even colder, she says. Apply to the closed, bruised eye two or three times a day for 5 to 10 minutes each time until the bruise goes away.

Calendula

Try a compress to help the healing. Calendula has healing properties similar to those of comfrey, and studies have shown that it fights inflammation and aids in the growth of healthy new cells. Janet Zand, N.D., O.M.D., a naturopathic doctor and doctor of oriental medicine in Austin, Texas, and Los Angeles, recommends making a calendula infusion. Put a tablespoon of the dried herb in 4 ounces of distilled, boiled water and steep for 10 to 15 minutes.

Let the mixture cool and strain it to remove any pieces of herb, then apply to the closed black eye using a clean cotton cloth. Hold it there for 5 to 10 minutes as often as you feel the need to, she says. Do not let the liquid enter your eye.

Witch Hazel

Use a cold compress three or four times a day. Witch hazel has anti-inflammatory properties and helps control bleeding.

To prepare a compress, Dr. Broadhurst recommends putting 10 to 12 drops of witch hazel tincture in 4 ounces of cold water. Soak a clean washcloth in the mixture, wring out the excess water, lie down, relax, and hold the cloth against your closed eye for 10 to 15 minutes.

You can prepare fresh witch hazel tea to use in this compress by steeping 3 tablespoons of the dried herb (bark, actually) in 8 ounces of water for no more than 5 to 10 minutes. Let the resulting brew cool with the herb in it, then strain it well—you don't want pieces of herb in your eye. Chill it in the refrigerator, then apply it in a compress as described for calendula.

BLISTERS

Striding out in a pair of new hiking boots or plunging into an afternoon of heavy yard work can rub you the wrong way. Literally. In fact, any activity that subjects your skin to pressure and friction can leave you with a painful blister. So can burns, contact with irritant plants, and certain diseases, such as chickenpox.

Blisters caused by rubbing are one of those first-aid "emergencies" that bring out the practical problem solver in many an herbalist, and the plant kingdom comes to the rescue with natural bandages and an abundant supply of antiseptics and skin soothers. Here are some herbal tips to make your next nature walk a pleasant, pain-free experience.

Plantain

Grab a fresh leaf or two to put in your shoe. "If you get a blister while you're out hiking and you don't have a bandage handy, you can use fresh plantain leaves as an emergency poultice," says Connie Catellani, M.D., medical director of the Miro Center for Integrative Medicine in Evanston, Illinois. The benefit is twofold: The soft leaves will cushion the tender spot and prevent further painful rubbing, and the antibacterial properties in the plantain will protect against infection should the blister burst.

Plantain is a common weed that you've probably seen in your yard. The plant starts out very low to the ground, but if left unchecked, it grows to be 6 to 18 inches high. It has wide, fanlike leaves that are dull green with wavy margins on the edges and have a parchmentlike texture. Eventually, it sprouts flower spikes that grow very long and thin and look something like pipe cleaners. The flowers are very tiny and reddish in color when they bloom.

Calendula

Drop some succus on the blister. For a burst blister, Mark Stengler, N.D., a naturopathic doctor in Oceanside, California, and author of *The Natural Physician: Your Health Guide for Common Ailments*, recommends calendula. "It's a natural disinfectant and also a vulnerary herb, which means that it speeds the healing of skin tissue."

Calendula tincture is fine to use, although it tends to run all over

Fast FACTS

Cause: Shoes that pinch and rub commonly cause blisters. You can also get these raised, fluid-filled areas on your skin if you are burned, come in contact with a chemical or a poisonous plant, or come down with a case of chickenpox. Eczema, herpes simplex, and shingles can also cause blisters.

Incidence: Virtually everyone gets a blister at some point.

When to see the doctor: See your doctor if you suspect that your blister is caused by a disease or if you notice redness or pus, which could be signs of infection.

---

the place. If you can lay your hands on a bottle of calendula succus, a low-alcohol tincture with a consistency somewhere between a liquid and a gel, it will stay in place better. The succus comes in a bottle with a dropper. Twice a day, let a couple of drops fall onto the blister, then cover it with a sterile dressing.

Tea Tree

Dab some oil on a burst blister four times a day for a week. With its antiseptic and germicidal properties, tea tree oil is a natural choice for preventing bacterial infection. "This is an excellent remedy for a blister that's popped," says Eric A. Weiss, M.D., assistant professor and associate director of emergency medicine at Stanford University Medical Center and founder of Adventure Medical Kits, an Oakland, California–based company that makes first-aid kits that include both conventional and herbal remedies.

It's best to dilute the tea tree oil with a vegetable oil, such as olive, safflower, or corn oil, before applying it to the blister, especially if the skin underneath is very painful and raw, says Dr. Catellani. Mix 3 parts vegetable oil with 1 part tea tree oil.

Comfrey

Saturate a bandage with oil and tape it over the blister. Whitney Miller, N.D., a naturopathic doctor who has a family practice in New London and Colchester, Connecticut, favors a comfrey dressing because this powerful herb is known to speed wound healing. Change the dressing as often as your level of activity requires.

BLOODSHOT EYES

City smog, smoke, dust, allergies, infections, sun, wind, lack of sleep—there are probably more potential sources of eye irritation in the world today than you can count.

"It isn't always easy to tell what's causing red, irritated eyes, even for a doctor," says Alice Laule, M.D., who practices holistic medicine and ophthalmology in Harrison, Arkansas. The classic signs of irritation are a burning sensation and some itching, she says. Severe itching usually suggests allergies. Discharge of pus or an aching type of pain could indicate an infection and should be checked out by an ophthalmologist, as should any eye problem that has an impact on your vision.

Sometimes, a vein in the eye bursts, causing a swatch of red in one spot on the eyeball. "It will look like someone took a red paintbrush to the eye," Dr. Laule says. Burst vessels by themselves are usually harmless, she adds, but they can be signs of a serious health condition, such as diabetes or high blood pressure. If this type of redness is recurrent or painful or you experience vision loss, see your ophthalmologist or general practitioner.

Good Witch Hazel Wash

Witch hazel provides the base for this herbal mixture, which cleans out irritants and soothes irritated eye tissues. This recipe, an old classic spruced up with some new touches, comes from C. Leigh Broadhurst, Ph.D., a nutrition consultant and herbal researcher based in Clovery, Maryland.

To make a compress, soak a washcloth or cloth napkin in the witch hazel mixture. Squeeze out the excess liquid until the cloth is wet but not dripping. Hold the compress over your closed eyes for 5 to 10 minutes twice a day.

4 ounces witch hazel (water extract, standardized form)
1 ounce pure aloe juice
10–12 drops total of any combination of extracts of echinacea root, thyme, lavender, and marshmallow

Combine the witch hazel, aloe, and herb extracts in a small bowl. Wash your eyes and face with plain water, then apply the mixture with an eye cup. If the eyewash is too strong—if it does not have an overall smooth, comforting effect—dilute it with water.

If plain old irritation is your problem, the best solution is to get away from whatever's causing it, Dr. Laule says. That may be easier said than done for anyone who lives or works in a city, but take heart: Eye irritation is a modern problem that some old-fashioned remedies can fix.

Potato

Make an eye-soothing poultice of fresh potato. Nobody knows exactly why, but the juice of a potato can do wonders for irritated eyes, says Nicholas G. Nonas, M.D., medical director of American WholeHealth, an integrative medical center in Littleton, Colorado.

The preparation couldn't be easier, although application can be a bit messy. Simply peel and finely grate a ripe baking potato (check that there are no green areas). Put the gratings in a piece of clean cloth that is strong enough to hold them but porous enough to let the juice run through. Gauze is ideal. Then lie back and hold the cloth on your closed eye for 5 to 10 minutes. Repeat as often as you like.

Eyebright

Make an eye rinse. Eyebright is aptly named: Its gentle anti-inflammatory properties can help make your red, irritated eyes bright and clear again. For a soothing eyewash, Dr. Nonas recommends buying something called euphrasia mother tincture at a health food store (*Euphrasia* is the botanical name for eyebright). Dissolve 10 drops of tincture in $\frac{1}{2}$ pint of warm water and add 1 teaspoon of salt. Salt-water solution has the effect of re-creating your natural tears, so it won't irritate your eyes.

Let the water cool to body temperature and then rinse your eyes thoroughly twice a day, using either an eyedropper, an eye cup, or a bulb syringe (an infant syringe with a blue bulb, used to suction mucus out of a baby's nose). Dr. Nonas recommends giving your eyes a good soaking with this solution by washing out each eye five or six times until it feels better. The recipe above makes about enough for one day, he says.

You can also make an eyebright rinse using the herb itself, says David Winston, a professional member of the American Herbalists Guild and an herbalist in Washington, New Jersey. Bring 4 ounces of water and a pinch of salt (about $\frac{1}{8}$ teaspoon) to a boil, then add about 2 teaspoons of dried eyebright. Let the mixture boil for 30 seconds in order to kill off any bacteria that may be in the herb. Remove the pan from the heat and let the mixture steep. When it cools, strain it through muslin or cheesecloth to get any particles out, so you don't add new sources of irritation while you're treating the old. Wash your eyes thoroughly twice a day, Winston says, using an eye cup. Refrigerate the mixture during the day

Cause: Any condition that might irritate the eyes can cause them to become bloodshot. Common irritants include air pollution, cigarette smoke, chemicals, dust, night driving, conjunctivitis or other infections, and allergies. Your eyes may also become bloodshot simply because they're too dry.

Incidence: People who live or work in polluted environments are more prone to eye irritation. Tear ducts become less efficient with age, which can cause dry eyes. Fair-skinned people with blue or green eyes tend to be more susceptible.

When to see the doctor: If the irritation is accompanied by severe pain or a decrease in vision, see a doctor immediately. If allergies cause year-round problems with irritated eyes, have a doctor test you to see if you have food allergies.

and make a fresh batch each morning to keep it completely bacteria-free.

Grape Seed

Take 200 milligrams of extract a day. If your eyes are red because of allergies, grape seed extract has properties that make it a natural antihistamine, Dr. Nonas says. It also has excellent anti-inflammatory capabilities, he adds, which make it perfect for irritated eyes. It is available in capsules.

Feverfew

Take 6 to 10 500-milligram capsules of extract or drink four to six cups of fresh tea a day. For red, swollen eyes caused by allergies, this hefty dose of feverfew can bring some much-needed relief, says C. Leigh Broadhurst, Ph.D., a nutrition consultant and herbalist based in Clovery, Maryland. Since this is a heavy dose, you should use it only when you need immediate relief, she says, and then only for a few days. If your allergies are less severe, however, take one capsule of feverfew extract three times a day or one to two cups of tea daily.

To make feverfew tea, boil some water, let it stand for a minute, then add 3 to 4 heaping tablespoons of the dried herb and steep for no more than 5 minutes. Strain out the feverfew before you drink the tea.

"This is a strong medicinal tea," says Dr. Broadhurst, "so don't expect it to taste very good." You can improve the flavor, she suggests, by adding dried chamomile, peppermint, or spearmint to the mixture in an amount equal to the feverfew.

THE BLUES

Long before Prozac was available, there were herbal remedies for depression.

Unlike prescription drugs of today, which are doled out only when a doctor decides that you are seriously depressed, herbal pick-me-ups can help you feel better when you're laboring with the basic blues and daily downers of life.

While herbs can help when you're down and out, there are other things that you need to do to shake off that melancholy, says George Milowe, M.D., a holistic physician in Saratoga Springs, New York. For starters, you have to address the underlying problem that is the source of your malaise.

You also need to be sure that you're getting enough sleep and eating properly, since exhaustion and poor nutrition can contribute to the blues. At the same time, you should be getting some regular mood-lifting exercise, Dr. Milowe says. And, of course, you ought to try one of these approaches.

St. John's Wort

Take 300 milligrams in capsule form three times a day or 20 to 30 drops of tincture two or three times a day, or drink a cup of tea three times daily. More than 20 carefully controlled studies have found that St. John's wort can help ease the blues and mild to moderate depression with fewer side effects than prescription drugs, says Dr. Milowe. Chemicals in this flowering herb seem to inhibit enzymes that break down the neurotransmitters, or brain chemicals, that make you feel good, he explains.

If you're taking St. John's wort capsules, look for a formula that's standardized to 0.3 percent hypericin, an active ingredient. Take 300 milligrams before or between meals three times a day, suggests Dr. Milowe.

Quality tincture is blood-red in color, adds Lise Alschuler, N.D., chair of the botanical medicine department at Bastyr University in Kenmore, Washington.

If you'd rather have your St. John's wort in a teacup, use 1 rounded teaspoon of dried herb, add 8 ounces of boiling water, cover, and steep for 15 minutes. Strain the tea before drinking. Check to be sure that the flowers you use in your brew have a little red color and that the leaves are green, not brown—that means they're fresh.

Like prescription antidepressants, St. John's wort (wort means "plant" in Old English) takes a few weeks to have full effect. You can take it as long as necessary. If you're already taking a prescription antidepressant, though, check with your doctor before adding St. John's wort.

Green Oats

Take 1 teaspoon of tincture in 1 cup of water twice daily. The invigorating effects of green oats are the inspiration behind the ex-

Fast FACTS

Cause: Stressful situations, such as trouble at work or problems in relationships, can contribute to the blues and depression. Nutritional deficiencies, certain prescription drugs, food allergies, and health
problems, particularly thyroid disorders, can also be culprits.

Incidence: Everyone gets the blues on the heels of life's disappointments.
About 17 percent of Americans will have a bout of severe, lingering
depression at some time in their lives.

When to see the doctor: You should see your physician if feelings of
melancholy linger for more than a couple of weeks or if they interfere with your personal or professional life. You should do the same
if you have telltale signs of clinical depression: feelings of melancholy or hopelessness, loss of pleasure or interest in favorite activities, changes in appetite or sleep habits, fatigue, feelings of
worthlessness and guilt, difficulty thinking, or thoughts of death or
suicide.

pression "sowing your wild oats," says Erik Von Kiel, O.D., a holistic
osteopathic physician in Allentown, Pennsylvania, who recommends
green oats to help shake off mild depression. You can find green oat
extract in tincture form at most health food stores.

Siberian Ginseng

**Take 15 drops of tincture each day or 400 milligrams in capsule
form two or three times daily before meals.** Ginseng can also alleviate
mild depression without causing the side effects associated with prescription drugs, says Dr. Alschuler. Look for a 25:1 tincture, meaning
that it was made with 25 parts plant to 1 part alcohol.

If you buy capsules, look for formulas standardized to contain 1
percent eleutherosides, suggests Dr. Milowe.

Ginkgo

Take 80 milligrams three times a day. Ginkgo is particularly helpful for the elderly, says Dr. Milowe. Among other things, it improves circulation to the brain, he says. Look for capsules standardized to contain 24 percent ginkgolides, an active ingredient.

BODY ODOR

*S*weat stinks.

Well, sometimes it does.

On a hot day or during strenuous exercise or emotional turmoil, a person may sweat several quarts a day. Even on a cool day devoid of exercise or stress, the body loses more than a pint of perspiration. This is typically unnoticeable, however, and it evaporates as soon as it reaches the surface of the skin. It's when sweat secretions aren't washed away and bacteria grow that a body can get a bit rank.

The primary function of perspiration is to maintain body temperature at a constant level. The skin is therefore cooled as sweat evaporates.

Cooling us off isn't the only benefit of sweating. Body odor contains pheromones, chemicals that may attract the opposite sex with their subtle smells. A Japanese entrepreneur even developed synthetic sweat-laced underpants for men in an effort to re-create the pheromone effect.

Still, if you sometimes reek like last week's cabbage when you sweat, you probably want to douse the smell, not savor it. Conventional solutions include washing regularly and diligently using deodorant or antiperspirant.

Fast FACTS

Cause: Body odor assaults our noses when bacteria form where perspiration has been secreted. The human body has about two million sweat glands, of which there are two kinds, apocrine and eccrine. The largest are the apocrine glands, located in the armpits and groin, that are responsible for body odor. The eccrine glands, whose function is to cool the body, are found all over the body, with the largest number on the soles of the feet and the palms of the hands.

Incidence: While there are no statistics on how many people have body odor, it's widespread enough to have been a source of concern to people for centuries.

When to see the doctor: Seeing a doctor because of your body bouquet is rarely necessary. If body odor is present at an early age, it could signal an enzyme deficiency. Sometimes, people with skin diseases such as psoriasis and eczema have an increase in skin bacteria and odor. If this is a concern for you and you aren't having the skin condition treated, see a doctor.

If you wash too often, however, you may irritate your skin, especially in dry or winter weather, says Kenneth Landow, M.D., a Las Vegas dermatologist and professor in the department of medicine and dermatology at the University of Southern California in Los Angeles. And in case you don't know the difference between a deodorant and an antiperspirant, it's this: A deodorant masks odor, while an antiperspirant limits the amount of sweat that comes to the skin's surface.

In addition to these conventional solutions, here are some herbal remedies.

Arnica

Apply arnica cream in place of a deodorant. Arnica doesn't mask the smell, it stops it at the source, says Terry Willard, Ph.D., a clinical herbalist, professional member of the American Herbalists Guild (AHG), and founder and president of Wild Rose College of Natural Healing in Calgary, Alberta. Arnica kills odor-producing bacteria for several days, so you need to apply it only about once a week. You can find arnica products in many health food stores.

Parsley

Eat 1 teaspoon of parsley with meals that contain odor-producing foods like garlic. Parsley is a natural odor fighter, Dr. Willard says. If you can't take it straight, try the herb in a 500-milligram capsule. You can also make a tea with 1 teaspoon of chopped fresh parsley and 1 cup of boiling water. Steep it for 5 minutes before drinking.

Witch Hazel and Sage

Make an herbal deodorant. Witch hazel is an astringent, so it has a drying effect that can help stop perspiration, says Mindy Green, a founder and professional member of the AHG, director of educational services at the Herb Research Foundation in Boulder, Colorado, and co-author of *Aromatherapy: A Complete Guide to the Healing Art*. She recommends creating a deodorant consisting of 1 ounce of witch hazel, 1 ounce of sage tincture, and 20 drops of your choice of bergamot, rosewood, lavender, sandalwood, tea tree, or rosemary essential oils. Mix the ingredients in a small spray bottle and use the concoction under your arms as you would a commercial deodorant. Let it dry before getting dressed. If you like, you can also use this on your feet.

Bergamot and rosewood are effective because of their antibacterial properties, Green says. If you like a floral-scented deodorant, use lavender. For a more earthy or spicy smell, add sandalwood, tea tree, or rosemary, either alone or in combination.

BOILS

*I*n biblical times, healing boils was a picnic, or at least, the method of healing boils included one of the contents of the picnic basket—figs. It's right there in the book of Isaiah: "Let them take a lump of figs, and lay it as a plaster upon the boil, and he shall recover."

European gypsies knew a thing or two about treating these infected hair follicles, too. Their traditional—and distinctly less appetizing—romany balm was an unctuous ointment made from 3 ounces of pig fat, 1 ounce of horse-hoof clippings, a leek, and 1 ounce of grated elder bark.

Also known as a furuncle, a boil begins when a hair follicle is infected by bacteria. The hairy parts of the body—the neck, face, buttocks, and armpits—are the likeliest spots for a boil to develop. The white or yellow pus in the center of a boil is actually made up of white blood cells that have rushed to the site to fight the infection, along with dead skin cells and bacteria.

A boil begins as a tender, warm, red lump that, over the course of a day or two, increases in size and becomes progressively more painful. It hurts because, as the pus collects underneath the skin, pressure builds up. Usually, a boil bursts on its own within 2 weeks, and as the pus drains out, the painful pressure is relieved and healing begins to take place.

It's no fun waiting for a boil to burst, but you can take steps to speed the process along. "Ultimately, you want to get fluids to drain, so they need to be gently drawn to the surface of the skin," says Marcey Shapiro, M.D., a family doctor in Albany, California, who combines natural healing with conventional medicine. Pressing a cloth soaked in hot water against the boil every few hours is one of the simplest remedies. Along with taking away some of the pain, it will hasten the draining of the boil, says Dr. Shapiro. Most of the herbal remedies for boils work along similar lines—and they're a little more appealing to use than mashed figs or pig fat.

Goldenseal and Echinacea

Take two 500-milligram capsules of each herb three times daily for 7 days and apply an herbal paste to the boil twice a day for 2 or 3 days. Mark Stengler, N.D., a naturopathic doctor in Oceanside, California, and author of *The Natural Physician: Your Health Guide for Common Ailments*, recommends these herbs because of their strong antibacterial properties. To launch an effective, all-out attack on boils, you should use the herbs both internally and externally.

To make the topical application, you'll need goldenseal and echinacea powders. If you can't find them in a health food store, buy 500-milligram capsules and break them open. Mix 1 tablespoon of each herb with enough egg white to form a thick paste. Spread it right on the boil. The paste will dry on the boil and help suck some of the bacterial poisons out, says Dr. Stengler. You should see some improvement after a couple of days of treatment.

Slippery Elm and Eucalyptus

Apply a hot poultice to the boil repeatedly. Penelope Ody, a member of Britain's National Institute of Medical Herbalists and author of many books about herbs, including *The Complete Medicinal Herbal*, recommends this traditional remedy for extracting the central core of a boil.

Add enough boiling water to 25 grams of powdered slippery elm to form a paste. Mix in three drops of eucalyptus oil. Once the mixture has cooled but is still quite warm, spread it on the boil and cover with gauze. Apply a fresh poultice when the mixture cools completely, repeating as often as you can until the pus begins to drain, says Ody. This may take a few hours or several days, she adds.

Fast FACTS

Cause: Boils can indicate poor resistance to infection, or they can be the result of poor hygiene. Other possible causes are diabetes, obesity, and a poor diet. Often though, a boil is simply a localized infection with no easily identifiable cause.

Incidence: Boils are very common; most people will experience one at some time. Football players, wrestlers, and other athletes seem to be particularly susceptible to recurrent boils.

When to see the doctor: Make an appointment to see your doctor if a boil does not burst on its own within 2 weeks. If you regularly get boils, you should see your doctor to rule out the possibility of an underlying disease such as diabetes.

Figwort, Honeysuckle, and Thyme

Brew a tea using equal portions of these herbs and drink it three times a day. Together, these herbs make an effective infusion that's easy to make at home and tastes fairly pleasant, says Ody. "The thyme has quite a strong flavor, so it helps to disguise the others," she adds.

The tea acts as an antiseptic. Chinese honeysuckle flowers are included because they are antibacterial. Cleansing and anti-inflammatory, figwort has a long tradition of use for suppurating skin complaints, says Ody.

Mix equal portions of the dried herbs and place 1 teaspoon of the mixture in a mug. Pour in a cup of boiling water, cover and steep for 15 minutes, then strain.

Ginger

Twice daily, grate 1 inch of fresh root and pack it on top of the boil. Dr. Shapiro calls this the counterirritant approach because instead of trying to soothe the inflammation, its purpose is to elicit a reaction—in this case, bringing blood to the surface and raising the boil from under the skin.

Simply grate an inch-long piece of ginger and heap it on top of the boil. Sit still for 20 minutes to let it do its work, then repeat later in the day. This remedy is especially good for deep boils that are painful and stubbornly refuse to surface, says Dr. Shapiro. Because ginger increases circulation, your skin will turn red, she adds.

Burdock

Make a paste from fresh seeds and apply it to the boil for 1 hour twice a day. If you have a dog, you probably know what burdock seed looks like, because the burrs are always getting caught in dogs' furry coats. "Burdock seed is fabulous for boils," says Dr. Shapiro. "It's very drawing and clearing."

About the size of a sesame seed, burdock seed may be a little hard to find, but you should be able to track it down as a specialty item, either in a local herb store or through an herbal catalog. Soak 1 tablespoon of seeds in 1 cup of water for 10 minutes. Strain off the liquid and mash the seeds into a thick paste. You can cover the paste with gauze, then wipe it off after an hour, or leave the gauze-covered paste on overnight for your second application.

BRONCHITIS

Get a bad case of bronchitis, and the first thing the doctor will try to figure out is "which kind?" An unpleasant symphony of hacking, coughing, and lung-clearing will tell your physician that it's bronchitis, all right—but then the task is to determine whether it's acute or chronic. To do that, any doctor will want to know whether you're a smoker. Chronic bronchitis is the version that's usually tobacco-induced. For that, the cure is clear: Stop smoking. Allergic conditions may also cause chronic bronchitis.

Anyone, smoker or nonsmoker, can get acute bronchitis, which is an infection of the bronchial tubes that connect the windpipe to the lungs. But smokers are more susceptible. "An ordinary cold is more likely to turn into bronchitis if somebody smokes," says Connie Catellani, M.D., medical director of the Miro Center for Integrative Medicine in Evanston, Illinois. "It is a frequent side effect of any viral respiratory infection that gets out of control." The inflamed bronchi produce a lot of airflow-restricting mucus; the wrenching cough is generated by your lungs to get rid of that mucus.

There's a natural healing progression for overcoming acute bronchitis, and herbal medicine works right along with it. "First, get the immune system up to fight the infection, then clear out the residue, and finally, heal the lung tissue," says Chanchal Cabrera, a member of Britain's National Institute of Medical Herbalists, a professional member of the American Herbalists Guild, and an herbalist in Vancouver. "Herbs basically do what the body is trying to do to heal itself."

Conventional medicine often uses antibiotics to curb the infection, along with cough suppressants. "Those will certainly work," Cabrera says, "but they won't strengthen the lung tissue, they won't support the immune function, and they do nothing to protect you against future attacks."

If anything, antibiotics weaken the immune system for the next attack, says Dr. Catellani. They tend to promote the growth of resistant bacteria, which means that the next infection may be more virulent and harder to treat.

On the other hand, the following home herbal remedies recommended by herbal experts for acute bronchitis will do all of those positive things. Plus, they should make you feel a lot better while you're on the way to recovery.

CHANCHAL'S TONIC TEA FOR THE LUNGS

Once herbal remedies have done their job on bronchitis, you'll still be a little weak in the lung department. Chanchal Cabrera, a member of Britain's National Institute of Medical Herbalists, a professional member of the American Herbalists Guild, and an herbalist in Vancouver, has created a tonic tea to rebuild bronchitis-damaged lung tissue and boost your immune system so you'll be less likely to get it again. Here's her explanation of what each of the ingredients does.

- Plantain leaf is a lung tonic.
- Horsetail is a connective tissue regenerator.
- Ground ivy leaf is a lung tonic.
- Gotu kola leaf or root is a connective tissue regenerator.
- Licorice root is a lung tonic, immune booster, and expectorant.
- Astragalus root is an overall immune booster.

All of these herbs are easy to find at well-stocked health food stores, with the possible exception of ground ivy, which may be omitted from the blend if necessary. Use equal parts of the dried herbs to make a tea blend, then simmer 1 ounce (by weight) of the blend in 1 pint of water for 10 minutes to make a strong tea. Strain and drink one to two cups a day for 6 weeks following a bout of bronchitis.

Echinacea

Take 500 milligrams in capsule form four times a day, or drink four to five cups of tea a day. A stimulator of infection-fighting white blood cells, echinacea root is the herb of choice for respiratory infec-

Fast FACTS

Cause: Cigarette smoking is by far the most common cause of chronic bronchitis, but it can also be aggravated by allergic conditions. Acute bronchitis usually starts when a viral infection such as a common cold reaches the bronchial tubes, with a bacterial infection sometimes following it and complicating the condition.

Incidence: Acute bronchitis is a common complication of the very common cold, and it generally clears up in 1 to 2 weeks. Chronic bronchitis, however, is a chronic obstructive pulmonary disease, or COPD, that affects about 14 million Americans, making it the seventh leading chronic condition in the United States.

When to see the doctor: A cold that turns into a cough but starts to subside with fluids, rest, and herbal remedies and doesn't include a fever may not require a doctor's care. If your cough is complicated by fever, chest discomfort, difficulty breathing, or bloody sputum, however, you should see a medical professional right away.

---

tions. Bronchitis is no exception. "The first thing to try is echinacea and rest," says David Field, N.D., a naturopathic physician, licensed acupuncturist, and president of the California Association of Naturopathic Physicians in Santa Rosa. For acute bronchitis, he recommends the freeze-dried root in capsule form at the very first hint of symptoms.

You can also sip echinacea tea. Cabrera recommends making a medicinal-strength echinacea decoction by simmering 1 ounce (by weight) of echinacea root (buy it already cut and sifted at a health food store) in 1 pint of water for 10 minutes. Strain the tea, then "drink four to five cups a day to get the results you're looking for," Cabrera says. "That's really a moderate dose."

That moderate dose will still taste pretty strong. Luckily, you can sweeten it up a bit. "When you're dealing with a lung condition like bronchitis, adding a little honey is fine," Cabrera says. "It's good in the lungs as an expectorant."

After the first few days, cut the dose in half, whether it's tea or capsules, and continue only as long as you still have symptoms.

Garlic

Sleep with a poultice of mashed garlic and wet socks. The allicin in garlic is a powerful antimicrobial for lung infections such as bronchitis. A great way to get it into your lungs is to make what Jacob Schor, N.D., a naturopathic physician in Denver, calls a garlic foot poultice. It's easy to do.

Just mash from two to six raw garlic cloves (depending on the size of your feet) and mix in enough small dabs of petroleum jelly to keep the goo from falling apart. Spread it on the bottoms of your feet, put plastic bags over them, and don wet socks. Add a layer of dry socks and snuggle into bed. Sure, it sounds goofy, but there's no better way to get garlic to your lungs than to let your blood circulation whisk it there after it soaks into your feet, Dr. Schor says.

Try this wet sock treatment early in the infection. Garlic can be irritating, so apply the mash to the bottoms of your feet, not the sensitive tops, and use it only if your feet are free of cuts or abrasions.

Usnea

Take 3 teaspoons of tincture a day. Usnea, sometimes called old man's beard, goes right to work on the infection component of bronchitis. "It has a lot of acids in it that are especially active against the type of bacteria that can cause bronchitis," Cabrera says.

Usnea is actually a lichen that is ineffective as a tea because the active chemical constituents aren't extracted well in water and need alcohol as a solvent. But tinctures are available in well-stocked health food stores or by mail order. Look for a 1:5 tincture—that is, 1 part of the dried herb to 5 parts liquid, 70 percent of which is alcohol. Take the tincture three times a day between meals until the infection is gone, says Cabrera.

BRUISES

$\mathcal{L}$ike a painter's palette, a bruise seems to span the whole color spectrum, from deep indigo through violet and vermilion to glowing, saffron yellow.

This parade of colors begins when a fall or blow hurts a blood vessel but doesn't break the skin. The blood seeps out of the injured vessel, making the skin around it black and blue. The ensuing color changes are the result of chemical changes in the pigment of the red blood cells as they break down and are absorbed back into the bloodstream.

Even though bruises are very rarely serious, they're uncomfortably tender and not very appealing to the eye. Thankfully, the human body is remarkably efficient at dealing with bruises. Although they usually fade without any treatment after 10 to 14 days, you can treat them with simple remedies, such as elevating the injured area and applying ice packs for a day or two to help lessen any swelling, says Pierre Brunschwig, M.D., a member of the American Holistic Medical Association who practices at Helios Health Center in Boulder, Colorado. The world of herbs also has some impressive solutions.

Arnica

Smooth gel over the bruise. "This is a must-have for your first-aid kit," says Marion Gladwell, a member of Britain's National Institute of Medical Herbalists who has an herbal practice at Bury Natural Health Center in Suffolk, England. Germany's Commission E, which evaluates herbs for safety and effectiveness, recommends arnica flower specifically for bruises and sprains. The more quickly you can get this anti-inflammatory gel on the bruise, the better, so be sure to always keep a tube handy, says Gladwell. Look for a homeopathic arnica preparation such as Traumed, which is widely available in health food stores.

Dr. Brunschwig suggests this treatment for a severe bruise: Rub in the arnica gel until it seems to be absorbed, then apply another thin

ADVENTURES IN HERBALISM

EVERYTHING IN ITS PLACE

*H*erbalists sometimes refer to a phenomenon known as the Doctrine of Signatures. According to this rule, herbs can actually offer clues to their medicinal use through their physical form or the way in which they grow, says Lorilee Schoenbeck, N.D., a naturopathic physician at the Champlain Center for Natural Medicine in Shelburne, Vermont.

The doctor found a telling example of the Doctrine of Signatures while hiking in Oregon's Columbia River Gorge. After a particularly arduous hike to a waterfall, Dr. Schoenbeck decided to brave the sharp, slippery volcanic terrain near the base of the waterfall. "I knew that just one slip would lead to a traumatic fall," she recalls.

As she got closer, she noticed that there were pretty yellow flowers growing on top of the rocks nearest to the pounding water. She discovered that the plants were a species of arnica, an herb prescribed by herbalists the world over for trauma and bruising.

layer and cover it snugly with a large bandage or a wrap. If you experience numbness or if the skin appears blue beyond the wrap, loosen it, he says. You may leave the bruise covered overnight, but change the wrap and reapply the arnica daily until the pain is gone. "It should improve all the symptoms—not just the color or appearance but also the tenderness," he says.

St. John's Wort

Gently smooth infused oil onto the bruise three times a day. St. John's wort oil is excellent for bruises, says Bradley Bongiovanni,

Fast FACTS

Cause: Bruises happen when a fall or blow damages blood vessels but doesn't break the skin. The blood leaks into the tissues, making the skin around it black and blue.

Incidence: Everyone on the planet has been bruised at some time or other. People who frequently take aspirin bruise more easily because aspirin reduces the blood's tendency to clot.

When to see the doctor: If a bruise doesn't go away or at least fade within about 2 weeks, or if bruises start appearing for no obvious reason, call your doctor.

N.D., a naturopathic doctor at Wellspace in Cambridge, Massachusetts. It works better on bruises the sooner you can apply it. "I've had patients tell me that they fell off a bike and knew they'd have a bruise, so they went home and put St. John's wort oil on the area," says Dr. Bongiovanni. "The next day, they had either no bruise or just a very slight discoloration." Make sure that you apply the oil only to unbroken or unscratched skin.

Comfrey

Wrap a poultice around the bruised area. "This one's great for those goose-egg-producing mountain bike spills," says Rena Bloom, N.D., a naturopathic physician in Denver.

A member of the forget-me-not family, this fuzzy-leaved plant has long been prized for its ability to help wounds heal. Comfrey's common names, knitbone and boneset, attest to its historical use as an aid to mending broken bones. Its wound-healing properties are at least partly due to a chemical in the herb called allantoin that helps speed healing. Germany's Commission E, which evaluates herbs for safety and effectiveness, endorses use of the herb for bruises.

Soak 3 to 4 tablespoons of dried comfrey leaves in a cup of boiled water for 10 to 15 minutes, then place the warm mass directly on the skin, holding it in place with gauze that you have soaked in apple-cider vinegar. Wrap the gauze around the bruised area, and, says Dr. Bloom, "you should be like new the next day." Comfrey itches when it's dry, so remove the poultice when it's no longer moist. Don't use this treatment on broken skin—only on bruises and mild abrasions.

Rose Hips and Hibiscus

Make an herbal tea to drink twice a day and an herbal compress to apply to the bruise. "These herbs are high in vitamin C and bioflavonoids, and they taste really good," says Dr. Bongiovanni of this winning combination that speeds up healing by strengthening the blood vessels and decreasing recovery time.

For the tea, mix $\frac{1}{2}$ tablespoon each of dried rose hips and hibiscus in 1 cup of boiling water. Steep for 10 minutes, strain, and drink. Use the same recipe for the compress, but let the tea cool, then soak a washcloth in it and press it against the bruised area for 30 minutes two or three times a day. Use both the tea and the compress for best results, says Dr. Bongiovanni, but don't apply the compress to broken skin. The tea can be quite astringent and painful, he says, so wait until the skin heals before using the compresses.

BURNOUT

A TV commercial a few years ago captured a painful truth about modern times. It showed a series of average folks looking stressed and miserable. The announcer explained matter-of-factly what the problem was: "Life got harder."

Burnout is what happens when life seems to get harder, when the normal stresses of modern life become overwhelming, says psychiatrist James Gordon, M.D., director of the Mind/Body Center in Washington, D.C., and author of *Manifesto for a New Medicine*. Often, it's the body's way of signaling mental and emotional distress, a sign that the pressure or unhappiness of a given situation is taking a toll on your health.

"The first question to ask is, why are you burned out?" Dr. Gordon says. "Burnout is a symptom—a sign that something in your life isn't working. That's what you have to address."

This is not to say that physical factors don't count in burnout—they do, tremendously. A holistic approach to the problem is what's needed, says Thomas Kruzel, N.D., former president of the American Association of Naturopathic Physicians, who practices in Portland, Oregon. Restoring physical, emotional, and spiritual balance is the goal, he says. Diet, exercise, nutrition, soothing activities such as yoga or meditation, and rest are all key. And while herbal remedies by themselves can't fix burnout, they can help.

Asian Ginseng

Take between 75 and 150 milligrams twice a day. Ginseng is one of the leading adaptogenic herbs, which means that it works in a variety of ways to help the body adapt to situations that are less than optimal.

"Ginseng has overall toning and strengthening properties that help give people a greater tolerance for stress," says Timothy Birdsall, N.D., director of naturopathic medicine at Midwestern Regional Medical Center in Zion, Illinois. One of its benefits is a restorative effect on the adrenal glands, which tend to be hit especially hard by burnout.

Dr. Birdsall recommends buying Asian ginseng—also called Chinese, Korean, or panax ginseng—that has at least 20 percent ginsenosides. Siberian ginseng is also an effective adaptogen, he says. Look for capsules that contain at least 0.5 percent eleutherosides and use the same dosage as for Asian ginseng. Take the capsules with meals, he suggests, starting with the lower dose and increasing it after 3 to 4 weeks if necessary. You can take it for 4 to 12 weeks.

Schisandra

Take 400 to 600 milligrams three or four times a day. Like ginseng, schisandra is an adaptogenic herb that is widely used in China, according to C. Leigh Broadhurst, Ph.D., an herbal researcher and nutrition consultant based in Clovery, Maryland.

"Schisandra is a bit more gung-ho than ginseng," she says, "which is why it's one of my favorite herbs for increasing athletic performance. When you're pushing yourself too hard, you have a lot of biochemical debris in your bloodstream. Schisandra can help flush the toxins out. It also helps the body process blood sugar more efficiently, so you don't feel that you have to keep pumping yourself up with sugar or coffee every couple of hours."

The dosage above is recommended for times of high stress, Dr. Broadhurst says. Once things calm down, you can take one-half to two-thirds of that dose on an ongoing basis.

Ashwaganda

Take one 400- to 600-milligram capsule three or four times a day. Ashwaganda is India's version of ginseng, according to Dr. Broadhurst. "Like other adaptogens, it helps increase resilience to stress," she says, "no matter what form the stress takes. Some people are hyper when they're burned out, while others are sluggish. Adaptogens like ashwaganda help return you to normal."

It's fine to take ashwaganda on an ongoing basis, Dr. Broadhurst says, but, as with schisandra, it's a good idea to reduce the dosage to two capsules a day once you're out of a crisis situation.

Fast FACTS

Cause: A combination of physical, emotional, and spiritual factors—from stress and insomnia to feeling unappreciated or spiritually adrift—can contribute to burnout.

Incidence: Given the stress and pressures of today's environment and the variety of contributing causes, burnout can affect anyone.

When to see the doctor: Any sign of a physical breakdown related to stress—exhaustion, sleeplessness, or frequent colds—suggests that a checkup may be in order. Psychological symptoms worth checking out include lethargy, excessive difficulty getting out of bed in the morning, changes in appetite, or marked passivity. Consult a therapist or a general practitioner.

Turmeric

Take one 400- to 600-milligram capsule of extract three times a day. Anyone who eats Indian food is familiar with turmeric, the bright yellow spice that's a principal ingredient in the cuisine. Besides being flavorful, turmeric is an excellent source of antioxidant vitamins, Dr. Broadhurst says, and upping your daily dose of antioxidants is a good idea when you're burned out. She suggests looking for a turmeric product with a standardized extract of curcuminoids, the active ingredients.

Oats or Passionflower

Drink a cup of tea before bedtime. Oats have antidepressant properties that can round off some of the sharp edges before you go to sleep, according to Dr. Kruzel. "This herb helps restore the nerve endings that are frayed, in the body and in the brain," he says. Passionflower has a similar ability to restore the central nervous system.

To make a nerve-soothing infusion of either oats or passion-

Burnout Blend

One of the more pleasant ways to fight burnout is with the soothing smells of aromatherapy. Here's a formula especially designed to counter burnout by aromatherapist Victoria Edwards, owner of Leydet Aromatics in Fair Oaks, California.

To use, sprinkle a few drops of the oil blend on a handkerchief, cotton ball, or tissue, then sniff. The formula is particularly effective for burnout that is exacerbated by exhaustion, Edwards has found. She often gives it to clients who are recovering from jet lag. Don't use this for more than 2 weeks at a time.

5 drops geranium essential oil
5 drops bay laurel essential oil
10 drops lavender essential oil

Combine the geranium, laurel, and lavender oils in a small, dark glass bottle and shake.

flower, Dr. Kruzel recommends pouring boiling water over a wire tea ball filled with 1 tablespoon of dried herb and steeping it for 5 minutes. Add 1 to 2 teaspoons of lemon and a little honey and use as needed.

Geranium or Bay Laurel

Use either scent as aromatherapy to help fight frazzled nerves. "These are the two best essential oils for fighting burnout," says aromatherapist Victoria Edwards, owner of Leydet Aromatics in Fair Oaks, California. "You can use them wherever you are—commuting on a train, in your car, or sitting at home in front of the TV. Just try a few drops sprinkled on a tissue or a handkerchief. You'll notice a calming effect immediately." Use as needed, but don't use bay laurel for more than 2 weeks at a time.

BURNS

*I*t's hard to stay cool when your skin has just been attacked by searing heat. If you're accident-prone, the kitchen can be a battleground. See that cast-iron pot of chili simmering on the stove? Grab the handle without thinking, and it will switch from comforting friend to dangerous foe in a flash. Many herbs will help, but if you want to know the truth, the ultimate relief for a minor burn is mere steps away. That's right, the cold water from your kitchen faucet.

Nothing stops the pain of a minor burn more effectively than plunging it under cold running water for at least 10 to 15 minutes. "Heat damage continues after the heat source is removed," says Pierre Brunschwig, M.D., a member of the American Holistic Medical Association who practices at the Helios Health Center in Boulder, Colorado. Making the skin cold fast minimizes this lingering effect, he says, because it carries the heat away from the skin.

If you have a first-degree burn—with redness and swelling but no blistering—go ahead and treat it at home. Second-degree burns, with significant blistering, are generally not serious if they're small (less than 3 inches across), but if the skin is broken, don't apply any lotions or creams, as this could increase the chance of infection. For the same reason, leave blisters intact.

Here are some herbal remedies to cool things down.

Aloe

Smooth aloe gel directly onto the burn as often as necessary while you have pain. Aloe is soothing and healing for the skin because it has both anti-inflammatory and antimicrobial properties, says Ian Bier, N.D., Ph.D., a naturopathic physician, licensed acupuncturist, and natural medicine researcher in Portsmouth, New Hampshire. Aloe also appears to stimulate the production of connective tissue cells, thus helping the healing process.

Ideally, says Dr. Bier, you should slice the leaf of a fresh plant to release some of the thick gel, then apply that directly to the burn. If that's not feasible, go to your health food store and try to find a brand of aloe lotion that's hypoallergenic and as natural as possible—not that bright green stuff that you often find next to the sunscreen. "Good aloe gel is basically just the clear plant gel with only a little bit of preservative," says Dr. Bier, "so you'll want to keep it in the fridge.

"The cold gel feels great on a burn, and because it's a gel, it stays put," he says. He should know. After a cooking accident that splattered hot oil over the entire left side of his face, he immediately reached into the fridge for a bottle of aloe and dabbed the icy gel onto his scorched skin. "Whenever the pain started to come back, I just kept putting more on until it stopped," he says. You should continue to apply the gel several times a day even after the burn is no longer painful. When you don't see any redness or discoloration, you can stop.

Calendula

Apply calendula gel directly to the burn as often as necessary to relieve the pain, or at least three times a day for 2 to 3 days even if you have no pain. One of the nice things about a gel is that it supports your skin's natural moisture layer, which is essential where burns are concerned, says Marcey Shapiro, M.D., a family doctor in Albany, California, who combines natural healing with conventional medicine.

"With a burn, part of the damage to the tissue arises simply from a loss of water. The skin dries out, so putting a gel on is really beneficial," she says. Stop using it when you haven't had any pain for 3 days or there is no inflammation. That means that the wound is on the way to healing. You can find calendula gel at many health food stores.

Witch Hazel

Dab on witch hazel water with a cotton ball. Witch hazel is another herb that's good for burns, says Bradley Bongiovanni, N.D., a

Cause: Burns happen when skin comes in contact with excessive heat, such as an open flame or a hot skillet handle. Other causes include chemicals, radiation, and electrical current.

Incidence: Anyone can be burned, but minor burns are more common among young adults. Teenage boys are most at risk for fireworks injuries, while small children have the highest incidence of scald burns from hot water or beverages or spilled cooking pots.

When to see the doctor: If you have a second-degree burn that is more than a couple of inches across, with pain, swelling, and blistering, or that is on your hands, face, or genitals, see your doctor. If you were burned by corrosive chemicals, electricity, hot liquids, or contact with fire, play it safe and seek medical attention. Third-degree burns are medical emergencies that require immediate attention. Often, the skin looks white or charred, and because the nerve endings have been destroyed, you may feel no immediate pain.

naturopathic doctor at Wellspace in Cambridge, Massachusetts. The diluted concentration that you can buy in any drugstore is fine. Dab on just enough to cover the burn. You can apply it as needed to relieve the pain, more frequently the first day and less often over the next few days as the pain diminishes.

Mint

Chop a couple of fresh mint leaves and lay them on top of the burn for 15 to 20 minutes. Mint has cooling qualities, and simply chopping up a few leaves and putting them in contact with the burn will calm the scorching pain, says Dr. Bongiovanni. You can keep the leaves in place by taping a piece of gauze over the area. Reapply a fresh preparation as needed for the pain, more frequently the first day, then tapering off over the next few days as the pain decreases.

Calendula, Aloe, and Witch Hazel

Make an herbal skin spray and spritz tender, burned skin as often as necessary when you feel pain. Skin sprays come in handy when the skin is too tender to be touched, says Allen Green, M.D., of the Center for Optimum Health, a holistic practice in Fountain Valley, California.

In a spray bottle, mix 2 parts calendula succus (a thicker tincture that's available in some health food stores) with 1 part each aloe gel and witch hazel water. Add the liquid from two vitamin E capsules to help minimize scarring. Keep the herbal spray in the fridge and use it as often as you like until the burn stops feeling tender.

St. John's Wort

Smooth St. John's wort oil on a first-degree burn twice a day until there is no pain or redness. With all the focus on St. John's wort as an antidepressant, some of its more traditional uses in herbalism have been overlooked, says Dr. Shapiro—but not by Germany's Commission E, which evaluates herbs for safety and effectiveness. That research body recommends St. John's wort specifically for first-degree burns. A beautiful, deep red color, St. John's wort oil is soothing and anti-inflammatory and has a long tradition of topical use.

BURPING

*O*n a May day in 1975, Peter Dowdeswell of Great Britain entered *The Guinness Book of Records*. His feat? In 5 short seconds, Dowdeswell put away a yard of ale. That's 3 whole pints.

In a glaring omission, what's not listed in the record book is the length of the belch that surely followed. Too much food or drink is one of the primary reasons that you live with chronic burping.

"A lot of people swallow air when they gobble their food down," says Yvonne Tyson, M.D., a physician in Long Beach, California, and a member of the American Holistic Health Association. The resulting eructations can even be worse when the beverage is carbonated, such as beer or soda.

So slow down, leave the world records intact, and you'll be more than halfway to solving your belching problems. Another hint—let hot beverages like coffee cool a bit before you drink them, says Dr. Tyson. Many people suck in air as they sip hot java so it doesn't burn their tongues. That air comes right back up.

If you still find burps slipping out more often than you'd like, give some of these herbs a try.

Papaya

Take one or two enzyme tablets after meals, or follow package directions. Papaya enzymes work by doing what your body has trouble doing for itself, says Dr. Tyson. They assist in the breakdown of foods that your gut has trouble digesting, thus reducing the amount of gas formed.

You can buy these enzymes in rolls of tablets similar to Tums or in bottles. They come in regular and extra-strength formulations, so check the package to see if the dose is appropriate for your symptoms.

Peppermint

Drink one cup of tea immediately after meals. Peppermint is a great all-around tea for burping, says Theresa MacLean, R.Ph., N.D., a naturopathic physician and pharmacist based in Berwick, Nova Scotia. It's a stomach soother and a mild carminative, which means that it helps expel excess gas. Pick up some real peppermint tea at a

Fast FACTS

Cause: Burping is commonly caused by swallowing air when you eat or drink. It can also occur when your body has trouble digesting food or because of food allergies, resulting in excess gas. Anxiety may also cause you to swallow more frequently, leading to increased air in your stomach that in turn leads to belching. Sometimes, chronic burping is due to a problem with your breathing. You draw a breath in, some air lodges in your esophagus, and you belch it right back out. This can become a vicious cycle.

Incidence: In days gone by, a hearty belch was seen as an appreciative gesture for a good meal. Although Victorian etiquette stripped belching of its respectability, occasional burping after a meal is normal and quite common.

When to see the doctor: If your belching is combined with symptoms such as pain, nausea, or a burning sensation, you should have a checkup. You may have an ulcer or some other condition. Also, if you try home remedies for a few weeks without success, make an appointment with a physician to check for problems such as a hiatal hernia.

---

health food store or grocery store. To be sure that it's not regular tea with peppermint flavoring, check the label.

If you have a bunch of fresh peppermint, that will work very nicely as well. Add 1 cup of boiling water to 1 tablespoon of chopped, fresh, clean leaves, steep for 10 minutes, and strain the herb out. Sip slowly when it has cooled somewhat.

You can also find peppermint in enteric-coated capsules. Look for 0.4 milliliters of essential oil per capsule. Take one capsule 30 minutes before eating three times a day.

Ginger

Drink one cup of tea immediately after meals. Like peppermint, ginger is a good digestive tonic, says Dr. MacLean. To make the tea, grate 1 teaspoon of fresh root, pour 1 cup of boiling water over it, steep for 5 minutes, and strain. Let it cool so you don't swallow air while drinking it and sip it slowly.

If you don't have fresh ginger, you can make tea from the powdered spice you probably have in your kitchen. Add 1½ teaspoons of ginger per cup of boiling water. Steep for 5 to 10 minutes, let cool, and drink.

Anise, Caraway, or Fennel

Drink one cup of tea with each meal. Aniseed and caraway and fennel seeds aid digestion, helping your body break down foods with less gas, says Dr. MacLean. To make tea, add 1 teaspoon of crushed seeds to 1 cup of boiling water, steep for 10 to 20 minutes, and strain. Let it cool and drink it slowly.

You can also get fennel in capsule or tincture form. Manufacturing methods vary, so just follow the label directions. For capsules, the dosage is usually one capsule with meals.

BURSITIS AND TENDINITIS

*T*rying to figure out whether you have a case of bursitis or of tendinitis is a bit like an anatomical whodunit. Whether the culprit is a fluid-filled bursa or a wiry tendon, your first clue is in the pain. Is it sharp or dull?

Although bursitis and tendinitis are often lumped together, they are actually two distinct types of inflammation. A dull, persistent pain nagging at a joint could signal bursitis—swelling and inflammation of bursae, small, fluid-filled sacs that help muscles and tendons glide smoothly and prevent them from being inflamed by the underlying bone. If you have bursitis, the more you move an afflicted joint, the more it hurts, says Andrew Cole, M.D., a Seattle physician and member of the American Academy of Physical Medicine and Rehabilitation.

If you experience more of a sharp pain triggered by movement, you may have tendinitis, or inflammation of the tough, elastic fibrous tissue that connects muscles to bone. Like bursae, tendons generally become inflamed from repetitive motion, says Dr. Cole.

Rest is the first order of treatment for both. It's important, though, to see a doctor to find out which condition you have. While bursitis responds better to moist heat, ice generally relieves the pain of tendinitis. No matter which brand of pain you have, though, adding a few herbal home remedies to your recovery plan will help you feel better faster.

Arnica

Rub on arnica two or three times a day. Arnica ointments and creams are available in health food stores and can be applied topically to the affected area, says Jill Stansbury, N.D., chair of the botanical medicine department at the National College of Naturopathic Medicine in Portland, Oregon, and author of *Herbs for Health and Healing*. For best results when treating bursitis, cover the arnica with heat, such as a heating pad or hot water bottle, for as long as is comfortable. Arnica is thought to contain anti-inflammatory compounds.

St. John's Wort, Rosemary, Juniper, Eucalyptus, and Chamomile

Use this combination of healing oils to rub away joint pain three times a day. If you are prone to bursitis or tendinitis, keep this blend of oils on hand to help alleviate swelling and pain, says Dr. Stansbury. Here's how to make it. In a dark glass bottle, mix 1 tablespoon of St. John's wort infused oil, 1 tablespoon of vegetable oil, 10 drops of rosemary essential oil, 6 drops of juniper essential oil, 5 drops of eucalyptus essential oil, and 4 drops of chamomile essential oil. Shake gently to mix. Rub it into the joint after you've applied a warm or cold compress. It's safe to use this remedy indefinitely. The best St. John's wort oil is bright red, Dr. Stansbury says.

Boswellia

Stop pain with 400 to 500 milligrams of boswellia three times a day. This extract from the frankincense tree can relieve pain from chronic inflammatory conditions like bursitis and tendinitis without causing unwanted side effects, says C. Leigh Broadhurst, Ph.D., a nutrition consultant and herbal researcher based in Clovery, Maryland.

Research suggests that certain chemicals produced in this tree prevent the production of chemicals in our bodies that start the pain process. According to researchers, boswellic acid extract has been shown to prevent tissue breakdown and reduce the production of biochemicals that cause inflammation. As pain lessens, take the above dosage twice and then once a day, says Dr. Broadhurst. It's safe to take boswellia for 6 to 12 months. If your symptoms haven't improved by then, seek professional care.

Turmeric

To relieve chronic pain and inflammation, take 400 to 500 milligrams of extract three times a day. Curcumin, the powerful anti-inflammatory substance in turmeric, isn't a drug, but it can act like one, says Dr. Broadhurst.

Although it has been used for thousands of years in India for cooking, dyeing, and medicinal uses, turmeric was largely overlooked in North America until the 1970s. When modern science finally took a closer look, the results were impressive. When compared to standard anti-inflammatory drugs, curcumin was found to be as effective or more effective in treating pain and inflammation. You can take turmeric for 6 to 12 months, she adds.

Fast FACTS

Cause: Injury, trauma, and overuse can cause inflammation and swelling of either the small, fluid-filled sacs in the joints, called bursae, or the tendons that attach muscle and bone.

Incidence: Because bursitis and tendinitis are related to overuse, men—who are generally more physically active—tend to be affected more often than women.

When to see the doctor: If you experience increasing pain, swelling, weakness, or instability in any joint, you should consult a doctor to see what's causing the problem.

Bromelain

Take 500 milligrams 1 hour after meals three or four times a day. Any type of inflammation heals faster when you take bromelain, says Jacqueline Jacques, N.D., a naturopathic physician in Portland, Oregon, who specializes in pain management.

An enzyme derived from the pineapple plant, bromelain helps you digest your food when you take it with meals. When taken on an empty stomach, it promotes circulation and reduces inflammation by inhibiting the release of inflammation-producing biochemicals called prostaglandins and thromboxanes. Patients who take bromelain report that they have less pain.

You won't get a healing dose of bromelain from a glass of pineapple juice. To get the right amount of the pineapple plant's healing enzyme, buy capsules of the standardized extract at a health food store. Bromelain strength is standardized in measurements called milk-clotting units (mcu) or gelatin-dissolving units (gdu), which indicate how much enzyme is needed to curdle milk or dissolve gelatin. Look for a product that has a strength between 1,200 and 2,400 mcu or between 720 and 1,440 gdu, says Dr. Jacques.

Bromelain, like other anti-inflammatory medications, is for acute injury. If you still have inflammation and/or pain after 2 to 3 weeks, consult a physician.

Grape Seed or Pine

Add a daily supplement of 30 to 60 milligrams of nature's antioxidants. With a daily dose of either of these botanical extracts, you will help strengthen and repair connective tissue between joints, an ability that makes them especially helpful for tendinitis, says Dr. Jacques.

Packed with antioxidant activity 20 times more potent than that of vitamin C and 50 times greater than vitamin E's, grape seed and pine bark extracts contain unique flavonols called proanthocyanidins. While it may take your mouth a few tries to pronounce this seven-syllable stumper, your body makes quick work of utilizing these powerful antioxidants to heal inflamed tissues.

Grape seed and pine bark extract are extremely safe and nontoxic. At the dosages recommended here, they are safe to take indefinitely, says Dr. Jacques.

CAFFEINE DEPENDENCY

*C*affeine is a vice we love to hate. Reports of caffeine causing high blood pressure and heart disease have given the stimulant a nefarious reputation. But the scientific fact is that a little caffeine, even on a daily basis, probably won't affect your overall health.

Yet, some experts still feel that caffeine is best avoided. That's because excessive caffeine intake (more than about three cups of coffee or five to six cups of tea per day) can cause insomnia, rapid pulse, and anxiety. Plus, coffee in particular has been linked to a condition known as fibrocystic disease that causes painful breast lumps.

If you are prone to any of these problems, it's wise to cut back on or eliminate caffeine from your diet, says William Page-Echols, D.O., an osteopathic physician at Full Spectrum Family Medicine in East Lansing, Michigan. If you've ever gone even a morning without your fix, though, you're probably familiar with the uncomfortable effects of caffeine withdrawal: headaches, fatigue, and increased tension and irritability.

If you're working your way off caffeine for any reason, herbs can help you wean yourself more easily, without all of the common cold-turkey side effects.

Green Tea

Drink green tea instead of coffee. Plain water may be the world's number one beverage choice, but green tea comes in a very close second. Pale, golden-colored tea has been popular for centuries in Asian countries. Today, it is quickly becoming favored even in places where coffee has long been the reigning drink.

Green tea is different from the more familiar black tea in a couple of ways. First, green tea leaves are green because they are not fermented, as black and pekoe leaves are. Second, while green tea does contain caffeine, the amount is relatively low—only about 50 milligrams a cup as compared to 85 or more milligrams in a cup of coffee.

Lighter caffeine content is what makes green tea a doctor-recommended coffee replacement. But there's even more reason to switch. "Green tea is also very good for you," says Dr. Page-Echols.

Substances in green tea called polyphenols are known to protect against certain cancers, tooth decay, and high cholesterol, as well as to stimulate immunity and kill viruses. While it may have a bigger caffeine kick, coffee certainly can't do all that for your health.

Fast FACTS

Cause: Caffeine-containing beverages like coffee and tea activate the central nervous system and deliver a feeling of energy. Going without caffeine after you've become used to it can cause withdrawal effects such as headache and fatigue, which make continuing the habit the preferred option for many.

Incidence: In the United States alone, caffeinated beverages, including coffee, tea, and soft drinks, are consumed by the gallon—more than 80 gallons a year per person, to be exact. On an average day, nearly half of all Americans indulge in a cup of coffee. Most go on to drink two more, for a total of three cups a day.

When to see the doctor: Quitting caffeine usually isn't as difficult as many people imagine, but the adjustment period for chronic tea or coffee consumers who go "cold turkey" may be a few days to a week—or even several weeks, in some cases. If you find that you absolutely cannot eliminate caffeine on your own, see your doctor or other qualified health practitioner for assistance. It may help to consider lifestyle issues that could be influencing your dependency.

To try green tea, start by drinking a cup instead of one of your usual cups of coffee. Then gradually wean yourself from coffee by increasing the ratio of green tea to coffee each day. Eventually, aim to have as many (or fewer) cups of green tea as you were of coffee. At that point, you'll be getting only about 60 percent of the caffeine provided by your former coffee habit, plus all of the benefits that only green tea can give.

Chicory

Quaff a chicory-based beverage. An integral part of the coffee culture is the ritual of indulging in a steaming cup of rich, brown brew. The secret to successfully kicking the caffeine habit is to do it without doing away with your daily hot mug.

Try substituting a stand-in herb for your standard cup of joe, says

Dr. Page-Echols. "There are coffee-substitute beverages, like one called Pero, that I find very satisfying."

The main ingredient in such drink mixes is a root called chicory. In colonial days, coffee was actually mixed with roasted and ground chicory root to stretch the supplies of expensive coffee beans. The unique flavor of chicory coffee has since earned it a reputation as a Southern specialty.

Besides being caffeine-free, chicory offers some healthy fringe benefits. The root is referred to as a bitter, that is, a digestive stimulant that benefits the liver. It increases bile production in the gallbladder, which may help lower cholesterol.

Look for coffee substitutes such as Pero in health food stores. Prepare the product you buy according to the directions on the package. Then, to make the switch most convincing, fix your chicory drink the same way you would coffee. You can enjoy as many cups as you like without worrying about the java jitters.

Wood Betony

Take 2 to 4 milliliters of tincture at the first sign of a withdrawal headache. Caffeine has a vasoconstricting effect, says Steven Rissman, N.D., a naturopathic physician at American WholeHealth in Cherry Creek, Colorado. That means that when you try to go without your usual cup of java, veins that are accustomed to being narrowed open wide instead. This flood of circulation is what leads to the typical throbbing caffeine-withdrawal headache.

Wood betony can make that first week of going caffeine-free a lot less uncomfortable, says Dr. Rissman. A trio of alkaloids in this flowering plant have a quieting effect on nervous headache, anxiety, and nerve pain.

Look for wood betony tincture in well-stocked health food stores. If the dropper in the bottle does not have measuring marks, purchase a dosing syringe at a drugstore. Then, when you feel a headache brewing, take the tincture by measuring the drops and adding them to a half-glass of water or juice.

You can safely do this up to three times a day for as long as withdrawal symptoms last, which shouldn't be more than a week.

CANKER SORES

Canker sores won't kill you. It just seems that way.

These small, ulcerous sores, which sprout on the tender flesh of your inner cheek, lip, or tongue, turn orange or tomato juice into liquid fire, a slice of cheese pizza into a shard of glass, and brushing your teeth into a truly bristling experience.

It is likely that there is more than one cause of canker sores, including a glitch in your body's immune system. Normally, it protects us from disease. For some reason, though, your immune defenses can suddenly attack what they are supposed to protect—in this case, the healthy cells of your mouth and tongue. Female hormones can also play a role, since canker sores afflict women more often than they do men, often during a woman's menstrual periods. Emotional stress or a mouth injury (biting the inside of your lip or cheek, for example) can trigger a sore.

Commonsense tactics can help take the sting out of a canker sore. Since eating is a major cause of canker pain, avoid foods with sharp edges and those that involve a lot of crunching and chewing, such as potato chips, and acidic foods such as tomatoes and citrus fruits, says Roy Page, D.D.S., Ph.D., professor of periodontics in the school of dentistry at the University of Washington in Seattle.

Two simple conventional treatments can also serve you well. Try crunching on chewable antacid tablets to reduce sting-causing mouth acids or drying the sore with a cotton swab and coating it with an over-the-counter protective gel such as Zilactin.

Thankfully, canker sores heal on their own, usually within 2 weeks. But herbs can help speed them on their way.

Calendula

Drink two cups of tea a day until the sore heals. The petals of this cheery yellow flower are rich in mucilages have been used to heal

Fast FACTS

sores and reduce inflammation, says Barry Sherr, a professional member of the American Herbalists Guild (AHG) who practices in Danbury, Connecticut. Europeans sip calendula tea to help treat mouth and throat infections. To make the tea, pour 1 cup of boiling water over 1 to 2 teaspoons of dried petals, steep for 10 to 15 minutes, and strain.

Calendula tea can also be used as a mouthwash. Rinse your mouth with the still-warm tea several times a day.

Echinacea

Apply tincture to the sore three or four times a day. Echinacea naturally stimulates your immune system, says Ed Smith, a professional member of the AHG and founder of Herb Pharm in Williams, Oregon. As such, it helps stimulate the body's own defenses to prevent or heal infections. Many components may be responsible for echinacea's healing power, including polysaccharides, substances that stimulate infection-fighting white blood cells.

Propolis

Apply propolis tincture to the sore with a cotton swab three to five times a day. Bees make this sticky substance to fortify their hives, but it can also fortify your mouth, reducing inflammation and killing viruses and bacteria that can make sores worse, says Smith.

Sage and St. John's Wort

Apply a mixture of equal parts of both tinctures to the sore with a cotton swab three or four times a day. "When people suffer from chronic canker sores, I recommend two tinctures: sage and St. John's wort," says Sherr.

Sage is an anti-inflammatory that soothes and helps the canker sore heal. In the past, St. John's wort was typecast as the depression herb, but "it's also a potent pain reducer and antiviral," says Sherr. While canker sores don't seem to be caused by viruses, St. John's wort can help prevent viruses from worming their way into your system through a canker sore, he says.

Use the herbal combination as recommended above until your symptoms are greatly reduced, then once daily for about one more week.

Echinacea, Calendula, Oats, Burdock, and Lomatium

Combine equal parts of these tinctures and take ½ teaspoon four or five times a day. This blend of herbal tinctures helps heal cankers by goosing the immune system, moving toxins out of the body, and killing viruses and bacteria, says Sherr.

Dried oats have traditionally been used to reduce emotional stress, one trigger of canker sores, while burdock soothes inflamed, irritated mucous membranes, says Sherr. Lomatium is used as a prime infection fighter and is thought to inhibit the growth of a variety of viruses and bacteria. If you are plagued by canker sores, a daily ¼-teaspoon maintenance dose may help to prevent recurrences.

CARPAL TUNNEL SYNDROME

*W*e've heard a lot more about carpal tunnel syndrome (CTS) since computers started to pop up on desks the world over, turning many of us into typists. But it's been around much longer than the information age has, and it's not limited to the office.

Any activity that involves repetitive hand motions or that keeps the wrist bent for an extended period of time can cause this injury. The source of the problem lies in the carpal tunnel, a passageway formed by the wrist bones and a tough band of tissue on the inside of your wrist called the carpal ligament. This narrow tunnel is a busy place; the tendons that bend your fingers pass through it, and so does the major nerve that relays signals between your brain and your hand.

Sometimes, repetitive motion isn't the only culprit. CTS strikes whenever tissues inside the tunnel become swollen and the nerve is pinched. Because hormone changes due to birth control pills, pregnancy, or menopause, as well as health conditions such as diabetes, arthritis, and thyroid problems, can cause tissue swelling or affect nerve endings, these are also possible instigators of CTS. If you have it, you're likely to feel numbness, tingling, and pain in your wrist, thumb, and first three fingers.

CTS should be diagnosed by a doctor, but you can calm the inflammation with these herbal remedies.

Bromelain

Take a 500-milligram capsule three times a day between meals. "For any kind of inflammation like this, I rely on bromelain," says Joan Haynes, N.D., a naturopathic physician based in Boise, Idaho.

Bromelain, an enzyme derived from the pineapple plant, reduces inflammation by inhibiting the release of inflammation-producing biochemicals. It also speeds healing. Take it between meals; otherwise, this enzyme—a principal ingredient in many meat tenderizers—will set to work breaking down the food you've eaten rather than addressing the problem at hand. It's safe to take until your symptoms subside.

Turmeric

Make a turmeric poultice for your wrist, and take 400 to 600 milligrams of curcumin extract three times a day on an empty stomach. Mix 2 tablespoons of turmeric powder with enough warm water to form a paste, advises Connie Catellani, M.D., medical director of the Miro Center for Integrative Medicine in Evanston, Illinois. Sandwich the paste between two layers of gauze, wrap it around your sore wrist, and hold it in place with a bandage. It's less messy doing it this way than daubing it directly onto the skin, says Dr. Catellani. Leave the bandage on all day. It's safe to do this periodically, but for no longer than 3 to 4 days at a time.

You can also take an extract of a substance called curcumin, which is believed to be one of the most active components in turmeric. It's been shown to be as effective as cortisone in reducing inflammation. Although this substance is derived from turmeric, it's specifically curcumin extract that you'll need to find at a health food store. "If you took just turmeric, you'd need about 60,000 milligrams to get enough curcumin," says Dr. Haynes. It's safe to take this until your symptoms subside.

Arnica

Rub oil into your wrist twice a day. Arnica, an ancient herb with anti-inflammatory properties, has been used for wounds and injuries since Greek and Roman times. Andrew Lucking, N.D., a naturopathic doctor in Minneapolis, recommends using arnica infused in olive oil

Fast FACTS

Cause: Repetitive hand motion and activities that involve prolonged bending of the wrist can lead to CTS. So can the fluid retention that often occurs during pregnancy and menopause and with the use of oral contraceptives. Diseases such as rheumatoid arthritis, diabetes, and underactive thyroid, as well as some wrist injuries, can promote CTS.

Incidence: CTS is most common among women ages 30 to 60.

When to see the doctor: See your doctor if you have any CTS symptoms—numbness, pain, or tingling—that cause discomfort as you go about your daily activities.

---

to soothe the pain of CTS. The herb, which is also known as leopard's bane, grows at high altitudes and has traditionally been used by mountain dwellers, he adds. You'll find it in most health food stores. Just make sure that you don't buy homeopathic arnica; since the bottles look similar, check the labels. Sometimes, you'll find arnica mixed with St. John's wort oil, which would work fine, too, says Dr. Lucking.

Rub ¼ teaspoon of oil into the soft tissue on the inside of your wrist and massage in a gentle motion from the center toward the bones at the base of your thumb and little finger. Continue for 3 to 5 minutes, then work up the wrist about 4 inches, rubbing laterally from the center as well as up and down. Do this once in the morning and once at night, advises Dr. Lucking. That way, you'll loosen your wrist up for the day and relax it again at night so that you can get a good night's sleep. It's safe to use this remedy until your symptoms subside.

Skullcap and Passionflower

Make iced tea with these herbs and drink a glass twice a day, with breakfast and dinner. Mildly anti-inflammatory, skullcap also acts as a nerve tonic and helps calm spasms, says Beverly Yates, N.D., a naturopathic physician with the Natural Health Care Group in Portland, Oregon, and Seattle. She suggests combining it with passion-flower, which is also a nerve tonic.

For each cup of water, use 1 tablespoon each of dried skullcap and dried passionflower. Steep for 10 minutes, then strain the tea and let it cool. Store in a covered pitcher in the refrigerator. Make enough to last 4 to 5 days, suggests Dr. Yates.

It's safe to take this tea until symptoms subside, but if you have no improvement after 1 month, consider other remedies.

Cabbage

Wrap a leaf around your wrist. You probably wouldn't want to go around all day with a cabbage leaf around your wrist, but this is a great anti-inflammatory remedy for the hours when you're in slumber, says Dr. Catellani. And it couldn't be simpler. Just cut the hard rib out of a dark green cabbage leaf, warm the leaf over a radiator or in the microwave until it becomes soft, and wrap it around your wrist. Hold it in place with a bandage. It's safe to use this remedy as often as you like.

Dandelion

Drink a cup of tea twice a day. If your CTS was brought on by the fluid retention of pregnancy, try a mild diuretic like dandelion leaf, says Anita Clay, a member of Britain's National Institute of Medical Herbalists who holds the British medical degree Bachelor of Medicine, Bachelor of Surgery and practices in Exeter, England. If you can't find it growing wild in your area, you may be able to track it down in the salad greens section of a specialty grocery store or farmers' market.

Finely chop a couple of leaves in a small bowl. Add 1 cup of warm water and steep for 5 minutes before drinking. Don't drink the tea too close to bedtime, warns Dr. Clay. You don't want the diuretic effect to take hold in the middle of the night and disturb your sleep. It's safe to use this remedy until your symptoms subside, but if you don't feel better after 6 to 8 weeks, see a doctor.

CHAFING

*Y*ou don't have to be a marathon runner to experience chafing. Bicycling can rub you the wrong way, too. So can being overweight. Whenever sweaty skin rubs against sweaty skin—the inner thighs, underarms, and groin are common trouble spots—friction builds up. Chafing can also happen when soft skin comes up against rough clothing.

At first, you may feel a little irritation, but before you know it, the skin is beet red, raw, and extremely tender to the touch. If left untreated, chafed skin may begin to ooze and develop a crusty surface.

Doctors tend to recommend friction-reducing powders and petroleum jelly to prevent chafing and hydrocortisone cream or zinc oxide paste to treat it. Herbalists look to the soothing herbs that have earned a reputation for healing wounds and calming irritated skin.

Comfrey and St. John's Wort, Calendula, or Usnea

Sprinkle natural baby powder on chafe-prone areas before you hit the jogging trail. As an alternative to talcum powder, use one of the natural baby powders that you can find in health food stores or

Fast FACTS

Cause: Chafing happens when the skin on an area of your body, such as your underarms or inner thighs, rubs against skin or fabric. The friction that's set up by the motion abrades your skin, making it inflamed and tender.

Incidence: Although it's common to all athletic pursuits, chafing is particularly prevalent among those involved in endurance sports such as running or bicycling. People who are very muscular or obese are also more likely to experience chafing.

When to see the doctor: If your skin is still irritated after 4 to 5 days, make an appointment to see your doctor or a dermatologist.

by mail order, says Whitney Miller, N.D., a naturopathic doctor who has a family practice in New London and Colchester, Connecticut.

These powders are non-talc-based. Fine white clay and arrowroot powder are the moisture-absorbing components, and finely ground comfrey and other herbs are added for their soothing qualities. Other ingredients to look for in a powder, says Dr. Miller, are St. John's wort, calendula, and usnea (sometimes known as old man's beard) as well as vitamins E and A.

Chickweed

Smooth on a thin layer of soothing cream twice a day. If your chafed skin itches, try a cream containing chickweed, says Mindy Green, a founder and professional member of the American Herbalists Guild and director of educational services at the Herb Research Foundation in Boulder, Colorado. Seventeenth-century herbalist Nicholas Culpeper recommended using chickweed boiled in hog's grease to calm itchy skin. Times have changed, thank goodness, and now you can just go to your local health food store and buy a tube of chickweed cream—no hog grease included—to ease the itchies.

CHAPPED OR DRY HANDS

Like snowmen in front yards or ski racks on the roofs of cars, dry hands are a sure sign of winter. While cold, dry air will certainly encourage chapping on hands and fingers, other factors can make dry hands a year-round concern. Culprits such as heavy scrubbing (think of the constant washing that doctors and nurses do) and harsh chemicals like paint or cleaning solutions can take their toll on our most-used tools.

Wearing gloves religiously in cold weather and avoiding drying soaps and chemicals are smart steps to take toward prevention. But when dryness strikes, certain herbal oils can help ease the soreness, redness, and scratchiness of chapped hands. Here's what the experts recommend.

Calendula

Use a homemade oil on your hands nightly as needed to heal cracked skin. Calendula is a relative of the familiar, sunny-faced marigold. This flowering herb has both anti-inflammatory and skin-soothing properties, according to Mercedes Cameron, M.D., family practitioner at The Woman's Place at St. Mary's Hospital in Grand Junction, Colorado. Using a calendula-infused oil is a way of delivering the healing power in an emollient base—the perfect thing to apply to reddened, chapped skin.

To make your own calendula hand oil, you'll need a slow cooker, about 8 ounces of almond oil, and 4 ounces of dried calendula flowers. Put the flowers in the slow cooker and pour the oil over them, making sure that all the buds are covered. Set the cooker on the lowest setting

Fast FACTS

Cause: Dry skin on your hands and fingers can come from exposure to sun, wind, or cold, as well as low humidity from heated or air-conditioned rooms. But soap and overwashing are by far the biggest causes of dry hands.

Incidence: Dry skin is a common—but luckily, mostly cosmetic—problem. People who work with their hands in water or who must frequently wash their hands are more prone to dry hands, as are people who live in cold or harsh environments.

When to see the doctor: If your dry hands are accompanied by itching or redness that is not alleviated by regular use of a moisturizer, see a dermatologist to rule out allergies or a more chronic dry skin condition.

and leave it overnight (or about 12 hours). In the morning, use a mesh strainer or colander lined with a layer of cheesecloth to strain the oil into a bowl. Then, using a funnel, pour the oil into a dark glass container. This will minimize its exposure to light so it doesn't become rancid.

Massage this oil into your hands every night. If you wear thin cotton gloves (available at beauty supply stores and some drugstores) while sleeping, your skin will absorb as much of the healing ingredients as possible. They will also keep your sheets from getting greasy.

Avocado

Rub oil from this fruit into your hands after every washing. This natural oil offers healing properties for hands that are so dry they hurt, says Diana Bihova, M.D., a dermatologist in New York City. The mild oil pressed from the luscious avocado is known to be soothing to the skin. Avocado oil is used for gourmet cooking, so look for it in well-stocked grocery stores as well as health food stores.

To magnify the moisturizing effects of the oil, use it when your hands are still a bit damp from washing, Dr. Bihova says. The oil will form a protective seal that will retain the moisture that your dry digits are so thirsty for.

CHAPPED LIPS

*I*t's a wonder that our lips aren't chapped full-time. They don't have oil glands to keep them lubricated, and they have very little pigment to protect them from the sun. This lack of natural protection makes them all too vulnerable to blazing sun, dry heat, and biting winds, or even our own nervous licking or biting.

Herbal preparations can help keep your lips soft and chap-free. Still, don't underestimate the protection of over-the-counter lip balms, says Roy Page, D.D.S., Ph.D., professor of periodontics in the school of dentistry at the University of Washington in Seattle. If you want to keep one on hand, pick a balm with added sunscreen, "especially if you're outdoors a lot or live in a sunny climate," he says. Also, opt for a balm formulated with lanolin. Petroleum-based balms coat your lips nicely, but they also draw moisture right out of them.

Certain herbs do offer the protection that our own kissers lack, says Ellen Kamhi, R.N., Ph.D., a professional member of the American Herbalists Guild (AHG), an herbalist in Oyster Bay, New York, and author of *The Natural Medicine Chest*. As you'll see, skin-soothing herbs such as jojoba and calendula, among others, contain essential oils and other substances that soothe dry, cracked lips and protect them while they heal.

Jojoba

Apply a balm directly to your lips as needed. Jojoba, an evergreen shrub whose seeds contain a waxy oil, "is the best herb for

Fast FACTS

Cause: Lips lack oil glands and contain very little natural pigment, so they're virtually defenseless against sun, wind, and indoor heat and air conditioning. All of these suck precious moisture from our lips. Sometimes, our own unconscious licking or biting is to blame.

Incidence: People who live in extreme climatic conditions—very sunny, very dry, or very windy, for example—are most likely to develop chapped lips.

When to see the doctor: If you have a crack in your lip, especially in the lower lip, that doesn't heal within 2 to 3 weeks, have it checked to rule out infection or a more serious illness.

chapped lips," says Dr. Kamhi. "Native Americans used it to protect their skin and lips when they were out on the plains, which were very windy."

Jojoba oil is expensive. "It takes a lot of seeds to make a small amount of oil," says Dr. Kamhi. Fortunately, most health food stores stock ready-made lip balms or salves formulated with the oil. If you can, select a balm made with beeswax, advises Dr. Kamhi. "Beeswax itself has protective properties for the skin and lips, and it smells delightful," she says.

Propolis

Apply directly to lips as needed. "Propolis is another excellent remedy for chapped lips," says Dr. Kamhi. This brownish resin is made by bees to fill cracks and holes in their hives. Opt for one of the many ready-made salves containing propolis that are available at health food stores, she says.

Calendula, Comfrey, and Lavender

Make a three-herb lip balm. "Calendula and comfrey are excellent herbs for chapped lips," says Barry Sherr, a professional member of the AHG who practices in Danbury, Connecticut. His quick-and-easy lip balm can help turn dry and scaly into moist and luscious.

In the top of a double boiler, place 1 ounce of coconut oil and ½ ounce (by weight) each of fresh or dried calendula petals and comfrey leaves. Place over boiling water in the bottom of the double boiler and simmer over low heat for about 1 hour. (The oil should have a vibrant orange hue.) Strain the hot oil and return it to the pan, then add ¼ ounce of beeswax. When the beeswax has melted, add 2 to 3 drops of lavender essential oil. Pour into a small jar and allow to set. Once it has hardened to a balmlike consistency, simply use it as needed. If you don't like the consistency, remelt it, adding more beeswax if it is too soft and more coconut oil if it is too hard.

Cold Hands and Feet

*C*old hands and feet can cause trouble when you want to snuggle with your sweetie on a chilly winter's night, but extremities that are chronically cold can signal health problems. These may be related to menopause, an underactive thyroid gland, low iron levels, or sluggish circulation.

Since even healthy fingers can turn frosty when winter sets in, and cold toes—even under a comforter—are common from September to April in some latitudes, try turning the heat up with herbs that increase circulation and generate gentle warmth.

Cinnamon and Cayenne

Use one or both spices liberally on food or take them in capsule form, following directions on the label. If you're trying to keep warm in a cold, wintry world, the two Cs—cinnamon and cayenne— are worth indulging in before heading out. In Traditional Chinese Medicine, cinnamon is known as a warming herb. Herbalists also believe that cayenne, commonly known as red pepper, increases circulation, says Steven Rissman, N.D., a naturopathic physician at American WholeHealth in Cherry Creek, Colorado.

Sprinkle a generous dusting of cinnamon on your morning oatmeal or chew on a cinnamon stick to help keep your toes and fingers warm. Then make lunch a cayenne-spiced bowl of chili or stow some cayenne capsules in your day pack (follow the dosage directions on the label of the bottle you buy). You can take cayenne indefinitely, but if your symptoms go away and your body constitution becomes warm, says Dr. Rissman, stop using it.

Ginger

Drink tea freely or take capsules according to the directions on the label. Ginger is an Asian medicinal herb known for its heat-gen-

Fast FACTS

Cause: Cold hands and feet are a normal response to a cold environment, but chronically cold extremities can be blamed on menopause, thyroid problems, low iron, less-than-optimal circulation, or a vascular disorder known as Raynaud's disease.

Incidence: Circulatory problems increase with age, making cold hands and feet more common in the elderly. Since women experience low iron levels, thyroid problems, and Raynaud's disease more often than men and because their blood vessels have poorer tone, women are more likely to have cold extremities.

When to see the doctor: If your fingers and toes turn white or blue when briefly exposed to cold, you may have Raynaud's disease. Also, tiny red lines that look like splinters under your nail beds could signify that all is not well in your circulatory system. See your doctor for diagnosis and treatment of any of these symptoms.

erating abilities, says Dr. Rissman. While dried ginger root is warming, fresh root is cooling, he says.

Hot ginger tea is a delicious way to warm up. Put about 1 teaspoon of dried root in a small teapot and cover with 1 cup of boiling water. Steep for 10 minutes, then strain the tea into a mug and sweeten it with honey, if you like. Wrapping your fingers around the steaming mug while you drink doubles the warming effect. Or try ginger capsules, which are widely available.

Ginkgo

Take 60 milligrams of extract twice a day. For warming over the long term, ginkgo gets the go-ahead. Its use as a memory herb stems from its circulation-stimulating effects on the tiny blood vessels above the neck. At the same time that ginkgo increases blood flow to the brain, however, it also boosts blood flow elsewhere, including the fingers and toes, according to Monique Martin, D.O., a doctor of osteopathic internal medicine at American WholeHealth in Littleton, Colorado.

The circulation boost from ginkgo doesn't happen immediately. Germany's Commission E, which evaluates herbs for safety and effectiveness, has determined that the effects take at least 6 weeks to build. Also, you won't have to take it forever. Try it for 6 to 8 weeks. If you notice improvement, you can continue to take it for 3 months, then discontinue use.

COLD SORES

*I*n ancient Rome, an outbreak of cold sores prompted one emperor to forbid kissing in public ceremonies. Unfortunately, his bussing ban failed to banish these fluid-filled blisters, which still occur in epidemic proportions, erupting around the lips, nostrils, chin, and cheeks.

Cold sores are caused by a highly contagious virus called herpes simplex type 1. (This type usually causes oral herpes, or cold sores, while type 2 is usually responsible for genital herpes.) Most people are infected with type 1 by the time they are 10 years old, even if they never develop a single sore. And once you get the virus, you have it forever.

Type 1 takes up permanent residence in a nerve near the cheekbone. It may lurk there forever, causing no trouble at all, or it may travel down the nerve to the surface of the skin, triggering a recurrence of blisters. Doctors aren't sure why some people get the blisters and others go unscathed.

Along with using the following herbal remedies, you can take other steps to prevent cold sores, says Flora Parsa Stay, D.D.S., a dentist in Oxnard, California, and author of *The Complete Book of Dental Remedies*. For example, do what you can to reduce the emotional stress in your life. Stress weakens the immune system, increasing the risk that you'll sprout a cold sore.

When you're outdoors, coat your lips and the area around your mouth with a lip balm that contains sunscreen, since sunlight, too, can trigger sores. Above all, don't pick at a blister. You may spread the virus from your lip to your eye or genitals—or to another person.

Cold sores usually heal within 2 weeks. Certain herbs can speed their healing or help to prevent them entirely, says Barry Sherr, a professional member of the American Herbalists Guild (AHG) who practices in Danbury, Connecticut. Some contain substances that build up the immune system, the body's defense against viruses and bacteria. Others may be able to slow the growth of the herpes simplex virus in particular. Still others soothe the pain and inflammation that accompany fever blisters.

Echinacea

Take 30 drops of tincture in a glass of water three times a day. Arguably the mother of all medicinal plants, echinacea was the best-selling medicinal plant in America into the 1920s. In recent years, Americans have rediscovered its healing powers. "Echinacea is a potent antiviral," says Ed Smith, a professional member of the AHG and owner of Herb Pharm in Williams, Oregon. While no one component is credited for echinacea's medicinal action, it is rich in polysaccharides, substances that have been found to stimulate infection-fighting white blood cells.

Lemon Balm

Swish your mouth with some tea three to five times a day. Place 1 heaping tablespoon of the dried herb into 1 cup of boiling water and steep for 20 minutes. Let the tea cool, then rinse your mouth with it, says Smith.

Cold-Sore-No-More Herbal Helper

When his clients complain of cold sores, Barry Sherr, a professional member of the American Herbalists Guild who practices in Danbury, Connecticut, offers them this combination of tinctures. The licorice, goldenseal, and echinacea jump-start the immune system; the lomatium, St. John's wort, and osha fight infections, including herpes simplex.

Take 1 teaspoon twice a day until your symptoms are greatly reduced, then take it once daily for about a week longer. But hold your nose: This mixture tastes foul. "I suggest taking it with a little bit of juice," says Sherr.

- **2 parts licorice**
- **1 part goldenseal**
- **2 parts lomatium**
- **2 parts St. John's wort**
- **3 parts echinacea**
- **2 parts osha**

Combine the licorice, goldenseal, lomatium, St. John's wort, echinacea, and osha in one bottle for convenience. Store any unused mixture in a cool, dark place.

Lemon balm contains tannins, which are antiviral and have been shown to hasten the healing of cold sores. Moreover, it acts as an astringent.

Myrrh

Dab the tincture directly on the sore with a cotton swab up to 10 times a day. This fragrant, resinous substance is the herbal remedy of choice for mouth inflammations, says Smith. It works by directly attacking infectious invaders and by stimulating the body's natural defenses to fight harmful microbes.

Fast FACTS

Cause: The formation of these annoying sores is one symptom of infection with the herpes simplex type 1 virus.

Incidence: An estimated 45 to 80 percent of Americans have suffered through at least one episode of these blisters. Each year, about 100 million Americans experience the annoyance and discomfort that they cause. Happily, recurrences tend to be less frequent after the age of 35.

When to see the doctor: If this is your first outbreak of cold sores, see your doctor immediately. You should also consult a doctor if you are plagued by frequent, severe cold sores or if they don't heal within 2 weeks.

Propolis

Apply tincture directly to the sore with a cotton swab three to five times a day. Also called bee glue, this sticky substance—made by bees to fill the cracks in their hives—"is extremely high in aromatic resins, essential oils, and flavonoids, all of which help to reduce inflammation and kill viruses and bacteria," says Smith.

St. John's Wort

Take ½ to 1 teaspoon of tincture in a glass of water once a day until your symptoms are gone. St. John's wort helps slow the growth of viruses while also quieting emotional stress, says Sherr. In some laboratory and animal studies, a substance in St. John's wort called hypericin has been shown to slow the replication of several viruses, including herpes simplex types 1 and 2.

Tea Tree

Apply a mixture of equal parts olive oil and tea tree oil directly to the sore with a cotton swab two or three times a day. As soon as you feel the telltale tingle of a cold sore about to erupt, dab the area with this mixture, says Sherr. Look for tea tree oil that's high in a substance called terpinen-4-ol and low in one called cineole; it's considered the highest-quality stuff.

Tea tree oil's reputation as an antiseptic harks back to the eighteenth century, when the aborigines of New South Wales were found painting their wounds with it. Research conducted in the 1920s found that it had up to 13 times greater antiseptic power than carbolic acid, which was then a common germicide.

COLDS

One cure for colds was invented by none other than Granny Clampett, the ornery but lovable doyen of the original *Beverly Hillbillies* TV clan. Granny guaranteed that if you partook liberally of her homemade concoction (ground possum innards and the like), you'd be cured within a week.

The joke, of course, is that the only "cure" for the common cold is to let it run its course—which it will usually do inside a week, with or without possum innards. What is hampering science's search for a cure is the constantly mutating army of about 200 viruses responsible for the respiratory tract infections that we know so well as colds. Unfortunately, we're also plenty familiar with the symptoms: congestion, cough, chills, runny nose, sneezing, watering eyes, and sore throat.

Conventional medicine can only offer symptom-hiders such as pain relievers, decongestants, expectorants, and other medicines that deal with the ills without curing the cause. Herbal medicine has a different idea—namely, to aid the body's natural healing powers while simultaneously easing the accompanying discomforts. Herbs are the cornerstone of an overall natural approach of helping the body to heal itself.

It's also important to heed what may be the most ignored piece of good advice in medicine. "You need to rest," says Gill Stanard, a member of the National Herbalists Association of Australia and an herbal practitioner in Melbourne. "Don't try to soldier on. Go to bed."

With bed rest, you'll give the herbs a chance to do their thing. And for the common cold, there are more herbal remedies than any single herbalist could ever catalog. Here are some of the best.

Echinacea

Take 1 teaspoon of tincture five times a day. From Alaska to Australia, echinacea has achieved superstar status as a cold remedy. "Almost everybody in this country has heard of echinacea," says Stanard. "It's now right up there with vitamin C in the arsenal that people choose when they have a cold."

An American native sometimes known as purple coneflower, echinacea is no cure-all, Stanard warns, but it does work wonders in rallying the immune system when you have a cold. Using numerous active constituents, the herb increases production of the white blood cells in your body that go after the cold virus. It also activates the killer cells that destroy virus-infected cells.

Use echinacea early, at the first hint that you're coming down with something, because it doesn't work well once a cold is full-blown. "If you jump on the infection soon enough, using lots of echinacea will really help," says David McLeod, an herbalist and acupuncturist and president of the National Herbalists Association of Australia in Sydney.

Because there's so much demand for this herb, it's easy to find at health food stores and drugstores in lots of forms. The highest doses are available in tinctures, and that's what you want, because you need relatively high doses to halt a cold, McLeod adds.

Look for a tincture made with 1 part echinacea to 5 parts alcohol, says Susan B. Kowalsky, N.D., a naturopathic physician in Norwich, Vermont. She recommends making a dose by putting 1 full teaspoon of tincture in $\frac{1}{2}$ cup of water.

Echinacea is a safe herb, but it may lose its effectiveness if you use it regularly for more than a few days.

Ginger-Garlic Super Soup

You think chicken soup is the sure kitchen cure for a cold? Then you haven't tried this doctor's ginger and garlic soup. "Both ginger and garlic are very boosting to the immune system," says Mary Bove, N.D., a naturopathic physician at the Brattleboro Naturopathic Clinic in Vermont and a member of Britain's National Institute of Medical Herbalists. "And garlic is just great for colds," she adds. The mung bean sprouts are added for extra doses of folate, potassium, and magnesium for overall good health. Here's Dr. Bove's recipe for cold relief.

- **4 cups chicken broth**
- **½ cup finely chopped fresh garlic**
- **½ cup finely sliced fresh ginger**
- **½ cup mung bean sprouts**

Place the broth in a large saucepan and warm over medium-high heat.

In a medium saucepan, sauté the garlic and ginger for about 3 to 4 minutes, or until soft. Add to the broth. Stir in the sprouts and simmer for 2 to 3 minutes, or until heated through. Keep any leftover soup in the refrigerator for later "treatments."

Goldenseal

Take 2 teaspoons of tincture or one 500-milligram capsule three times a day between meals. Goldenseal rivals echinacea's effectiveness as a cold medicine. "It's a very potent antibiotic herb," notes Lorilee Schoenbeck, N.D., a naturopathic physician at the Champlain Center for Natural Medicine in Shelburne, Vermont. The alkaloids in goldenseal root (notably berberines and hydrastines) are thought to reduce inflammation, thus restoring the ability of the mucous membranes to immobilize microbes, including the cold virus.

Because they work differently, goldenseal and echinacea make a great cold-fighting team, Dr. Kowalsky says. For goldenseal, find a tincture with an herb-to-alcohol ratio of 1 to 5. Goldenseal is an acquired taste, to say the least, she warns. "I definitely recommend the 'shooting' method. Mix it with a little water in a shot glass, shoot it down, and chase it with fresh water."

Alternatively, you can take capsules of the powdered root. "Standardized capsules of 8 to 12 percent alkaloid content can be taken at a dose of 500 milligrams three times a day," Dr. Kowalsky says. Goldenseal is generally nontoxic, but don't take it for more than a week or two.

Sage

Drink ½ cup of tea twice a day between meals. A few years ago, several leading herbalists were sitting around talking shop when the subject of cold remedies came up. Interestingly, neither echinacea nor goldenseal won by consensus. The winner? Sage.

"Sage is antiseptic and astringent," says Cascade Anderson Geller, an herbal educator and consulting herbal practitioner in Portland, Oregon. That means that it helps fight infections while drying up problems like postnasal drip.

Steep 1 teaspoon of dried medicinal sage leaves in ½ cup of water and drink it slowly—it's strong and bitter. The tea will make you feel better, but sage's drying effects are not something that you want to expose yourself to for more than a day or two, according to Geller.

Echinacea, Elder, Usnea, Wild Indigo, and Clove

Take 1 teaspoon of this formula three times a day. Mary Bove, N.D., a naturopathic physician at the Brattleboro Naturopathic Clinic in Vermont and a member of Britain's National Institute of Medical Herbalists, offers this immune-boosting adult cold formula that combines the well-known benefits of echinacea with those of several other hard-working herbs.

"The wild indigo works very well in combination with echinacea on the upper respiratory tract for congestion from colds," Dr.

Cause: Viruses cause colds, but they need a vulnerable host in order to create an infection. Many factors make you vulnerable, including stress, radical temperature changes, and poor nutrition.

Incidence: Colds are the most commonly occurring infectious diseases. Few are spared, but people such as schoolchildren and their teachers, who spend winter days in closed, crowded, virus-breeding conditions, are at higher risk.

When to see the doctor: A cold with a fever above 101°F for more than couple of days warrants a doctor's attention. So does a cold accompanied by a new or worsening cough, especially one that produces green, yellow, or bloody phlegm. Earache, facial pain, or swollen glands with a cold also call for a professional checkup.

Bove says, "while elder flowers support the entire immune system, not just specific parts of it as echinacea does." Usnea, a lichen sometimes called old man's beard, is also an immune stimulator, while clove is included for its antimicrobial as well as its aromatic qualities.

All of the herbs in this formula are available in tincture form at some health food stores or by mail order. Dr. Bove suggests combining 2 parts echinacea tincture with 1 part each of the elder, usnea, and indigo. Add a smaller amount of the clove tincture.

Yarrow, Elder, Peppermint, and Catnip

Drink three to four cups of this tea blend daily. Drinking pots and pots of hot yarrow tea is a time-honored folk remedy for colds. "The classic formula is yarrow, elder flowers, and peppermint," Stanard says.

A fourth ingredient, catnip, is recommended by Dr. Bove as a decongestant that also helps you relax. "Each individual herb brings its own strength," she says, "but basically they're all diaphoretic herbs, meaning that they stimulate the immune system by raising the body's temperature." Since turning up your temperature is one of your body's natural defense mechanisms against foreign invaders, it will help fight off the cold virus. It makes your body's environment inhospitable to germs because bacteria, parasites, and viruses replicate more slowly at high temperatures.

Combine equal parts of elder and yarrow flowers and peppermint and catnip leaves, all in dried form. You may want to skimp a bit on the bitter catnip and add a little extra peppermint to improve the flavor, Dr. Bove suggests. Make an infusion by steeping 1 heaping teaspoon of the blend in 8 ounces of water in a covered pan for 5 to 10 minutes. Drink it while it's nice and warm at least three or four times a day, starting as soon as you feel the onset of a cold. "Take the last cup with a warm bath in the evening," Dr. Bove says. "Then put yourself to bed."

COMMUTER FATIGUE

*Y*ou know the feeling. Either the stop-and-go of rush-hour traffic or the stress of trying to make your flight or train on time has fried your nerves and worn you out.

Most of us commute by car, and the number of us who are tired while we do it is as scary as a tenacious tailgater. The federal government estimates that 100,000 police-reported car crashes each year are caused by tired motorists. Those crashes result in 1,500 deaths and 71,000 injuries annually. The true numbers may be even higher.

In several states, police don't even list fatigue as a cause on accident reports, says Darrel Drobnich, director of government and transportation affairs for the National Sleep Foundation. And many motorists don't realize that they've had a 2- or 3-second "microsleep" while at the wheel of a car, he adds.

"A sleepy driver is equivalent to a drunk driver," says John P. Galgon, M.D., medical director at the Sleep Disorders Center at Lehigh Valley Hospital in Allentown, Pennsylvania. And while the number of crashes caused by drunk drivers has declined, there has been no change in the number caused by dozing drivers, he adds.

There is no substitute for simply getting enough sleep. If you didn't, though, and you know that you'll be sleepy on your drive, Dr. Galgon says that taking a 20-minute "power nap" before your trip may help you avoid the sleepiness. Or try conventional coping mechanisms such as drinking a caffeinated beverage, keeping the temperature cool inside your car, and tuning the radio to a talk program rather than music to stimulate, not lull, your brain, he says. If you use a caffeinated drink to help keep you alert (coffee has the most caffeine), sip it gradually throughout your drive so you don't have a letdown later, Dr. Galgon adds. If caffeine isn't your cup of tea, however, herbalists recommend the following.

Siberian Ginseng

Take two 200-milligram capsules or ½ to 1 teaspoon of tincture three times a day. This popular herb helps restore energy, and it can be used safely for prolonged periods, says herbalist Rosemary Gladstar of the Sage Mountain herbal education center in East Barre, Vermont, author of *Herbal Healing for Women*.

Peppermint

Spray your car interior with oil and water. Buy a 4-ounce spray bottle, fill it with water, and add a couple of drops of peppermint oil.

Fast FACTS

Cause: Lifestyle, and the fact that so many people burn the candle at both ends, account for most commuter-related fatigue. Three-quarters of Americans get less than 7 hours of sleep nightly; one-third snooze for fewer than 6 hours. All told, that's bound to affect some commutes.

Incidence: A survey conducted for the National Sleep Foundation found that 57 percent of respondents said that they had driven while drowsy in the previous year, and 23 percent had fallen asleep at the wheel. Young adults, business travelers, shift workers, and people who drive long distances, experience sleep disturbances, or take sedating medications are most likely to drive while sleepy or drowsy. Statistics show that the number of fatigue-related car collisions is at its lowest between 10:00 P.M. and midnight and highest between 2:00 and 8:00 A.M. and 1:00 and 4:00 P.M.

When to see the doctor: If you are habitually sleepy when driving, see a doctor to determine if you are suffering from a sleep disorder.

Give your car a few spritzes to help invigorate you on your next grueling commute, Gladstar suggests.

You needn't confine the use of aromatic sprays to your car commutes, though. "When I fly, I take my spritzers and spray the area," Gladstar says. Just be sure not to get any in your eyes, she says.

Don't want to tote water bottles? Look for dispensers for relaxing or stimulating aromatic oils; they plug into a vehicle's cigarette lighter, Gladstar says. A variety of scents is available in most health food stores; you can find the dispensers at health food stores and bath shops.

Guarana

If you're truly exhausted or have a particularly long drive, take ¼ teaspoon of guarana powder mixed in some water. Gladstar suggests using this herb sparingly because it is fairly high in caffeine, which can become addictive and contribute to the anxiety of your commute. "Like coffee, guarana should not be used to create everyday energy," she says. "It should be used only when you absolutely need it."

CONCENTRATION PROBLEMS

*C*ongratulations!

Many readers who a few minutes ago were scanning the table of contents in search of this chapter have forgotten by now what it was that they were looking for and have wandered off to do something else. The fact that you found your way here is worthy of some praise, and it's also a good sign that your concentration concerns can be licked.

Concentration problems can have many sources, including stress, fatigue, and depression, says William Warnock, N.D., director of the Champlain Center for Natural Medicine in Shelburne, Vermont. Potential remedies vary accordingly. Nonetheless, if you want to get yourself focused—either for a big meeting tomorrow or for better mental acuity in general—herbs can definitely help.

Green or Black Tea

Drink a cup for a quick pick-me-up. For the most part, herbs are not quick-fix solutions—they take time to take effect. That's generally good: It means that they won't pump you up only to bring you crashing down later, as stronger stimulants do. Still, there are times when you need a quick jolt, and tea can deliver one.

There's no secret to where the boost in tea comes from, says Andrew Weil, M.D., director of the program in integrative medicine at the University of Arizona College of Medicine in Tucson and author of *8 Weeks to Optimum Health*. Per cup, tea contains about 40 milligrams of caffeine, about half the amount found in coffee. A half-dozen or so studies have suggested that both green and black tea have protective effects against heart disease and cancer.

Dr. Warnock feels that green and black tea are safe if they're not abused. "Sometimes, if I need to read something and I just can't focus, I'll have a cup of tea, and that's fine," he says. "I don't drink it every day—maybe a couple of times a month."

Another, stronger herbal remedy is also quite safe to use under similar circumstances, Dr. Warnock adds. It's called coffee.

Asian Ginseng

Take extracts that provide 10 to 15 milligrams of ginsenosides, the active ingredients, three times a day. One of the biggest enemies of concentration is fatigue. "A person who's tired all the time can't concentrate," says Dr. Warnock. Ginseng has been used for centuries to address just that problem, among others.

If you want to use ginseng for more than 6 to 8 weeks at a time, Dr. Warnock suggests that you stop taking it for a week, then use it again for 6 to 8 weeks. Continue cycling on and off in this way if you need to continue taking it.

According to master herbalist Steven Foster in his book *Herbs for Your Health*, a Chinese herbalist lauded ginseng's powers for "enlightening the mind and increasing wisdom" more than 2,000 years ago. More recently, Germany's Commission E, which evaluates herbs for safety and effectiveness, described ginseng as "a tonic for invigoration and fortification in times of fatigue and debility, for declining capacity for work and concentration."

Finely Focusing Aroma

Here's an aromatherapy formula to help with concentration problems, designed by aromatherapist Victoria Edwards, owner of Leydet Aromatics in Fair Oaks, California. She calls it Cassandra's Blend, after her daughter.

Edwards came up with this formula to help her study for a chemistry final, which she says it helped her pass. She describes the aroma as spicy and lemony, with an "energetic and stimulating" effect, particularly for those who tend to be nervous when they're on the spot.

You can either sniff the formula directly from the bottle or place some in a diffuser. Do not apply it to the skin, because the black pepper can cause irritation.

4 drops black pepper essential oil
2 drops cistus essential oil
6 drops may chang essential oil

Mix the pepper, cistus, and may chang oils in a clean glass dropper bottle. Shake well before using.

Cistus (*Cistus ladaniferus*) and may chang (*Litsea cubeba*) may be difficult to find, but you should be able to locate them at well-stocked health food stores and through some mail-order suppliers.

Brahmi

Take 100 to 200 milligrams of standardized extract daily. A staple of India's ancient form of medicine, Ayurveda, brahmi is the perfect herb for people who have problems concentrating because they're nervous, says C. Leigh Broadhurst, Ph.D., an herbal researcher and nutrition consultant based in Clovery, Maryland. The botanical name for brahmi is *Bacopa monniera*, but in some parts of India, gotu kola (*Centella asiatica*) is also called brahmi, so check the label to be sure you're getting the right herb.

Tension can cause changes in brain chemistry that interfere with its ability to retain and access information. In extreme cases, it's experienced as "freezing up" in trying situations. According to Ayurvedic medical tradition, brahmi helps thaw that freeze, Dr. Broadhurst says.

Studies to determine exactly why the herb works haven't produced definitive answers yet, but it seems to help the neurons in the brain remodel themselves into coherent memory patterns. It's thought that such remodeling is necessary to encode fresh memories into our mental data banks, and stress makes it more difficult for that process to occur, Dr. Broadhurst says.

Tests have shown that anxiety-prone people significantly increased their performance on memory tests after taking brahmi for at least 2 weeks, she says. The improvement was even greater after 4 weeks. That's not to suggest that there's any reason to exceed the 100- to 200-milligram recommended dose, however.

"This isn't an herb that will give you more benefit the more you take," Dr. Broadhurst says. "A little too much may produce anxiety, restlessness, or, alternatively—with drastic overdose—sedation." Once you've experienced relief from the acute symptoms of anxiety, you may want to cut back to taking it just once every 3 days, she says. That seems to do the job for most people. Not only that, she adds, but taking it less frequently saves money.

Ashwaganda

Take one 500-milligram capsule two or three times a day for as long as needed. Ashwaganda is another staple of Ayurvedic medicine—it's called the Indian ginseng, according to Dr. Broadhurst. Like brahmi, ashwaganda is thought to help the neurons of the brain remodel themselves so that they can "learn" and retain new memories, although even prior to modern research, it had been used for centuries to help counteract concentration problems.

As exotic as it may sound, ashwaganda has very familiar relatives. It's a member of the nightshade family, Dr. Broadhurst says, as are

Adventures in Herbalism

A Stomach for Herbs

*L*egend has it that the first-ever printed compilation of herbal remedies was the *Pen-T'sao*, said to have been assembled by Shen Nung, the Red Emperor of China, somewhere around 2800 B.C. That would date it about 1,300 years before the Egyptians began using herbs such as myrrh and castor oil.

In truth, the *Pen-T'sao* may be based on oral traditions that go back that far, but the written version has probably been around only since 200 B.C. or so. It's old, but Egyptian and African herbals are considerably older.

Still, the Red Emperor must have has tremendous powers of concentration: He was certainly nothing if not thorough. The *Pen-T'sao* contains some 350 herbal remedies, each of which he is said to have tried out personally. One story has it that he cut open his abdomen and stitched a window in it so that he could observe the action of the plants he was testing. Few herbalists today can claim that degree of dedication.

tomatoes, potatoes, and peppers. It's widely available and safe for regular use.

Kava Kava

Take 70 milligrams two or three times a day for as long as necessary. The effect of kava kava is relaxing—too relaxing if you need to be at your peak for a meeting or a test, says Dr. Warnock. Still, if you're prone to worry, and worry is interfering with your ability to concentrate on an important task, a moderate dose of kava can help you focus.

Fast FACTS

Cause: A broad range of physical and psychological factors can contribute to concentration problems, among them stress, fatigue, anxiety, depression, hormone imbalances, attention deficit disorder, and simple lack of interest. Other factors, such as vision and hearing problems, can make it seem as if you have a concentration problem.

Incidence: Because of the range of possible causes, just about anyone can develop concentration problems.

When to see the doctor: When you or those around you notice a change in your ability to focus that lasts more than a week or two, see a psychologist who's trained in testing for memory disorders, or visit your family physician.

"In Polynesia, where kava originates, they brew up big pots of it," says Dr. Warnock, "and the average dose of a cup there is about 210 milligrams of kavalactones, the active ingredients. For most people who want to accomplish things in the world, that's pretty high, but in lower doses, kava can soothe anxiety without putting you to sleep." Research has also shown that the relaxing and slightly euphoric effect of kava may be due to its activation of certain neurotransmitter sites in the brain.

The body doesn't adapt to kava, Dr. Warnock adds, so it can be taken for long periods of time without losing its effectiveness. For concentration problems, though, he recommends taking it for only as long as the specific situation demands.

Gotu Kola

Take 100 milligrams twice a day. Gotu kola has long been popular in India, says English herbalist Andrew Chevallier, a member of Britain's National Institute of Medical Herbalists, in his book *The Encyclopedia of Medicinal Plants.* There, it's used as a revitalizing herb that's useful for strengthening nervous function and memory.

Like kava kava, gotu kola helps you concentrate by easing anxiety, but its effects are more subtle than kava's. "It doesn't lead to the drowsiness or relaxation that kava often does," Dr. Warnock says, "but for some people, it seems to be able to clear the mind equally well."

He recommends taking an extract standardized for 40 percent asiaticoside, the active ingredient. If you want to use it for more than 6 to 8 weeks at a time, he suggests that you stop taking it for a week, then use it again for 6 to 8 weeks. Continue cycling on and off in this way if you need to continue taking it.

Rosemary

Drink three cups of tea a day. Rosemary has been known for centuries as "the herb of remembrance," and modern science has been finding out why. According to Dr. Broadhurst, rosemary contains a number of antioxidant compounds that can help prevent the breakdown of the brain's neurotransmitters, which are key in storing memories. A cup of rosemary tea can also help your ability to concentrate by helping you to relax, she says.

To brew a cup, simply add 1½ tablespoons of dried rosemary to about 8 ounces of boiling water. Simmer with a lid on for 5 minutes, then take it off the heat and let stand for 5 minutes. Strain and drink.

CONSTIPATION

*H*erbs were custom-made by nature to cure constipation. How? Well, herbs, as you know, are plants. Plants, as you may not know, are largely responsible for keeping your plumbing functioning smoothly and regularly. In fact, doctors say that most cases of constipation could be avoided simply by adding more plant-based foods to your diet. The opposite, a diet full of meats and dairy products, is a surefire recipe for plugged bowels.

Poor diet isn't the only cause. Some medications, some illnesses, and even trying a new food can leave you straining fruitlessly. Once again, plants can help you out, this time in the form of herbal medicine. What's more, herbal treatments for constipation stack up nicely against the conventional kind, says Carolyn DeMarco, M.D., a physician in Winlaw, British Columbia, and member of the advisory board of Dominion Herbal College in Burnaby.

With prolonged use, some conventional constipation remedies, such as over-the-counter laxatives, can impair the normal function of the colon and lead to dependence over the long term. Herbs don't do that as often. In fact, herbs usually address the reason that you're constipated, not just the very obvious symptom.

Before you open your herbal medicine cabinet, though, there's something you need to do, says Theresa MacLean, R.Ph., N.D., a naturopathic physician and pharmacist based in Berwick, Nova Scotia. Drink like a fish.

"Your best friend, initially, is water," she says. That means six to eight 8-ounce glasses a day. Many people, Dr. MacLean says, are in chronic states of dehydration. When that happens, your bowels draw as much water as they can out of your food as it's being digested. This leaves the stool hard and difficult to pass. Another reason to start drinking lots of water is that some of the herbal remedies offered here require it to work properly. Here they are.

Cascara

Take 15 to 20 drops of tincture once daily. If you want to, er, get moving right away, you should know about cascara. Also called cascara sagrada, it's probably the world's most popular laxative, says Dr. MacLean. It's even an ingredient in several over-the-counter laxatives.

Cascara contains compounds known as anthraquinones, which

ADVENTURES IN HERBALISM

A MOVING TRIBUTE TO A SACRED HERB

*W*hen sixteenth-century Spanish explorers came ashore in northern California, they were carrying a lot of extra baggage. They were constipated, you see, most likely as a result of a seafaring diet low in fresh produce and fresh water.

The local Native Americans had what the Spaniards needed—an effective constipation remedy consisting of a tea made from dried bark. The herb worked nicely, and after the Spaniards relieved their bowels, they named the herb the most appropriate thing they could think of—*Cascara sagrada*, which means "sacred bark."

For a long time, cascara remained only a West Coast remedy, as the Spaniards were more interested in finding gold than in spreading the word on a new laxative. Ironically, it was gold that helped introduce a new group of people to cascara's moving effects.

During the Gold Rush period of the mid 1850s, the "Forty-Niners" made use of cascara for their own constipation. Presumably because they didn't speak Spanish, the roughshod gold seekers named the herb chittem bark—a polite variation on a word that sounds similar to *chit*.

---

stimulate the intestinal contractions that we recognize as nature's call. You shouldn't use cascara for long periods of time, though, warns Dr. MacLean. Two weeks is the maximum.

Senna

Take 20 to 40 drops of tincture at bedtime. If cascara doesn't get you going, you can bring in the big guns. Senna fits that description, notes Dr. MacLean, and because it's so powerful, it should be used only as a last resort. It should work in about 8 hours, so if you take it before you go to bed, it should start working by morning, she says.

Senna, like cascara, should never be used for more than 2 weeks, and you should never take more than the recommended amount. The resulting cramps and copious diarrhea will make you sorry that you did.

You'll see senna in various forms, but Dr. MacLean suggests the tincture to make it as palatable as possible. Look for one that's made with 1 part senna to 5 parts alcohol/water mixture.

Lemon

Squeeze half a fresh lemon into a glass of water 15 minutes before meals. Lemon juice is a gentle laxative that is best used for prevention, says Dr. MacLean. And it's cheap. If you find yourself in need and unable to get to an herb store, simply go to any grocery store or produce stand and pick up a handful of lemons.

Castor Oil

Take 1 to 2 teaspoons on an empty stomach. As with cod-liver oil, your mother was right to make you take your castor oil—at least in the case of constipation.

Castor oil is pressed from the seeds of the *Ricinus communis* plant and is slightly yellow or sometimes colorless. Its lingering aftertaste leaves something to be desired, but it works, says Varro E. Tyler, Ph.D., Sc.D., distinguished professor emeritus of pharmacognosy at Purdue University in West Lafayette, Indiana, and co-author of *Tyler's Honest Herbal*. That's because a component in the oil breaks down into a substance that goes to work on both the small and large intestines. You can expect results in about 8 hours.

Fast FACTS

Cause: Although constipation has many causes, a low-fiber diet is probably the primary factor. Others can include dehydration, a change in diet, a fever, some types of medications, and even cancer.

Incidence: Just about everyone goes through a period of constipation at one point or another. For some, though, it's a condition that becomes an uncomfortable way of life. About 4.5 million Americans put up with chronic constipation. Senior citizens who take several medications are more susceptible than others.

When to see the doctor: If constipation lingers for more than 2 weeks, with less than one bowel movement every 3 days, and is accompanied by abdominal pain or blood in the stool, have it checked out. While it's probably easily remedied, it may be a symptom of something more serious, such as inflammatory bowel disease or other bowel disorder.

Psyllium

Take 5 to 10 grams daily. Since a low-fiber diet is a primary cause of constipation, psyllium's high levels of fiber can address that over the long term, says Dr. Tyler.

You may not have heard of psyllium, but you have probably heard of Metamucil. It and products like it are psyllium. This seed-derived herbal product adds bulk and fiber to your digestive tract. It also absorbs a lot of water as it passes through the body, which is why it's important to drink generous amounts.

Psyllium and other fiber additives have double action. First, they add bulk to the stool, and your body responds by moving it through your digestive tract more quickly. Second—and this may surprise you—they help restore a normal balance of bacteria in your intestines.

Your colon is inhabited by more than 400 bacterial species that make up the normal flora of your gut. In fact, bacteria make up more than 50 percent of the total dry weight of your stool. When those bacteria become unbalanced, you get constipated. Fiber provides a platform for these normal bugs to grow. Although it may be a bit gruesome to think about, the right level of the right kind of bacteria is essential to having regular bathroom visits.

You may find psyllium in more than one form, so check the label when you're shopping. The above dosage is for the seed form. The husks have three times more fiber than the seeds, so if you use them, reduce the dose to 3 grams a day. Either type should start to work within 12 to 72 hours.

Flaxseed

Take 1 tablespoon of ground seeds two or three times a day. Also known as linseed, flaxseed is a bulk-forming agent like psyllium. As with psyllium, you need to drink lots of water in order for it to work properly, says Dr. MacLean.

To make taking flaxseed more pleasant, adds Dr. MacLean, try adding it to applesauce or sprinkling it on your cereal in the morning. With its long tradition of treating chronic constipation, it should get you moving within 3 days, she says.

CORNS AND CALLUSES

*W*hen abused, the human body will try in various ways to protect itself. Sometimes, though, our self-defense mechanisms themselves can become a problem. Corns and calluses are cases in point.

Both are buildups of dead skin in places where repeated friction and pressure of skin against bone cause irritation. The usual cause of that irritation, according to William Rossi, D.P.M., a doctor of podiatric medicine based in Marshfield, Massachusetts, is poor-fitting shoes. Sometimes, he says, there can be an underlying bone deformity that makes irritation more likely. In either case, your foot senses a need for padding and creates its own. Corns usually form on the tops of the toes or between them and are painful to the touch. Calluses are most common on the bottoms of the feet and are not tender.

This natural padding can create problems instead of solving them, however. The buildup of skin to combat the effects of tightness only increases the tightness. Your body is smart, Dr. Rossi says, but it operates according to natural laws that evolved long before the high heel or the wing tip.

Home remedies for corns and calluses generally aim to soften the hardened skin so that the dead skin gradually wears away by itself or so that it can be more easily removed by rubbing it with a pumice stone, an emery board, or a pedi-wand, all available at drugstores.

Foot doctors caution, however, that any treatment to remove corns and calluses, whether herbal, pharmaceutical, or surgical, will be wasted if the problem that caused them to form in the first place isn't addressed. You need to buy more foot-friendly shoes, have your feet examined by a podiatrist, or both.

That said, there are a number of ways to herbally encourage the corns and calluses you already have to do a disappearing act.

Bloodroot

Apply tincture once a day to soften and remove corns. According to Beverly Yates, N.D., a naturopathic doctor with the Natural Health Care Group in Portland, Oregon, and Seattle, bloodroot was used by Native Americans to deal with all sorts of skin problems, from warts to tumors. The extract is available in tincture form at health food stores, she says, but be careful: It's potent stuff that should be diluted 50 percent with water.

Apply the diluted mixture directly to the corn, avoiding the surrounding skin. It's also a good idea to cover the area with a sock when you're finished, Dr. Yates says, because bloodroot can stain sheets and clothing. Two weeks of nightly applications should be plenty.

According to Dr. Yates, this remedy may also be used on calluses,

Dr. Duke's Celandine Corn Remover

Here's a corn-killing recipe from James A. Duke, Ph.D., an herbalist and ethnobotanist in Fulton, Maryland, and author of The Green Pharmacy. *Its central ingredient is celandine, which has a worldwide reputation as a corn remover. Apply it to corns twice a day, such as before you leave for work and before you go to bed.*

> **6 cups water**
> **1 teaspoon potassium chloride (available at supermarkets as a salt substitute)**
> **4 ounces fresh celandine, chopped**
> **1 cup glycerin**

Put the water in a medium saucepan and add the potassium chloride. Heat and stir until the potassium chloride dissolves. Remove from the heat, add the celandine, and let stand for 2 hours.

Return the pan to the heat and bring the mixture to a boil. Reduce the heat and simmer for 20 minutes. Then, using a sieve or wire strainer, strain the liquid into a medium bowl. Discard the plant material.

Return the liquid to the pan and simmer until it is reduced to 1½ cups. Add the glycerin and continue simmering until reduced to 2 cups. Strain the liquid, place it in a bottle, and store in a cool place.

but the treatment may take longer—about 3 or 4 weeks, depending on the depth of the callus.

Castor Oil

Apply directly to corns once or twice daily. You might not think of castor oil as an herbal remedy, but in fact, it's derived

Fast Facts

Cause: Poor-fitting shoes or bone problems in the foot trigger formation of corns and calluses.

Incidence: It's estimated that 150 million new corns grow on American feet each year. Calluses are universal. Women's shoe fashions, including high heels, mean that they have more problems with corns and calluses than men do.

When to see the doctor: Persistent, painful corns or calluses may indicate underlying bone problems that could require special shoes or surgery. See a podiatrist.

from the seeds of the castor bean and therefore qualifies as plant-based, at least.

You can use castor oil right out of the bottle as an excellent solvent for corns, according to John Hahn, N.D., a naturopathic and podiatric physician in Bend, Oregon.

To apply, first surround the corn with a felt, adhesive-backed corn aperture pad (available at drugstores). Once it's in place, the pad will create a little cup to hold the castor oil on the corn.

Place a drop of oil directly onto the corn, then cover it with a piece of hypoallergenic silk tape, says Dr. Hahn. "This will soften the corn enough that a pumice stone will take it right off," he says. He cautions, however, that the oil will stain just about anything it comes in contact with, so cover your foot with an old sock when you're done. The castor oil will be most effective if it's allowed to soak into the corn for a while, so leave it on overnight.

Olive Oil

Apply nightly to soften calluses. Calluses are tough, but they can be softened by simply rubbing olive oil, or any other oil you prefer, on your feet, says Kathi Head, N.D., a Sandpoint, Idaho, naturopathic physician and an editor of *Alternative Medicine Review*. Once softened, the calluses can be filed down with an emery board or pumice stone.

For a slightly more aggressive approach, try adding some salt to the olive oil, says Stephanie Tourles, an herbalist, aromatherapist, and licensed aesthetician in Hyannis, Massachusetts, and author of *Natural Foot Care*. The salt will act as a natural abrasive to help remove the callus. She recommends 1 tablespoon of salt for each tablespoon of olive oil (almond oil is fine, too). "After you've softened your feet by soaking in the shower or in a foot bath, apply this mixture to the bottoms of your feet, anywhere you have calluses, and scrub really vigorously with your hands for a few minutes," she says.

The mixture can be scented aromatically by adding a drop of essential oil, Tourles says. She recommends peppermint or spearmint for a boost in the morning and orange or lavender at night, when you need to relax.

COUGH

A cough is usually there for a reason—and that reason isn't just to keep you up at night or bother everybody around you in a movie theater. Indeed, most herbal practitioners don't see a cough as something to be suppressed.

"Coughing is useful," notes Chanchal Cabrera, a member of Britain's National Institute of Medical Herbalists, a professional member of the American Herbalists Guild, and an herbalist in Vancouver. "It moves the mucus up out of the lungs, so if you have an infection in the lungs, you want to be coughing."

ADVENTURES IN HERBALISM

LESSONS FROM ARONA

*V*ice president of the American Herbalists Guild Roy Upton calls Soquel, California, home these days, but his vocation has led him to some of the world's most idyllic spots. He spent 4 years in the U.S. Virgin Islands, studying the traditional uses of medicinal plants, practicing herbal medicine, and—this was the Caribbean, after all—spear fishing.

"I was lucky enough to learn about herbs from some wonderful native West Indian people," says Upton. Most notable was Arona Petersen. Widely known throughout the Caribbean, Petersen was loved and respected by all who knew her, both for her wonderful Carib cooking and for her knowledge of plants.

One day during Upton's visit, Petersen was brewing some cough syrup on the kitchen stove. The heavy iron pot was filled with herbs: sweetly scented hibiscus flowers, lime leaves, some passionflower, the juice of the soursop fruit, and a few spoonfuls of honey. The fragrant mixture simmered and bubbled as it cooked down to a thick syrup.

"We got to talking and watching the Super Bowl and completely forgot about the herbal brew," recalls Upton. That is, until the smoky smell of the burning botanicals came wafting through the room at half-time. By the time Upton reached the kitchen and turned off the fire, the syrup was a brown, gummy mess.

"After the game, we went to clean the pan and found that the herbal mixture had solidified into a chewy, taffylike, aromatic mass of delicious hardened herbal candy," remembers Upton. "I don't know if it was medicinally effective, but it sure tasted good. I guess making mistakes like this is one way we learn about herbs."

"No, I don't," you say. Well, no matter how you feel about coughs, rest assured that herbal medicine does indeed have ways of dealing with them, including lots of home remedies. Your home herbal strategy is threefold: first, to aid your body's natural healing ability in overcoming the infection that's causing the cough in the first place; second, to help convert a dry, hacking cough into a more comfortable and productive (i.e., mucus-expelling) one; and third, to assist that productive cough in doing its job so it can quickly go on its merry way.

Marshmallow

Drink three cups of tea a day between meals. To get rid of that initial dry cough, you need what herbalists call a soothing expectorant, such as marshmallow. The mucilage in this herb can trigger a nerve reflex into the lungs, which makes all the mucus there thinner and easier to expel. Your miserable hack becomes a less unpleasant, productive cough.

Use the cut-and-sifted root of dried marshmallow to make a strong decoction by simmering 1 ounce (by weight) of herb in 1 pint of water for 10 minutes, says Cabrera. Take it at the earliest stage of your infection, when your cough is dry.

Elecampane

Drink three cups of tea a day between meals. Elecampane is another excellent soothing expectorant with lots of mucilage. It acts just like marshmallow. In fact, Cabrera says, you can easily combine the two by making a half-and-half tea mix. The result isn't bad-tasting, but it's too gummy to be considered pleasurable.

Alternatively, decoct 1 ounce (by weight) of cut-and-sifted dried elecampane root by simmering it for 10 minutes in 1 pint of water. You should take mucilaginous herbs like marshmallow and elecampane when mucus is thick and sticky and there is an unproductive cough.

Fast Facts

Cause: A cough is a reflex triggered by irritation or excess mucus. It's part of your immune system's effort to overcome an infection.

Incidence: A cough is a symptom, not a condition; it can accompany a number of ailments, often respiratory infections such as a cold or flu but also more serious conditions such as asthma, chronic obstructive pulmonary disease, or tuberculosis.

When to see the doctor: Seek professional medical care if you don't know why you're coughing, if you cough up blood, or if your cough or any other symptom associated with a cold lingers for more than a week or continues after other symptoms have subsided.

Licorice

Drink two to three cups of tea a day between meals. "Once your cough actually starts to bring stuff up, it's time to switch to another kind of expectorant, a stimulating one," Cabrera says. Stimulating expectorants include lobelia and grindelia, but a much safer (and better-tasting) choice is medicinal licorice. An expectorant like licorice is slightly irritating rather than soothing, so it will stimulate your cough to move the phlegm up and out faster.

Licorice tea is made from the dried root (or the rhizome, the underground part of the stem), and it's naturally quite strong. Cabrera suggests finding a strength that you can handle, somewhere between 1 teaspoon and 1 tablespoon of herb per cup of water. Simmer, covered, for 10 minutes and strain before drinking.

You'll get some bonuses with licorice, according to Cabrera. "It's also immune-supporting and helps regulate mucus production in the lungs," she says. "It will help build back some of the energy you've exhausted from prolonged coughing. If you only took one herb for a cough, this might be the one." It's best to take licorice while your cough is productive, and you can take it until coughing symptoms subside.

Echinacea, Elder, Usnea, and Thyme

Take ½ to 1 teaspoon of this tincture formula three times daily between meals. If you're coughing a lot from irritation associated with a cold or allergy, here's a formula from Mary Bove, N.D., a naturopathic physician at the Brattleboro Naturopathic Clinic in Vermont and a member of Britain's National Institute of Medical Herbalists. The cough-specific ingredient in the mixture is thyme leaf, which contains a volatile oil called thymol that's not only highly antiseptic but also relieves coughs. The other herbs help take care of the cold that's causing the cough in the first place.

The formula calls for 2 parts echinacea to 1 part of each of the rest of the herb tinctures, so you might go to your health food store and buy a 2-ounce bottle of echinacea tincture and 1-ounce bottles of elderflower, usnea, and thyme. Mix them together, and you'll have plenty of cough-with-cold formula.

CUTS AND SCRAPES

We may be the most highly evolved creatures on the planet, but with no thick hide or pelt of fur to protect us, we're at a distinct disadvantage when it comes to skin injuries. Clothes help, but even so, throughout history, our fragile skin has succumbed to dangers great and small—sharp rocks, the slings and arrows of cruel fate, a careless flick of the razor.

The ancient Romans made compresses out of spiderwebs to heal their cuts and scrapes. Native Americans used sphagnum moss. Now drugstores stock a whole arsenal of creams and ointments to fight off infection and speed healing.

Although nature's medicine chest is well-stocked with herbs to help your skin heal, don't overlook basic first-aid. When you nick your finger while cutting tomatoes, your first instinct is probably to clasp your other hand over the cut. That instinct's right on target. Applying pressure to the wound with a cloth, a T-shirt, your finger—whatever you have handy—helps to stop the bleeding, says Pierre Brunschwig, M.D., a member of the American Holistic Medical Association who practices at the Helios Health Center in Boulder, Colorado.

The next order of business is to clean the cut thoroughly, says Dr. Brunschwig. "That's especially important if it's a dirty wound—if you fell off your bicycle, for example," he adds. "The biggest danger with cuts is infection." Here are some herbs that can help cleanse and soothe a cut or scrape.

Shepherd's Purse

Let a few drops of tincture fall on the cut to stop the bleeding. Bleeding is the body's natural response to being cut, and letting a little blood flow helps to clean out the wound. If you have a small cut and it's still oozing blood after 5 minutes, stem the crimson tide with shepherd's purse, says Marcey Shapiro, M.D., a family doctor in Albany, California, who combines natural healing with conventional medicine. Just a few drops right on the cut will do the trick. As a bonus, the alcohol in the tincture is antiseptic.

Calendula

Cleanse a cut with tincture; soothe a scrape with salve. Used in the seventeenth century as a cure for "plague or pestilence," calendula has an even stronger reputation as a wound healer and is endorsed for this use by Germany's Commission E, which evaluates herbs for safety and effectiveness. Calendula extract is anti-inflammatory and antibacterial and stimulates the formation of new tissue at the wound site.

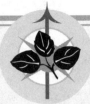

ADVENTURES IN HERBALISM

OF GUNS AND GOLDENSEAL

*N*ative Americans used the bright yellow root of the goldenseal plant to make dyes as well as medicines. In recent times, the herb has become popular because of its antibacterial and anti-inflammatory properties. It's so popular, in fact, that it is now endangered.

Goldenseal is often used to treat colds, sore throats, and sinus infections, but Rita Bettenburg, N.D., has all the proof she needs that the herb is also a powerful wound healer. A naturopathic doctor in Portland, Oregon, Dr. Bettenburg isn't in the habit of treating gunshot wounds, but one day she found herself doing just that.

Dr. Bettenburg's patient had taken a bullet in the upper arm 6 weeks earlier when he got in the way of a shootout on the public transportation system. The bullet was still in his arm, lodged against the bone. The doctors at the hospital were afraid of causing neurological damage by trying to remove it, so they had decided to wait for it to heal over.

"The wound was still open and draining when he came in," recalls Dr. Bettenburg, "and they had him on antibiotics to keep it from getting infected. He was having some trouble with all the antibiotics he was taking and also some difficulty with the tenderness of the wound. It just wasn't healing."

Dr. Bettenburg took matters in hand and, over the course of several weeks, regularly sprinkled goldenseal powder on the wound to prevent infection. "It really helped with the healing process," she says. The last time Dr. Bettenburg saw her patient, his wound was completely healed.

It may take some scouting, but look for a calendula succus, which is a low-alcohol tincture formula, says Rita Bettenburg, N.D., a naturopathic doctor at the Natural Childbirth and Family Clinic in Portland, Oregon, who uses calendula succus frequently to clean out wounds. Of course, if you can't find a succus, a regular tincture will do, but dilute it with a little water, says Dr. Bettenburg.

After washing the cut with soap and water, let a few drops of succus fall onto it from the dropper. You don't need to swab it off; just leave it there to do its job. Reapply every few hours as needed to keep the wound clean, Dr. Bettenburg advises. When it has dried, you can apply one of the herbal lotions or creams described below.

For a superficial scrape, Susan Allen, N.D., a resident naturopathic physician at the National College of Naturopathic Medicine in Portland, recommends a calendula salve to help heal the skin. You can find it in health food stores, and it's perfect if you fall and scrape your knee. After cleaning the scrape with soap and water, dab the salve right on the scrape and cover it with a bandage. Stop using it as soon as a scab starts to form, since the moisture will interfere with this healing stage. Often, one application is enough, says Dr. Allen.

Rosemary

Bathe an infected wound with an herbal wash. Rosemary makes a wonderful topical antiseptic, says Dr. Shapiro. Simply break off a few twigs of the herb, pour boiling water over them, and steep until the water is cool. Dab the wash on with a cloth or pour it directly over the cut. Reapply two to four times a day until the redness disappears, she says.

Dr. Shapiro recommends this wash if you notice that a cut is becoming a little red around the edges or if any pus is visible. "I'd more often choose an herbal antiseptic than something like a neomycin-type ointment," she says. "The ointment is oily, and it covers the wound and won't let it breathe, whereas the antiseptic

Fast FACTS

Cause: Falling down a flight of steps, opening a can of cat food, deboning a chicken breast—living an active life is bound to lead to cuts and scrapes sooner or later.

Incidence: Superman is about the only person who isn't vulnerable to cuts and scrapes. They are pretty universal problems.

When to see the doctor: If blood is spurting from a wound or flowing so fast that you can't stop it after applying pressure for a few minutes, seek medical treatment immediately. You'll also need swift professional attention if the cut is deep enough to expose fat, tendon, or muscle, or if it's more than $\frac{1}{2}$ inch long, has jagged edges, or is in a place where you'd rather not have a scar. (Even small cuts on the face can leave scars if they're not treated promptly.) For scrapes, you should see a doctor if the damaged area is the size of your hand or larger. If any cut or scrape becomes hot to the touch, red, or swollen or is leaking pus, or if you have a fever following the injury, see a doctor to treat the possible infection.

herb washes penetrate well, and the wound can still breathe after it has dried."

Myrrh

Clean a cut with this antimicrobial wash. Myrrh is a fantastic herb for warding off infection, says Marion Gladwell, a member of Britain's National Institute of Medical Herbalists who has an herbal practice at Bury Natural Health Center in Suffolk, England. The Chinese clearly agree: They began using this resinous gum to treat wounds in the seventh century. An antimicrobial herb, myrrh works by stimulating the production of white blood cells, which gather at the wound site to fight off infection, says Gladwell.

Mix 1 teaspoon of myrrh tincture with $\frac{1}{4}$ pint of water and slosh it over the cut or scrape. Let it air-dry before applying any kind of lotion, recommends Gladwell. You can use a myrrh rinse twice a day, she says, or whenever you change the bandage.

Aloe

Apply gel directly to the cut. The gooey gel from the interior of the aloe vera plant has strong anti-inflammatory properties, says Dr. Brunschwig, and numerous studies have backed up its long history of use in folk medicine. By dilating the blood vessels, aloe gel helps flood the wound site with blood, thus speeding up the healing process. Aloe is also antimicrobial and is thought to stimulate the formation of connective tissue cells, thus helping to heal the wound.

Aloe gel is one of the easiest herbal remedies to find, but the quality is not always consistent, says Dr. Brunschwig. If aloe is the first name you see on the label's ingredients list, you can be sure it's the primary ingredient.

Carefully dab the gel on the cut or scrape right after you have cleaned it and again each time you change the bandage—at least twice a day. If the cut is on your face or in another place where it won't become dirty or come in contact with clothing, you can leave it open to the air, but apply the gel twice a day. Not only will it soothe your poor, damaged skin, it will also help minimize the possibility of infection and scarring, says Dr. Brunschwig.

Oregon Grape

Sprinkle a pinch of root powder on the cut twice a day. After cleaning a cut with antibacterial soap or a rosemary wash, stave off infection by dusting it with Oregon grape root powder, advises Dr. Shapiro. Any of the yellow, bitter roots—goldenseal, barberry, or Oregon grape—will prevent the spread of bacterial infection, she says. That's because they all contain berberine, a constituent that has an antibiotic action.

Dandruff

*I*t's myth-dispelling time: Contrary to what the people who make television commercials would like us to believe, dandruff isn't caused by using the wrong shampoo, and it's certainly nothing to be embarrassed about.

The unfortunate scalp flakiness associated with dandruff is usually due to accelerated skin cell growth. Often, a yeastlike organism is responsible.

Dandruff can often be managed with over-the-counter hair products, says Diana Bihova, M.D., a dermatologist in New York City. Ingredients like salicylic acid, sulfur, selenium sulfide, tar, and zinc have been shown to be effective at ending accelerated scalp sloughing.

Ready-made dandruff shampoos can be harsh and drying to hair, though. If you'd prefer to go the natural route, there are helpful herbal products to look for as well as homemade cures to try.

Tea Tree

Look for hair products containing tea tree oil at health food stores, or add 10 to 20 drops of essential oil to an average-size bottle of regular shampoo. Tea tree oil has been called nature's antiseptic, but it could be just as well-described as nature's antifungal. That's because the clear to pale yellow, eucalyptus-smelling oil of the Australian *Melaleuca quinquenervia* tree inhibits the growth of fungi, including the one responsible for some cases of dandruff.

Tea tree essential oil is highly toxic if taken internally, but it is safe and gentle for external use. Its antifungal and antiseptic properties, combined with its scalp-safe strength, make it an ideal herbal treatment for dandruff, says Dr. Bihova.

When you use a tea tree shampoo, the tingling sensation invigorates your scalp while scales are swept away. Dr. Bihova suggests

Fast FACTS

Cause: Dandruff is really a mechanical problem—the overzealous shedding of scalp cells. More serious flaking that resembles dandruff but is harder to treat can come from skin problems that affect the scalp as well as the rest of the body, such as sebborrheic dermatitis, psoriasis, and eczema.

Incidence: Everyone sheds scalp cells as a matter of course, but there are so few that they simply go unnoticed. Roughly 20 percent of the population has the excess of scalp flakes that signals dandruff.

When to see the doctor: Using over-the-counter treatments or herbal home remedies for dandruff should provide some improvement within 2 weeks. If you still have flaking after that time, or if you have intense itching combined with a red, irritated scalp, see your doctor.

---

using this shampoo only once a week, though, because one of the ingredients in tea tree oil, d-limonene, can be a cause of allergic dermatitis.

Soak your scalp in pure olive oil for 15 to 30 minutes before shampooing with a tea tree oil product. If your dandruff is accompanied by a dry, scaly scalp, the emollience of natural olive oil can help. Before shampooing, part your hair in several places and use your fingers to coat your scalp with enough olive oil to do the job. Don't worry about reaching the ends of your hair—concentrate on the roots and scalp, suggests Dr. Bihova. Cover your hair with a shower cap or plastic bag for up to a half-hour, then wash it thoroughly with a dandruff shampoo. You can do this every other day or as often as needed.

Nettle, Horsetail, Johnny Jump-Up, and Lavender

Make a strong four-herb tea and use it as a final rinse after your daily shampoo. Make your very own herbal finishing rinse as a crafty, home-brewed way to handle dandruff, suggests Mercedes

Cameron, M.D., family practitioner at The Woman's Place at St. Mary's Hospital in Grand Junction, Colorado. This combination of herbs is especially suited for dandruff that feels oily.

Mix equal parts of the following four dried herbs: nettle, for its astringent properties; horsetail, for its high silica content, thought to regenerate and strengthen connective tissue (it has traditionally been used in baths to treat eczema and other skin conditions); Johnny jump-up, also known as heart's ease, for its saponoid content, which is known to heal skin and is frequently used for eczema; and lavender, for its soothing aromatherapeutic scent as well as antiseptic, scalp-healing oils.

Use 1 tablespoon of the dried herb mixture and 1 pint of boiling water to make a strong tea, steeping the brew for up to 15 minutes. Strain it into a clean glass bottle for use in the shower, says Dr. Cameron. After shampooing your hair, squeeze out the excess water, then douse your tresses with the herbal dandruff treatment. There is no need to rinse.

DIABETES

*D*iabetes has been called the disease of civilization. Although our basic nutritional needs have not evolved in the past 100,000 years, our palates have, and diabetes is closely related to diet.

While our ancient ancestors may have dined on fruits and vegetables, nuts and seeds, and an occasional kill of wild game, we're more partial to double cheeseburgers with a side of fries. Wash that down with a large soda, and you have the recipe for diabetes. Our civilized appetite for foods that are high in sugar and fat can cause metabolic changes that result in chronically high blood sugar, or diabetes. Like the complex civilization in which we live, this pervasive disease is not easily understood or easily treated.

To start with the basics, the cells in our bodies need energy to function. They get that energy from glucose, also called blood sugar, which is absorbed when we eat carbohydrates. As the level of glucose builds in your bloodstream, your body secretes a hormone called insulin. Like a key unlocking a door, insulin unleashes the stored energy in the blood and allows it to enter the cells.

There are two main types of diabetes. In both, glucose fails to enter the cells and accumulates in the blood. Over the long term, elevated blood sugar levels can damage the eyes, kidneys, blood vessels, and nerves. Because bacteria thrive on the glucose-rich blood and urine, people with untreated diabetes are also more prone to urinary tract infections.

In type 1, or insulin-dependent, diabetes, the pancreas loses its ability to produce insulin. Without the hormone, the glucose absorbed from food remains in the blood, even though the cells are starved for energy. A person with this type of diabetes must inject insulin regularly to help the cells absorb glucose.

About 90 to 95 percent of all people with diabetes have type 2, or non-insulin-dependent, diabetes. With this type, your body may produce enough insulin in early stages of the condition, but in time, your cells aren't able to respond to it, and they become insulin resistant. Blood sugar levels rise, but the energy-starved cells are unable to tap into their fuel supply, so they trigger the body to produce more insulin. When repeated continuously, this process eventually overworks and depletes the supply of special insulin-creating cells in the pancreas until they can no longer function. In an endless merry-go-round of symptoms, the disease perpetuates itself.

While both types of diabetes are serious diseases that require a doctor's care, you can use herbs to help regulate your blood sugar, says Robert Rountree, M.D., a holistic physician at the Helios Health Center in Boulder, Colorado.

Herbs aren't substitutes for the fundamental changes in diet and lifestyle that you need to make in order to control your diabetes. You still have to eat right, control your weight, and exercise regularly, says Nancy Welliver, N.D., director of the Institute of Medical Herbalism in Calistoga, California. Medicinal herbs can complement

Stevia: Sweeter Than Sugar

*W*ith virtually no calories and no effect on blood sugar levels, stevia is a safe herbal alternative to sugar or artificial sweeteners, says C. Leigh Broadhurst, Ph.D., a nutrition consultant and herbal researcher based in Clovery, Maryland, and a diabetes researcher with the USDA Human Nutrition Research Center in Beltsville. You won't find it next to aspartame or saccharin in your grocery store, though. Because of Food and Drug Administration restrictions, it is sold only as a dietary supplement.

Derived from the leaves of a wild shrub, *Stevia rebaudiana*, that grows in the mountains of Paraguay, stevia is estimated to be 150 to 400 times sweeter than sugar. You need to use just a drop or a pinch, not a spoonful.

Dr. Broadhurst recommends using stevia extract, which is sold by the ounce in health food stores as a liquid or white powder, but remember to use only a small amount. To get accustomed to the taste, Dr. Broadhurst suggests blending it with sugar to get the level of sweetness you want with less sugar.

Finely powdered, dried stevia leaf is also sold in bulk or packaged like tea bags. The distinctive flavor of the greenish powder is similar to that of licorice and blends well with cinnamon and ginger.

those efforts by lowering blood sugar levels, helping your body use insulin effectively, and protecting you from diabetes-related damage.

It's crucial for people with diabetes to take a daily multivitamin supplement to correct any nutritional deficiencies and to take at least 200 micrograms of chromium daily, says Dr. Welliver. Studies of people with diabetes have shown that supplementing the diet with this trace mineral can lower fasting blood sugar levels, improve glucose tolerance, and lower insulin levels. If you have diabetes, don't exceed 400 to 600 micrograms a day, and be sure to have your doctor carefully monitor your blood sugar levels.

It's safest to work with a practitioner who can develop a protocol specifically for you. Many nutrients and herbs can affect drug doses and regulation. Here's an idea of the types of herbs you can use to manage this complex problem.

Bitter Melon

Drink 2 ounces of juice twice a day. Because it works on so many levels, bitter melon is the best herb to start with to help control diabetes and its complications, says Dr. Welliver. This Asian food has been used traditionally as a remedy for diabetes. Eating bitter melon increases the insulin-secreting cells in the pancreas, called beta cells. It is thought to help regulate blood sugar levels by slowing the absorption of glucose. According to Dr. Welliver, studies suggest that bitter melon is most effective for type 2 diabetes and possibly early type 1.

Cultivated throughout the tropical regions of the world, bitter melon is used as an anti-diabetes remedy in China, India, Sri Lanka, and the West Indies. It's available in the United States at Asian markets. You can make the juice by running the fruit through a juicer or by blending it with a little water until it is thin enough to drink. You can take bitter melon indefinitely at these dosages. Looking farther down the road, a daily shot of bitter melon juice may reduce the risk of developing diabetic retinopathy, a complication of diabetes caused by damage to blood vessels of the retina, says Dr. Welliver.

Asian Ginseng

Take a daily dose of 200 milligrams in capsule form. Known as a feel-good herb to boost vitality, ginseng can help stabilize blood sugar levels if you have type 2 diabetes, says C. Leigh Broadhurst, Ph.D., a nutrition consultant and herbal researcher based in Clovery,

Maryland and a diabetes researcher with the USDA Human Nutrition Research Center in Beltsville.

For centuries, practitioners of Traditional Chinese Medicine have used ginseng to treat diabetes. Now, Western practitioners are catching on. In a study in Finland, researchers found that a daily dose of 200 milligrams of ginseng for 8 weeks improved mood, diet, and activity, which reduced weight and helped lower blood sugar levels.

Gymnema sylvestre

Take 400 milligrams in capsule form twice a day. The leaves of this climbing vine (also known as gurmar) have been used in traditional Ayurvedic medicine as a treatment for diabetes, says Dr. Welliver. "It seems to enhance the production of insulin, possibly through the regeneration of beta cells of the pancreas," she says. That would make it appropriate for people with type 2 diabetes and even those with early type 1.

"It has the unusual property of blocking sugary taste. Sugar is no longer pleasant," according to Dr. Welliver. The herb is safe to use on a regular basis, she says.

Cinnamon

Drink 1 quart of cinnamon water every day. Cinnamon contains a phytochemical that helps those with both type 1 and type 2 diabetes utilize blood sugar, says Dr. Broadhurst. In the past 10 years, researchers at the USDA Beltsville Nutrient Requirements and Functions Laboratory in Maryland have tested 60 other medicinal and food plants looking for the same anti-diabetes effect.

"Nothing has come close to the consistently excellent results of cinnamon," says Dr. Broadhurst. "Since the first report on cinnamon, hundreds of people have contacted the laboratory to say how cinnamon has helped them reduce their insulin or medication dosages."

A quart of cinnamon tea every day sounds like a lot, doesn't it? One way to make sure you get the recommended dosage is to make up a batch of this pleasant-tasting beverage and substitute it for part of your daily water intake. Add 3 tablespoons of cinnamon and 2 teaspoons of baking soda to 1 quart of boiling water. Reduce the temperature and simmer for 20 minutes, then strain the tea and store it in the refrigerator.

The flavor and quality of cinnamon vary according to the quality of its volatile oils. Since the active ingredient is a water-based chemical, it doesn't matter what type you use to make this tea, says Dr. Broadhurst. It will be just as effective with a cheaper, less aromatic spice. If you find that cinnamon helps you, you can use it regularly.

Prickly Pear

Eat 1 cup of cactus a day. The soluble fiber in this traditional Latin American food slows the absorption of glucose from the intestines, says Dr. Welliver. Studies began on the anti-diabetes activity of prickly pear (also known as Nopal cactus) in the 1920s. Researchers now theorize that it may improve the effectiveness of available insulin in people with type 2 diabetes by stimulating glucose to move from the bloodstream into body cells. "You have to eat the real thing," says Dr. Welliver. "All the studies showed that using capsules had no effect."

Don't worry if you don't live in the desert, though. Canned cactus is available in health food stores and some grocery stores, and it's safe to enjoy on an ongoing basis.

Flaxseed

Eat 2 tablespoons daily. Ground flaxseed is one of nature's richest sources of soluble fiber. It improves your body's ability to metabolize blood sugar in type 1 or type 2 diabetes, explains Dr. Broadhurst. Stir it into a glass of water or sprinkle it on your cereal. Your daily allotment can also be added to blender drinks, oatmeal, or baked goods on a regular basis, she says.

Fast FACTS

Cause: Diabetes is a chronic disease in which the body does not produce or does not properly use insulin, the hormone that allows glucose to be turned into energy. The cause is still a mystery, but several risk factors have been identified.

With type 1 (insulin-dependent) diabetes, the body does not produce any insulin. People who have this less common form of diabetes—most often children—must take daily insulin injections.

Type 2 (non-insulin-dependent) diabetes is a metabolic disorder that results from the body's inability either to make enough insulin or to properly utilize it. It is associated with lifestyle factors.

Incidence: Of the 15.7 million Americans who have diabetes, nearly one-third are not aware of it. Each day, 2,200 people learn that they have the disease, often after developing one of its secondary complications, such as blindness, kidney disease, nerve damage, or heart disease. It is the sixth leading cause of death from disease.

Only about 5 to 10 percent of people with diabetes have type 1. Siblings and children of those with this type are at greatest risk for developing it. The risk of type 2 diabetes increases after age 40, especially for people who are overweight, do not exercise regularly, and have a family history of diabetes.

When to see the doctor: Contact your doctor if you have any symptoms of diabetes, including excessive thirst, frequent urination, unusual weight loss, and ravenous hunger. If you have already been diagnosed with diabetes, work closely with your doctor when making any changes in your diet, exercise regimen, or nutritional and herbal supplement regimen. Even small changes can profoundly affect your blood sugar levels.

Bilberry

Take 80 milligrams of extract twice a day to reduce the risk of retinopathy. French doctors have used bilberry since 1945 to prevent diabetic retinopathy. While the leaves of this European version of the blueberry lower blood sugar levels, the flavonoid-rich fruit provides potent antioxidant effects that improve the circulation of blood in the eyes for those with both types of diabetes, says Dr. Welliver.

Ginkgo

Take 80 milligrams in capsule form three times a day. Known for its ability to improve memory, ginkgo can also improve circulation and help reduce your risk of complications such as eye problems or ulcers on the hands and feet, says Dr. Welliver. Native to China, the ginkgo tree is thought to be the oldest tree on the planet, originating more than 190 million years ago.

DIARRHEA

*I*s there anything as humbling as an attack of diarrhea? Since early childhood, we've taught ourselves that when nature calls, we put that call on hold until we're ready to deal with it.

Not so with diarrhea. A bout of diarrhea will *not* be ignored, and nature reminds us abruptly and clearly that she's back in charge. Acute diarrhea usually lasts from a few hours to 2 to 3 days; in some cases, it can go on for as long as 3 weeks. It is marked by more than three trips daily to the bathroom to give vent to liquid or semi-liquid stool. Chronic diarrhea lasts longer than 3 weeks and may be a symptom of any of several disorders.

When diarrhea strikes, the first thing you'll want to do, advises Carolyn DeMarco, M.D., a physician in Winlaw, British Columbia, and a member of the advisory board of Dominion Herbal College in Burnaby, is to replace the fluids that you're rapidly

ADVENTURES IN HERBALISM

A CURE AT HER FEET

*W*hen you're miles from the nearest town, let alone the nearest bathroom, a bout of diarrhea can be inconvenient, to say the least. Cathryn Flanagan, N.D., knows that only too well.

The Connecticut-based naturopath used to work for the U.S. Forest Service in Colorado's Rocky Mountains, identifying plant species, signs of animal presence, and loss of timber due to insects and disease. One morning, Dr. Flanagan developed the telltale symptoms of a stomach in turmoil. Luckily, she has a good memory and sound training in plant identification.

"I remembered reading about cinquefoil, a readily available scrubby plant that's supposed to be good for treating diarrhea," she explains. Searching the ground, she spotted this hardy relative of the rose family and added it to the thermos of tea that she was carrying.

The addition improved the taste of her tea, and within minutes of sipping, her stomach rumblings subsided. "This experience really increased my enthusiasm for herbal medicine, which had been a hobby up until then," she says. "It was very satisfying to find a cure literally at my feet."

losing. She advises drinking things like vegetable or chicken broth and clear juices. Dehydration can be a potentially dangerous result of diarrhea.

Dr. DeMarco recommends steering clear of solid food, milk products, and foods that are greasy, high-fiber, or very sweet for the first 48 hours of a diarrhea attack to give your disturbed innards a rest. From there, you can try some of these herbal remedies.

Fast FACTS

Cause: There are many reasons that you could find yourself doubled over with a bout of diarrhea. If it's acute diarrhea (lasting up to 3 weeks), it's usually caused by an infection of some type. Or it could be that something you ate disagreed with you. If it's chronic (lasting more than 3 weeks), it could be a symptom of something like inflammatory bowel disease or an undiagnosed food allergy.

Incidence: Everyone has an occasional round of diarrhea. It's an inevitable part of having a digestive tract.

When to see the doctor: If your diarrhea doesn't go away within 3 days, you need to seek medical help. Remember, diarrhea is not a disease, it's a symptom. If it lingers, it indicates an underlying disorder that needs to be diagnosed. If you begin having signs of dehydration from diarrhea—thirst, dry skin, dry mouth, fatigue, and lightheadedness—see a doctor immediately.

Cinnamon

Drink one cup of tea as needed. Cinnamon tea will stop the flow pretty quickly, says Dr. DeMarco. This recipe comes from an herbalist she works with. Add 1 teaspoon of powdered cinnamon to 1 cup of boiling water and steep for 10 to 15 minutes. Pour the tea through a paper towel to strain out the cinnamon, then drink.

Green and Black Tea

Drink one to five cups daily. Both green and black teas are high in tannins, says Varro E. Tyler, Ph.D., Sc.D., distinguished professor emeritus of pharmacognosy at Purdue University in West Lafayette, Indiana, and co-author of *Tyler's Honest Herbal*.

That's important because tannins help your bowel form a protective film that prevents the absorption of the toxins that are causing your diarrhea. The only difference between black and green tea is the way the leaves are prepared. Green tea, because it is dried immediately after harvesting, retains a higher amount of tannins. Black teas, such as Earl Grey and Orange Pekoe, are produced by allowing the leaves to ferment slightly before drying.

Whichever type you choose, let the tea bag steep for 15 to 20 minutes, says Dr. Tyler, to release as much tannin as possible. Be prepared, though, for a more bitter taste than you may be used to because of the extra steeping time.

Slippery Elm

Take 30 to 40 drops of tincture every 2 hours, or take ¼ teaspoon of powder three or four times daily, until the diarrhea stops. One of the unfortunate side effects of diarrhea, says James S. Sensenig, N.D., distinguished visiting professor at the University of Bridgeport College of Naturopathic Medicine in Connecticut and founding president of the American Association of Naturopathic Physicians, can be very uncomfortable rumbling in your bowels.

Slippery elm tincture can help. Pick up a prepared tincture at a health food store and add the appropriate dose to a small glass of water or juice. "Slippery elm doesn't do much to get at the cause of the problem, but it's good for soothing the gut," says Dr. Sensenig.

Slippery elm powder may work even better. Add it to a small glass of juice or water.

Carrot

Eat ¼ to ½ cup of puree every hour. Carrots are rich in pectins, substances that can soothe your war-torn small intestine and slow down the passage of stool through your colon. To get these benefits, Dr. Sensenig recommends eating pureed carrots for as long as you have diarrhea. Prepare the puree by cooking some washed carrots until they are slightly soft, then put them in a blender with some water. Add small amounts of water as you blend until the mixture is the consistency of baby food. Dr. Sensenig adds that you can take the same amount of applesauce every hour until the diarrhea stops. It is also very soothing to the bowel.

DRY HAIR

*G*lossy, enchanted, flowing, silken . . . it seems that poets and writers never run short of romantic ways to describe our crowning glory. But one type of hair that you can bet you'll never hear mentioned in a sonnet or a love letter is dry hair.

The reason that some people's tresses are shiny and soft and others' are brittle and dull is often simply a matter of moisture. Harsh shampoos and styling products, too-frequent perms, drying climates, sun exposure, and blow-dryer heat all conspire to steal suppleness from hair. Once the moisture's gone, it has to be replenished, says Diana Bihova, M.D., a dermatologist in New York City.

To restore moisture to dry hair, you must deliver it from the outside in. One smart way is to use an instant conditioner regularly. When you do, be sure to apply it to the entire length of the hair shaft, especially to the ends, says Dr. Bihova. Rubbing conditioner only into your scalp won't deliver the overall hair-softening effect that you're hoping for. Then, once a week, try a more intensive method of mane management that incorporates natural moisturizing ingredients.

Jojoba or Sweet Almond

Once a week, treat your hair to a hot oil pack for 30 minutes to an hour. Dry hair is dry in part because it lacks oil. You can replace that oil with a spa-style hot-oil compress. "The oil will actually penetrate and soften the hair shaft, lubricating it while it seals in moisture," says Dr. Bihova.

Generally, any kind of oil will do for restoring luster to crispy tresses, but Dr. Bihova recommends sweet almond or jojoba, both of which have excellent emollient properties. Used by Native Americans as a hair restorer, jojoba oil is extracted from the seeds of a desert shrub, but it is readily available in health food stores.

Depending on the length of your hair, pour $\frac{1}{2}$ to 1 cup of the oil

Cause: Dry hair is usually a result of harsh treatment with styling tools such as brushes, blow dryers, and curling irons and overuse of styling products like hair sprays, gels, and mousses. Exposure to arid weather, sun, and chlorinated swimming pool water can also contribute to the problem.

Incidence: Dry hair is probably more prevalent among people who rely on hair dryers and those who rarely condition their tresses.

When to see the doctor: In almost every case, dry hair is nothing more than a cosmetic concern. If your scalp or other areas of skin also feel excessively dry, itchy, and scaly, however, consult a doctor or dermatologist.

of your choice into a bowl. Dampen your hair, then use your fingers to gently part it into sections and massage the oil in from the roots to the ends.

Heat an old or dark-colored towel (it may become oil-stained) in the dryer for a few minutes, then use it to wrap your hair turban-style. Leave it in place for at least 30 minutes, says Dr. Bihova. If you have the time and the inclination, you can extend the oil treatment for up to 2 hours. When the time's up, shampoo once or twice with a mild shampoo to remove all traces of oil.

Lavender, Rosemary, or Sandalwood

Add up to 10 drops of the essential oil of your choice to your hot-oil treatment. Aromatherapy can add a sensual side to your dry hair remedy, says Connie Catellani, M.D., medical director of the Miro Center for Integrative Medicine in Evanston, Illinois.

Choose one of three commonly available essential oils that are associated with healthy hair: lavender, rosemary, or sandalwood. Since different essential oil aromas have different effects on the body and mind, selection is highly personal. "You should add an oil that is appropriate for you systemically," says Dr. Catellani. Lavender is calming, for example, while rosemary is invigorating, and sandalwood's woody-sweet scent is considered soothing.

Dry Skin

Children learn about bravery and perseverance from the tale of the little Dutch boy who discovers a small leak in the wall of the dike that keeps the icy waters of the North Sea from flooding his town. Knowing that even a small leak means danger, the boy plugs the hole with his finger until help arrives.

There's a lesson in that fairy tale for older folks, too. With age, the cellular structure of the skin develops microscopic leaks similar to those in the crumbling walls of the fictional dike. The top layer of skin becomes thinner, less compact, and less able to hold in moisture, explains Marcey Shapiro, M.D., a family doctor in Albany, California, who combines natural healing with conventional medicine. With less moisture stored, your skin becomes dry and flaky.

To save your skin, start on the inside. Sure, skin is the outside layer of your body, but as with the water behind the dike, most of the moisture in skin comes from "behind" it—from your bloodstream, not from showers or baths. You need lots of water in your system to keep skin healthy and moist. Thus, the first step in alleviating dry skin is to drink eight 8-ounce glasses of water each day, says Dr. Shapiro. In addition, lotions, creams, and ointments can work on the surface and help to plug the leaks by sealing in moisture. Use these products on still-wet skin right after bathing.

Using products with alpha hydroxy acids is one of the most effective ways to get rid of dry, flaky skin. "They're my first, second, and third choices for moisturizers," says Dr. Shapiro. "They remove the loose, dead skin layer and make the remaining layer more compact. Instead of loosely adhering layers of dry skin, you have a better barrier that is naturally able to hold onto moisture more effectively."

Dr. Shapiro recommends trying a product that contains at least 8 percent fruit acids. Before using it on your face, try a patch test by applying a little on your inner arm for a couple of days to be sure that it doesn't irritate your skin.

Here are some other remedies offered by experts.

Flaxseed

Start with 1 tablespoon of oil every day. Certain kinds of oil, like flaxseed, that are rich in omega-3 essential fatty acids have been shown to help many skin conditions, including dryness, says Alan M. Dattner, M.D., a holistic dermatologist in New Rochelle, New York.

Your skin is a reflection of your diet. To keep it healthy, you need to eat the proper balance of essential fatty acids—fats that your body needs but cannot make. The typical American diet is often lacking in these crucial fats.

Buy fresh, cold-pressed, refrigerated flaxseed oil packaged in an opaque dark bottle. The oil spoils quickly when exposed to light or heat, so keep it in the refrigerator. Good flaxseed oil has a pleasant, nutty flavor. Stir it into a glass of juice in the morning or drizzle it on salad or vegetables. This remedy is especially good to use during the cold months of winter. You should see results within a couple of months.

Rose

To hydrate and soften, massage a glycerin-and-rosewater lotion into your skin twice a day. An old-time remedy, glycerin and rosewater is the perfect moisturizer, particularly for people with dry skin, says Dr. Shapiro.

Happy Hands Oil

This recipe to soothe and nourish dry, sore, irritated hands was developed by Dina Falconi, founder of Falcon Formulations, a line of herbal skin- and hair-care products in New York state, and is described in her book Earthly Bodies and Heavenly Hair. *Massage it into slightly moist hands.*

- 1 ounce almond oil
- 2 ounces peanut oil
- 1½ tablespoons avocado oil
- 1 teaspoon wheat germ oil
- 20 drops birch essential oil
- 20 drops lavender essential oil
- 7 drops chamomile essential oil

Pour the almond, peanut, avocado, and wheat germ oils into a 4-ounce, small-mouth blue or amber glass jar. Add the birch, lavender, and chamomile oils drop by drop. Cap the jar and shake well.

"It's probably the most elegant light moisturizer that you'll ever find," she says. Glycerin is softening because it is soluble in water, while the fragrant volatile oils in rosewater are soothing. Apply it with your fingers to clean, wet skin.

Calendula

Use an oil, lotion, or salve twice a day. Also known as pot marigold, calendula is above all a remedy for the skin. Its mild antiseptic action soothes red, inflamed skin and speeds healing, says Dr. Dattner. He often gives patients with dry skin a calendula ointment formulated by an herbalist he works with. "By using an ointment, you avoid all the chemicals that are in creams," he says.

Fast Facts

Cause: As you age, glands under your skin produce less of the protective oils that help it stay moist. At the same time, the skin becomes thinner. With less fat and collagen holding skin together, the loosely adhering cells become less able to hold moisture. The result? An accumulation of dry, flaky skin.

Incidence: Everyone is prone to drier skin as they move through middle age and beyond.

When to see the doctor: If regular moisturizers don't provide relief, see your doctor. You may need a stronger prescription cream. If your dry skin is so severe that you're constantly scratching, or if it actually cracks and bleeds from ordinary activity, you may have a skin problem such as eczema or contact dermatitis that requires a doctor's care.

It's easy to make your own. Place $\frac{1}{2}$ cup of dried calendula blossoms (available in health food stores and herb shops) in a blender with 8 ounces of olive oil or almond oil. Blend for 1 minute, then pour the mixture into a jar with a tight lid. Let it stand for 2 weeks, until the oil becomes a dark yellow color. Then, over a large bowl, squeeze the oil from the plant pulp. Pour the oil back into the jar, close tightly, and store it away from heat and sunlight.

You'll see results within a few days. You can use the ointment for a few weeks at a time as needed.

Olive Oil

Seal in moisture with a protective layer of oil right after you bathe. No, you don't need expensive moisturizers from the cosmetics counter to keep your skin soft and supple, says Dr. Dattner. Look in your kitchen cupboard. Externally, olive oil is a good, basic moisturizer when your oil glands start to slow down. Use it as needed, and you'll see results in a couple of days.

Dry skin tends to become irritated easily, so Dr. Dattner prefers single-ingredient, simple remedies. That way, if itching or redness occurs, you know the cause. If you want to be sure that the olive oil you buy is totally pure, buy kosher oil, he says.

Chamomile, Peppermint, or Lemon Balm

Spritz away dryness when you travel with any of these herbal teas. The relative humidity can be less than 10 percent inside an airplane cabin—or even in your own house in the dead of winter. Like a dry sponge, the air soaks moisture and oils right out of your skin, says Dr. Dattner. To replace them, use a small spray bottle filled with your favorite herbal tea—such as lemon balm, peppermint, or chamomile—to hydrate and soothe. The volatile oils in the tea also have an anti-inflammatory effect. Remember to keep your eyes closed when you spray, and steer clear of teas such as raspberry, which can stain clothing.

Eczema
and Dermatitis

*T*he lexicon of skin disease can get pretty confusing, especially since some terms, such as eczema and dermatitis, tend to be used interchangeably. Dermatitis is actually just an umbrella term—it simply means "inflamed skin"—that covers a slew of skin ailments. Dandruff and diaper rash are both types of dermatitis. So is poison ivy rash.

Two common and irksome varieties of dermatitis are atopic dermatitis (often called eczema), a skin condition that's usually inherited, and contact dermatitis, which happens when your skin rubs up against something that it finds irritating. Both conditions can make your skin red, scaly, and itchy enough to make you want to jump out of it. Contact dermatitis usually clears up soon after the source of irritation is identified and taken out of the picture.

Eczema, which usually develops during infancy or childhood, can stay with you for life, flaring up sporadically after exposure to irritants, allergens, stress, or heat. "It belongs in the same spectrum of allergic diseases as asthma and hay fever," says dermatologist Nia Terezakis, M.D., clinical professor of dermatology at Tulane University School of Medicine and Louisiana State University School of Medicine, both in New Orleans.

The single most important thing you can do for yourself if you have eczema is to use a bland moisturizing lotion at least twice a day, Dr. Terezakis adds. This accomplishes two things: It prevents dry skin from cracking and letting in irritants, and it soothes the itch.

Herbally, remedies for contact dermatitis focus on calming and softening the skin topically. For eczema, there are also some remedies that aim to heal from the inside out. Try them and see which approach works for you.

Chamomile

Smooth a cream on irritated skin twice a day, or take an herbal bath. Looking to Europe, where chamomile is widely used for skin irritations, Marcey Shapiro, M.D., a family doctor in Albany, California, who combines natural healing with conventional medicine, recommends chamomile cream as a simple remedy that will help soothe inflammation.

Dr. Shapiro also advises her patients to soak in a calming chamomile bath. Put 2 tablespoons of dried chamomile flowers in a bowl. Add 1 cup of boiling water and let stand until cool. Strain out the plant material and pour the liquid into a warm bath. Try this remedy until the itchiness of the eczema or dermatitis goes away.

Chickweed

Smooth this cream onto the affected area twice a day. Chickweed is excellent for getting rid of the itchies, says Christopher Robbins, a member of Britain's National Institute of Medical Herbalists who practices herbal medicine in Ross-on-Wye, Herefordshire, England, and has written several books, including *The Natural Pharmacy*.

You can find chickweed cream at health food stores. Use it whenever you need to ease itching, following the instructions on the label. You can continue using it until the itchiness of the eczema or dermatitis is relieved.

Oats

Soak in an oatmeal bath to soothe the itch. Most forms of dermatitis seem to be more itchy at night, says Scott Norton, M.D., chief of dermatology at the R. W. Bliss Army Health Center in Fort Huachuca, Arizona, and assistant professor of medicine at the University of Hawaii in Honolulu. "When you're busy during the day, working, playing with your kids, cooking dinner, you're distracted. When you lie down in bed, the itch tends to be magnified."

To make an oatmeal bath, simply take 1 cup of edible oats and put them in a handkerchief. Tie it over the faucet and let the water run through it. At night before you go to bed, soak in the tub for 20 to 30 minutes.

When you soak in an oatmeal bath, two things happen, says Dr. Norton. First, the intrinsic soothing properties of the oats calm the itch. Second, the oats modify the skin somewhat to improve roughness and irritation, and a natural oil in the oats softens the skin and serves as a protective barrier. Applying a moisturizer to your damp skin after leaving the tub will also help soothe the eczema.

Be warned, though, that oatmeal makes your skin very slippery. "I always tell my patients to be careful when they step out of the tub," says Dr. Norton. Use this remedy until the itchiness of your eczema or dermatitis abates.

Calendula and Lavender

Add essential oil of lavender to calendula cream and smooth onto irritated patches twice a day. Lavender oil helps soothe the skin because of its calming effect on the nervous system, says Robbins. Calendula is an anti-inflammatory and antifungal herb that has been used for centuries in Indian, Arab, and Greek medicine. So much is grown in Russia for medicinal use that it's known as Russian penicillin.

Calendula cream is readily available in health food stores. Add five drops of lavender essential oil to 3½ tablespoons of the cream and smooth it on affected areas twice a day until the irritation diminishes.

Evening Primrose

For eczema, take 4,000 to 6,000 milligrams of oil daily in divided doses with meals. The yellow flowers of the evening primrose supposedly open only after 6 o'clock in the evening and bloom just once. What has herbalists excited, though, is the fatty acid obtained from the small, reddish-brown seeds, says Dr. Shapiro.

One of the most widely prescribed plant medicines in the world, evening primrose oil contains a highly absorbable form of gamma-linolenic acid, a substance that tends to decrease inflammation. Governments of countries around the world, including Great Britain, Germany, Denmark, and Greece, recognize it as an eczema treatment. Use it until your dermatitis or eczema flare-up subsides.

Gentian

For eczema, take 10 drops of tincture three times a day before meals. Herbalists tend to see eczema as an external sign of an internal

Fast FACTS

Cause: Some types of dermatitis remain a mystery to doctors. Others, such as atopic eczema, are thought to be hereditary and involve allergies to things such as pollen, animal dander, and certain foods or medications. Contact dermatitis is a temporary reaction caused by physical contact with irritating substances such as nickel, cleaning agents, detergents, fragrances, rubber, or latex.

Incidence: Atopic eczema usually appears first in childhood. It is very common in all parts of the world and is thought to affect 1 in 10 people at some time in their lives. Men and women of all races are affected equally. The incidence of this type of eczema has risen steadily over the past 30 years.

When to see the doctor: If your eczema does not respond to self-treatment or if it becomes widespread or recurs, seek the help of a doctor.

problem, so they often treat eczema internally as well as with external creams, says Robbins. They believe that stimulating the circulation and the liver helps clean the blood and remove waste materials that can aggravate the skin.

Bitter herbs like gentian help the liver and stimulate digestion. The French eat bitter green salads of radicchio or endive at the beginning of a meal, Robbins points out, to stimulate the liver and digestive system. Gentian extract will have much the same effect, revving up sluggish digestion and helping the body to rid itself of toxins, including skin irritants. You can continue to take this until the irritation goes away.

Oregon Grape and Chamomile

For eczema, brew a tea and drink it in the morning. You may have to take it for a year or more before your condition clears, says Douglas Schar, a medical herbalist in London, editor of the *British Journal of Phytotherapy*, and author of *Backyard Medicine Chest*, but Oregon grape root can really help improve eczema.

Two of its active components—berbamine and berberine—have antihistaminic and anti-inflammatory properties and may stimulate the immune system and liver function. Add 1 tablespoon of dried root to 1 cup of boiling water. Boil for 10 minutes and strain before drinking. To improve the flavor, add a handful of dried chamomile flowers.

ERECTION PROBLEMS

*H*aving erections on demand is something that every guy takes for granted—until his first bout with impotence, that is. And the likelihood of erection problems only increases with age. According to a study on sexual dysfunction in the United States, men ages 50 to 59 experience difficulty with erections more than three times as often as men ages 18 to 29.

"Problems with potency can be traced to emotional factors, physical factors, any number of things," says Steven Rissman, N.D., a naturopathic physician at American WholeHealth in Littleton, Colorado. "It's always a good idea to check with your doctor to pinpoint exactly what's going on."

Here's the inside story: The penis is a finely tuned device, designed to expand and hold blood when it rushes in. If the arteries leading to the penis are clogged, the valves that hold the blood in are leaky, or the tissue and muscles that usually expand are creaky from disuse, erectile capability will be diminished. Fatigue or depression can also contribute to the condition.

Exercise, regular erections, and a healthy diet are important parts of a pro-erection lifestyle. If the cause appears to be psychological, talking with a licensed therapist can help as well. But for mild to moderate cases, herbs may be just the ticket for getting over the, ahem, hump. Here's what experts suggest.

Ginkgo

Take an 80-milligram capsule twice a day. Ginkgo is widely used in Europe for all sorts of circulatory problems. It increases blood and oxygen flow to the extremities and penis, exactly what is needed for a powerful erection, says Steven Margolis, M.D., an alternative family physician in Sterling Heights, Michigan. In one study, 60 men with erectile dysfunction who didn't respond to injection treatments with a prescription medication were given 60 milligrams of ginkgo daily for 12 to 18 months. After 6 months, 50 percent of the men who took the ginkgo reported that they had regained potency. Dr. Margolis advises taking ginkgo phytosome, which is absorbed well.

Asian Ginseng

Take capsules providing 15 percent ginsenosides daily. Asian ginseng (also called panax, Korean, or Chinese ginseng) is a traditional Chinese virility tonic that has been shown in several studies to boost sexual activity. The effect builds over time, which means that you'll have to take it for a few months before seeing the benefits.

"Check the label to make sure you know how many ginsenosides you get in each capsule," says Dr. Rissman. "If it's a 100-milligram capsule but contains only 5 percent ginsenosides, you'll know you have to take three capsules a day."

Muira Puama

Take capsules containing 300 milligrams once a day. Also known as potency wood, this herb derived from a Brazilian shrub has a long history as an herbal treatment for impotence.

"In my experience, this ingredient is particularly effective, with no notable side effects," says Dr. Margolis. A landmark study at the Institute of Sexology in Paris found that 51 percent of men who had

Fast FACTS

Cause: Any disorder that impairs penile blood flow can lead to erection difficulties. The reasons can include physical factors such as injury, disease, or side effects from medication as well as psychological factors such as depression, stress, or low self-esteem.

Incidence: Researchers speculate that as many as 15 million American men experience impotence. The likelihood of erection problems increases with age, from 5 percent at age 40 to 25 percent by age 65.

When to see the doctor: All men have occasional erection problems. If you have difficulty over a period of months, however, have it checked out. It could be a sign of a serious health condition such as diabetes or high blood pressure.

difficulty attaining or maintaining erections claimed some improvement after receiving a daily dose of muira puama for 2 weeks.

Damiana

Take a tincture dose of 2 to 4 milliliters, or drink one cup of tea daily. Used in the United States since the late nineteenth century as a sexual aid, damiana leaves are thought to work by causing slight inflammation of the urethra, thereby increasing penile sensitivity. It may also work as a mild antidepressant, which can be helpful if the erection problems are linked in any way to emotional difficulties, says Dr. Rissman.

Saw Palmetto

Take two 160-milligram capsules daily. Saw palmetto is best-known as a treatment for prostate troubles, but that can also have a positive impact on erections. The reason? An enlarged prostate can impair blood flow, thus interfering with sexual performance. In addition, having an enlarged prostate can necessitate getting up several times throughout the night to urinate, and fatigue can play a role in impotence. By returning the prostate to its normal size, saw palmetto may eliminate these erection obstacles.

"Research shows that saw palmetto has revitalizing effects for the prostate and possibly throughout the entire urinary system," says Dr. Rissman.

EYESTRAIN

When you think about all the work your eyes do almost every day, from the moment you open them in the morning till the moment you go to sleep at night, it's no wonder that they get tired on occasion. Watching TV, driving, reading, even the imperceptible flickering of fluorescent lights can all result in vision fatigue. In the computer age especially, eyestrain is reaching epidemic proportions.

Symptoms of eyestrain include red, watery, or dry eyes, fatigue, an aching heaviness in the eyelids, and difficulty focusing. There's no evidence that staring at a computer monitor, a television screen, a book, or a highway will actually damage your eyes, but you don't have to put up with the irritation, either.

Remembering to blink frequently and taking regular breaks can help, says Jay Cohen, O.D., professor of optometry at the State University of New York College of Optometry in New York City. Computer monitors can be adjusted to reduce glare.

In addition, going back to Mother Nature can help you cope with this common side effect of high-tech life.

Fast FACTS

Cause: Overuse of the eyes in a wide variety of ways, including staring at computer screens, TV screens, printed matter, or the highway at night, can lead to eyestrain.

Incidence: Almost everyone experiences eyestrain at one time or another.

When to see the doctor: Eyestrain that lasts a week or more should be checked by an optometrist or ophthalmologist.

Bilberry

Take one 80- to 100-milligram capsule three times a day. Bilberry is a fruit-bearing shrub that grows throughout Europe. The fruit is similar to the blueberries grown in the United States, but bilberry has more pigments that may be beneficial to the eyes, says Andrew Weil, M.D., director of the program in integrative medicine at the University of Arizona College of Medicine in Tucson and author of *8 Weeks to Optimum Health.*

During World War II, it was discovered that pilots who ate bilberry jam could see better than those who didn't. It turns out that bilberries are rich in anthocyanosides, nutrients that help your eyes adapt to the dark and fight fatigue, according to Dr. Weil.

It's best to look for capsules of standardized bilberry extract that contain 25 milligrams of anthocyanosides, says Janet Zand, N.D., O.M.D., a naturopathic doctor and doctor of oriental medicine who practices in Los Angeles and in Austin, Texas. If you know that you're prone to eyestrain and want to avoid it, take one capsule a day as a preventive measure, Dr. Zand says.

Grape Seed

Take 50 milligrams of extract twice a day. Grape seed extract helps improve circulation to the eyes. It's also high in nourishing vitamins and has anti-inflammatory properties. In sum, it's a great natural restorative for the eye, says Dr. Zand. She suggests that you look for an extract that is standardized to 95 percent proanthocyanosides. For severe cases, she suggests increasing the dosage to 200 milligrams a day. For ongoing preventive use, try 25 milligrams a day.

Eyebright

Bathe your eyes twice a day. As its name implies, this herb can be very soothing to eyes dimmed by overuse. To make the wash, first brew some eyebright tea, Dr. Zand says. Bring 4 ounces of distilled water to a boil, then remove from the heat and add 1 tablespoon of dried eyebright. Steep for 5 to 10 minutes, then strain. Once the tea cools to room temperature, pour a little into an eye cup (you can get one at a drugstore). Place the cup over one eye and tilt your head back, then repeat with the other eye. Keep your eyes open so the solution can bathe them.

FATIGUE

*E*very person on the planet experiences fatigue at one time or another. But when fatigue refuses to disappear no matter how restful your life has been, it can begin to overshadow practically everything else.

"I see patients who suffer from fatigue every day," says Stephen Sinatra, M.D., a cardiologist in Manchester, Connecticut, who has done research on botanicals and dietary supplements and is author of *Optimum Health*. It can result from any number of factors, from the widely reported chronic fatigue syndrome (a constant sense of overwhelming fatigue, possibly related to a virus, a defect in the immune system, or toxins in the environment) to lousy eating habits, high stress, insomnia, and anything in between.

Fatigue can also be an early warning sign of serious health problems such as heart disease, depression, diabetes, or a thyroid problem, so your first step should be to see a doctor if you are fatigued most of the time, have difficulty concentrating, or find that formerly simple activities have become difficult.

There are a number of lifestyle choices that you can make to beat fatigue. Primary among them is simply to get more sleep. Exercise also helps by increasing your endurance and pumping a bit more oxygen-rich blood to your brain. Even short bouts of stretching or walking can help.

It's also a good idea to look at the fuel you're putting into your body. High sugar intake can cause what Dr. Sinatra calls a blood sugar spike. Here's how it works: After having a doughnut and a soft drink for breakfast, you have a temporary energy boost as the sugar courses through your system. Soon, however, your body adjusts to the increased sugar level by cutting back on blood sugar. After 30 minutes, your blood sugar levels are lower than they were in the first place, and your energy level has nose-dived. Instead of repeating the cycle over and over, eat a diet that includes healthy fats (omega-3's from fish or a monounsaturated fat such as olive oil) and is low in carbohydrates (preferably high-fiber, low-glycemic carbohydrates like legumes, yams, and broccoli) to ensure a steady stream of energy, says Dr. Sinatra.

Herbs can also be helpful tools in overcoming fatigue. Here are the top suggestions from the experts.

Gotu Kola

Take 60 to 100 milligrams in capsule form each day. This Indian herb contains no caffeine but has other stimulant properties that make it an effective treatment for fatigue, says Dr. Sinatra. In addition to simply providing an energy boost, gotu kola may help lift your spirits, since fatigue can lead to depression.

Licorice

Take 150 to 200 milligrams a day in capsule form. Many people with fatigue don't produce enough adrenal hormone, and licorice

Fast FACTS

Cause: Fatigue can be caused by a huge number of factors, such as an underactive thyroid, side effects of medication, poor nutrition, insomnia, overwork, depression, stress, heart disease, or diabetes. Another cause could be chronic fatigue syndrome (CFS), which doctors speculate may be related to a virus, a defect in the immune system, or environmental toxins.

Incidence: Everyone experiences fatigue at one time or another. CFS is much more rare, however, affecting an estimated 200,000 to 500,000 adults in the United States.

When to see the doctor: It's important to see an expert if you're fatigued more often than not. If fatigue habitually turns simple tasks into chores or makes it difficult to concentrate in important situations, you should visit your physician.

---

root is the closest herbal equivalent to that hormone that you can get, says Steven Margolis, M.D., an alternative family physician in Sterling Heights, Michigan. Look for a product that is standardized to contain 12 percent licorice root to ensure that you're taking a safe dose. Licorice root can raise blood pressure, which is why you shouldn't take it in large doses. That said, though, a slight boost in blood pressure might be just what you need if you're fatigued.

Ginger

Drink a cup or two of tea a day. Ginger effectively increases energy, perhaps by stimulating the immune system. "Most herbs that rev up the immune system seem to have a positive effect on energy," says Dr. Sinatra. It may be that if your immune system is functioning at full efficiency, your body doesn't have to siphon off as much energy to constantly battle illness.

To make ginger tea, grate 1 teaspoon of fresh root, pour 1 cup of boiling water over it, and steep for 5 minutes. Strain the tea and drink it when it's comfortably warm.

American, Asian, and Siberian Ginseng

Take 400 milligrams of this blend daily. "Ginseng has helped quite a few of my older patients with fatigue," says Dr. Sinatra.

According to Dr. Margolis, these different types of ginseng attack stress fatigue at different levels while also providing a nice circulatory boost, so the sum is greater than the individual parts. This blend is available at health food stores.

Don't take ginseng with caffeine, however, says Dr. Sinatra. Doing so may give you too much of an energy boost and cause the jitters.

Blue-Green Algae and Wheat Grass

Take in capsule form according to package directions. Both algae and wheat grass are naturally high in magnesium, says Dr. Margolis, which can help to correct a deficiency of the mineral that's often linked to fatigue.

FIBROCYSTIC BREASTS

*F*inding a lump—or lumps—in a breast is an experience that most women have at some time in their lives, but only about one-fifth of breast abnormalities turn out to be cancer. The rest are most likely fibrocystic lumps, which are harmless, fluid-filled cysts that can cause a lot of discomfort but not much else. In some women, they are as small as peas, while in others they grow to the size of grapes or even golf balls. Normally, lumps found in fibrocystic breasts are harmless, and they don't appear to raise a woman's risk for breast cancer.

Nevertheless, any and all lumps should be examined by your gynecologist, advises Larry Kincheloe, M.D., chairman of the department of obstetrics and gynecology at the Central Oklahoma Medical Group in Oklahoma City. And monthly breast self-exams are a must. Learning to tell what's normal and what's not is extremely important for preventive breast health—and that's even more true for a woman with lumpy breasts.

If you have fibrocystic breasts, you know that they can be painful. For premenopausal women, the 2 weeks before each period can be especially sore times. But there are some simple things you can do to make a difference, says Dr. Kincheloe.

Avoiding caffeine is the number one, most effective "treatment" for fibrocystic breast soreness, says Dr. Kincheloe. "Caffeine is one of those really interesting things," he says. "I can show you scientific data suggesting that caffeine is not related to fibrocystic breast disease, but in my practice, avoiding caffeine cures more fibrocystic breasts than anything else." To see if this works for you, Dr. Kincheloe recommends eliminating all sources of caffeine—including chocolate—from your diet for at least three full menstrual cycles.

Another expert-recommended home remedy for breast soreness is plain old vitamin E, which seems to be able to reduce the size and actual number of breast lumps. Dr. Kincheloe suggests taking 600 to 800 international units (IU) daily for 3 months to see if it helps. (You need to consult your doctor before taking more than 400 IU a day, though, since low-dose supplementation may increase risk of hemorrhagic stroke.)

There are also do-it-yourself herbal approaches to easing fibrocystic soreness. Dr. Kincheloe recommends the following herbs for their ability to balance out hormone fluctuations, thus making benign cysts feel better.

Chasteberry

Take one 175-milligram capsule of standardized extract once a day for 2 weeks before your period. The berries of the chaste tree have a natural hormone-balancing effect in the body. "The herb shifts the body from estrogen to progesterone production," says Dr. Kinch-

Fast Facts

Cause: Most breast lumps found in premenopausal women turn out to be cysts—fluid-filled sacs that feel soft and movable under the skin. It's thought that they are caused by changing levels of female hormones. Other types of benign lumps can develop from connective tissue or scar tissue, from abscesses caused by an infection in the breast, or from fat necrosis, which happens when a clump of fat cells dies due to surgery or injury.

Incidence: Harmless breast lumps occur in up to 90 percent of women at one time or another. Fibrocystic changes, in which there are multiple cysts, happen to at least half of all women at some point in their lives but are most common in women of childbearing age.

When to see the doctor: Your gynecologist should perform a breast exam during your yearly visit. If she says that you have fibrocystic or "lumpy" breasts, it means your breasts are naturally lumpy. Keep track of their normal state by doing a breast self-exam each month. If you notice anything unusual for you—a new lump or an old lump that has gotten bigger—call your doctor for an appointment to have it looked at, but don't panic. The vast majority of lumps turn out to be nonmalignant (not cancerous).

eloe. Tipping the balance in favor of progesterone helps because a relative overabundance of estrogen is what stimulates the monthly swelling of fibrocystic lumps.

If you prefer to take a liquid extract, follow the dosage recommendations on the label. It will probably take three to six menstrual cycles to see an improvement with chasteberry, but this isn't a problem, since it's considered a very safe herb.

Dandelion, Corn Silk, or Uva-Ursi

Take two 400- to 600-milligram capsules of dandelion or corn silk or two 250- to 500-milligram capsules of uva-ursi three times a day after meals. Premenstrual breast tenderness is often due to fluid being retained throughout the body—otherwise known as bloating.

"That's what makes women's rings feel tight, their ankles look swollen, and their bellies pooch out a little bit," says Dr. Kincheloe. It can also put pressure on your breasts, making them feel inflated and sore to the touch. If you have fibrocystic breasts, premenstrual water retention can make them even more painful.

Prescription medicines that help the body shed excess water are known as diuretics—but herbs can be diuretics, too. Dr. Kincheloe recommends dandelion, corn silk, or uva-ursi as good candidates for relieving water retention. Try them one at a time, if you like, or go for a combination approach. "All of these herbs do the same thing, so taking them together can be quite synergistic," says Dr. Kincheloe.

Try taking the herbs daily for the 2 weeks before your period. If you want to take all three, alternate them for the three daily doses—for example, take dandelion after breakfast, corn silk after lunch, and uva-ursi after dinner. Once your period begins, stop taking the herbs until you need them again.

FIBROIDS

*F*ibroids (also known as leiomyomas) are noncancerous tumors that grow on the outside, the inside, or within the walls of the uterus. While that may sound deadly serious, fibroids are actually very common and are usually symptomless. For every woman who has trouble due to fibroids, there are many others whose fibroids never make themselves known and never cause problems. Science can't yet explain what causes them, but it is known that once they occur, the female hormone estrogen can stimulate their growth.

When fibroid symptoms flare, take note. If fibroids are causing you severe pain, heavy bleeding, or bladder problems, or if you're planning a pregnancy, it's important to see your doctor. There are medications and surgical steps that are known to help.

Some fibroids cause only mild symptoms such as heavy periods or stronger-than-normal cramps. For women whose doctors have told them that they have that type of fibroids, taking an herbal approach like the ones outlined below can help.

Burdock, Dandelion, Yellow Dock, Red Clover, Cleavers, Nettle, Milk Thistle, and Vervain

Drink two cups of tea made from these liver-strengthening herbs every day. You can get fibroid growth under control by reining in the excess estrogen that may be stimulating them, says Aviva Jill Romm, a professional member of the American Herbalists Guild, certified professional midwife in Bloomfield Hills, Michigan, and author of *The Natural Pregnancy Book*. Since your liver is one of the primary organs of hormone regulation, Romm says, strengthening this part of your body with herbs can mean that hormones are processed and moved out of the body more quickly.

"We know that reducing estrogen levels will definitely shrink fibroids," says Larry Kincheloe, M.D., chairman of the department of obstetrics and gynecology at the Central Oklahoma Medical Group in Oklahoma City. That's the mechanism behind fibroid-shrinking prescription drugs like leuprolide acetate (Lupron) or nafarelin acetate (Synarel). While it's possible that herbs may be able to help reduce estrogen levels, however, Dr. Kincheloe notes that there are currently no medical studies proving that they can actually eliminate fibroids.

To ease mild symptoms or to keep small fibroids from growing bigger, making a tea with the dried leaves of burdock, dandelion, yellow dock, red clover, cleavers, nettle, milk thistle, and vervain is worth a try, says Romm. Their liver-friendly effects bump up hormone processing in that organ.

Put equal parts of all of the herbs in a large bowl and mix them well with your hands. Put 1 ounce (by weight) of the mixture (approximately an eighth of the total) in a large teapot or saucepan.

Fast FACTS

Cause: Fibroid growth can be stimulated by the female hormone estrogen, but what causes them to occur in the first place is unknown.

Incidence: Fibroids are very common. Up to a one-quarter of women over age 35 have them, with or without having symptoms. African-American women have a higher risk of developing fibroids than Caucasian women.

When to see the doctor: If your periods are suddenly heavier and more painful than normal, or if you begin experiencing pelvic pain or a frequent need to urinate, ask your doctor to check you for fibroids. If you have already been diagnosed with fibroids, and you develop symptoms of anemia from heavy menstrual bleeding or experience pain, see your doctor for treatment options.

Cover the herbs with 1 quart of boiling water and steep for 2 hours, then strain. You can refrigerate the extra tea for up to 2 days and re-heat it before drinking if you like.

Take this remedy for 4 weeks, then take a 1-week break. After three of these cycles, have yourself re-evaluated by a midwife or physician, says Romm.

Castor Oil

Make a soothing castor oil pack and drape it over your abdomen for up to 1 hour. Fibroids tend to cause an increase in abdominal cramps, especially around the time of menstruation. To help ease the pain, try an old-fashioned castor oil pack.

"This trick was one of my herb teacher's favorites," says Mercedes Cameron, M.D., medical director at The Woman's Place at St. Mary's Hospital in Grand Junction, Colorado. "The heat will certainly help the pain, while the castor oil may have an effect on shrinking small fibroids."

Fold a clean cotton diaper or a piece of cotton flannel so that the fabric forms a square or rectangle at least 2 to 4 inches thick. Pour 4 to 6 ounces of castor oil (which you can find at any drugstore or health food store) into the cloth and fold it over once or twice. Place the pack directly on the skin of your abdomen and cover it with plastic wrap and a thin towel. Use a heating pad set on low or a hot-water bottle to keep the pack warm as you lie back and relax. If this feels good to you, Dr. Cameron says, you can leave the pack in place for 20 minutes to an hour.

FLATULENCE

We're not going to spend a lot of time covering the symptoms of flatulence here. You know what they are. And so do your neighbors.

Herbal medicine is ideally suited to treat this most ancient of problems, says Yvonne Tyson, M.D., a physician in Long Beach, California, and a member of the American Holistic Health Association. Gas complaints have been with humanity for a long time, and many herbs have been plucked from the wilds to help banish the bugling. Here are some of them.

Peppermint

Drink tea as needed. Peppermint is one of the oldest known remedies for gas, says James S. Sensenig, N.D., distinguished visiting professor at the University of Bridgeport College of Naturopathic Medicine in Connecticut and founding president of the American Association of Naturopathic Physicians. So are other members of the mint family, such as spearmint and catnip.

Five-Herb
Gas-Blasting Tea

Perhaps you drink coffee or tea on a regular basis already. Since you're used to having hot beverages over the course of the day, why not drink something that can relieve excessive flatulence? This tea is packed with powerful carminatives, compounds that can blast that extra gas.

This particular mixture comes from the German Prescription Formula Index, *courtesy of Varro E. Tyler, Ph.D., Sc.D., distinguished professor emeritus of pharmacognosy at Purdue University in West Lafayette, Indiana, and co-author of* Tyler's Honest Herbal. *Drink it warm after every meal.*

- **I part dried chamomile**
- **I part dried peppermint**
- **I part dried valerian root**
- **I part caraway seeds**
- **I part aniseed**

Combine the chamomile, peppermint, valerian, caraway, and anise in whatever amounts you choose. To make a cup of tea, place 1 to 2 teaspoons of the mixture in a cup and add about 1 cup of boiling water. Steep for 10 minutes, then strain out the herbs.

Pick up some real peppermint tea at a health food store or grocery store. Just check the label to be sure it's not regular tea with peppermint flavoring.

If you have a bunch of fresh peppermint, that will work very nicely as well. Add 1 cup of boiling water to ¼ to ½ cup of fresh, clean leaves. Steep for 10 minutes, then strain out the herb. Sip slowly after it has cooled somewhat.

Papaya

Take one or two enzyme tablets after meals, or follow the package directions. Papaya enzymes work by helping your body do the digestive tasks that it has trouble doing for itself, says Dr. Tyson. The enzymes help break down foods that your gut has trouble digesting, thus reducing the amount of gas that forms.

You can buy these enzyme tablets in rolls like Tums or in a bottle. They come in different formulations, so check the package to see if the dose is appropriate for your symptoms.

Activated Charcoal

Take four to six capsules with problem foods. Activated charcoal is a substance that's usually made from specially treated wood, says Carolyn DeMarco, M.D., a physician in Winlaw, British Columbia, and a member of the advisory board of Dominion Herbal College in Burnaby.

You can find this type of charcoal at almost any drugstore or health food store. Use it only when you have flatulence following a meal. It's best used on an as-needed basis such as while traveling, says Dr. DeMarco, and is very effective, safe, and without side effects.

Psyllium

Take 1 tablespoon once daily with 8 ounces of water. Psyllium is a fiber supplement, sold under brand names such as Metamucil and Konsyl, that's used to keep bowel movements regular. Because it may take a few weeks to a few months to adjust, depending on how fiber-deprived your body is, fiber products can initially cause increased flatulence, Dr. Tyson says.

Regular bowel movements are important if you have chronic flatulence, because backed-up bowels can lead to unwanted flatus and abdominal discomfort, says Dr. Tyson. Look at it this way: if you pump air into a balloon, it will stretch only so far before it lets go with a loud bang. The same principle applies to you.

Make sure you take fiber supplements with lots of water, she warns. If you don't, you could end up even more constipated than before. It's also important to eat lots of fruits and vegetables and drink plenty of water every day.

Fast FACTS

Cause: There are as many causes of excess flatulence as there are unwanted outbursts over the course of a day. Some medications may cause it, and so may food allergies or lactose intolerance. Perhaps you swallow too much air when you eat, and it passes out the other end. Some gastrointestinal disorders—things like irritable bowel syndrome, inflammatory bowel disease, or gallbladder problems—can also be responsible.

Incidence: Flatulence is one of the most common symptoms encountered by family physicians. It's fair to say that virtually everyone has bouts of unwanted flatulence at some point.

When to see the doctor: If there's no apparent cause for your gassiness, if you can't trace it to a particular food, or if it stays with you for several weeks, have yourself checked out by a health-care practitioner. The doctor will want to rule out the possibility of any serious disorder.

Acidolphilus

Take 1 teaspoon daily. Acidophilus belongs to the category of probiotics, says Dr. Tyson. Probiotics work by normalizing the amount of good bacteria in your intestines that help your body break down tough-to-digest foods. When they're out of sync, gas buildup results.

Acidophilus is made from either carrots or dairy products, and you can buy it in liquid or powdered form. Both work in similar fashion, so it's your choice.

Fennel

Chew 1 teaspoon of seeds after meals. Fennel is classified as a carminative, says Varro E. Tyler, Ph.D., Sc.D., distinguished professor emeritus of pharmacognosy at Purdue University in West Lafayette, Indiana, and co-author of *Tyler's Honest Herbal*. That means that it's a compound that expels gas and soothes the stomach.

To get the gas out of your system, eat fennel seeds after trouble-some meals or simply after every meal if you're constantly plagued by gas. Chew the seeds thoroughly before swallowing. You can find them at health food stores and well-stocked supermarkets.

FLU

*Y*ou know how more boomer-age folks claim to have at-tended Woodstock than could have possibly fit into the state of New York, let alone the little farm where the event took place? Well, it's the same story with influenza. "When people tell me they have the flu, I'm suspicious," says Gill Stanard, a member of the National Herbalists Association of Australia and an herbal practitioner in Mel-bourne. "They tend to think a cold is the flu."

Two reasons come to mind. One is that even "a touch of the flu" sounds much more convincing than "a bad cold" when you need to ex-plain why you'll miss a day of work. The other is that the two really are similar. Both are viral infections, and they share many symptoms. Mild cases may be hard to tell apart, so a bad cold can seem a lot like the flu.

If you actually have the hard-core flu, though, you'll know it. "With a cold, you may feel bad, with things like a runny nose and sore throat," notes Stanard. "But the flu will absolutely knock you out, with muscle aches and chills and a good fever."

Another thing that colds and flu have in common is that both lack cures, although there is a flu vaccine, plus antiviral agents such as ri-mantadine that can help lessen the impact and shorten the course of some types of flu. Once you have the flu, however, conventional medicine is usually helpless to do much more than minimize bothersome symptoms.

On the other hand, herbal remedies such as the following—along with rest and vitamins—can assist your body's natural healing processes and leave your immune system in better condition for the next time the flu starts "going around."

Elder

Take 1 teaspoon of tincture three or four times a day. Research from Israel has provided some exciting information about the flu-fighting prowess of elderberry. It appears that the berry extract actually keeps the virus from replicating itself in your body. "Elderberry can decrease the duration of flu symptoms," says Rena Bloom, N.D., a naturopathic physician in Denver. "If someone calls in with the flu, I almost instantly put them on elderberry."

Dr. Bloom recommends taking the basic dose above for about 3 days, beginning with the first sign of the flu. She notes, however, that demand has spawned a booming business in commercial elderberry extracts such as Sambucol. Most of these products are effective, Dr. Bloom says, but dosage and strength can vary. "Follow the directions on the label," she advises.

Linden, Elder, Yarrow, and Peppermint

Drink three or four cups of tea blend a day. Linden flower is specifically effective against the influenza virus. That's why Mary Bove, N.D., a naturopathic physician at the Brattleboro Naturopathic Clinic in Vermont and a member of Britain's National Institute of Medical Herbalists, recommends adding it to the classic yarrow-elder-peppermint blend to create a powerful flu tea. What really makes this tea work is its sweat-inducing qualities, which help your immune system do its work by pushing up your body temperature, she says.

The elder is in flower form for this tea, as are the yarrow and linden. You can buy the dried flowers, along with dried peppermint leaves, in bulk at well-stocked health food stores. Mix enough of each in equal parts to have a good batch of tea ready for the winter. At the onset of flu symptoms, Dr. Bove suggests steeping 1 heaping teaspoon of the blend in 8 ounces of water for 10 minutes, then straining it. Drink it as warm as is comfortable. "Try to drink at least three or four

ADVENTURES IN HERBALISM

CURE OF THE COUNTESS

The European explorers, soldiers, and missionaries who "discovered" the New World in the seventeenth and eighteenth centuries also "discovered" a host of medicinal herbs long used by native healers there. Among these was the bark of a Peruvian tree called cinchona, which proved to be a miracle cure for what was then one of the world's most deadly diseases: malaria.

Cinchona was named for a Spanish countess, Anna del Cinchon, who was said to have been cured of a life-threatening fever with the bark. Another name that cinchona acquired was Jesuit's bark, because in 1633, Jesuit missionaries in Peru noticed its effectiveness and began shipping it home by the boatload.

Scientists later discovered the active ingredient that made cinchona such an effective medicine: quinine. But that name is something of a misnomer, taken as it is from the quina-quina plant. Quina-quina was often mistaken for cinchona, and unfortunately so, since it had no effect whatsoever on malaria.

cups a day," she says. "Do this for a few days, and it will help your body mount its own responses so the flu won't linger or be as severe."

If the yarrow's a little strong for your taste, Dr. Bove suggests adding a little honey or ¼ cup of apple juice. This tea is not recommended for pregnant women.

Echinacea, Elder, Usnea, and Wild Indigo

Take 1 teaspoon of this flu formula three times a day. Echinacea is famously effective for any respiratory tract infection, including in-

Superstar Flu Decoctail

Echinacea is the captain of a team of immunity-boosting all-stars that also includes ginger, licorice, astragalus, and cinnamon. "This is a good cold or flu tea blend for right when you're getting sick," says Cascade Anderson Geller, an herbal educator and consulting herbal practitioner in Portland, Oregon.

All of the players in this decoctail—a combination decoction and cocktail— help your body's defenses overcome the infection in different ways. For example, echinacea is a short-term stimulator of white blood cells, astragalus aids the entire immune system, and cinnamon provides a better immune environment by warming you up.

Echinacea and astragalus are not the worst-tasting herbs known to medicine, but even with the cinnamon, ginger, and licorice, this is no pleasure tea. It's strong herbal medicine. "It's better to drink small amounts of it frequently than large amounts infrequently," Geller says. Her recommendation is to drink ¼ to ½ cup four or five times a day from the onset of symptoms.

For maximum effectiveness, all of the ingredients should be in cut-and-sifted form.

3 parts echinacea
2 parts ginger
2 parts licorice
1 part astragalus
1½ parts cinnamon

Combine the echinacea, ginger, licorice, astragalus, and cinnamon. To make the decoction, use 1 heaping tablespoon of the blend per cup of water. In a saucepan, add the tea to cold water and bring it to a boil. Simmer, covered, for 10 minutes, and strain before drinking.

fluenza. Its various active ingredients help your white blood cells do their work when they're needed the most—right when invading viruses need to be neutralized. For flu, Dr. Bove recommends using echinacea as the chief herb in an immune-boosting formula that helps your body defend itself in more ways than echinacea could do alone.

You'll probably buy each of these tinctures in 1-ounce bottles from

Fast FACTS

Cause: When the influenza virus, in its many strains, mutations, and types, finds a host whose immune system isn't up to snuff, infection occurs.

Incidence: Influenza often hits in "outbreaks" and spreads rapidly via coughing and sneezing. Children ages 5 to 14 are most likely to catch it, and since schools are ideal virus breeding grounds, all members of families with school-age children are at higher risk.

When to see the doctor: Influenza can be life-threatening if you also contract a bacterial infection such as pneumonia. Consult a physician if you are coughing up thick yellow or green sputum or if you have symptoms such as high fever (over 102°F), vomiting, dizziness, or generalized weakness for more than 1 to 2 days. See a doctor immediately if you have difficulty breathing.

---

a health food store or by mail order. Dr. Bove's formula calls for 2 parts echinacea to 1 part each of elder, usnea (also known as old man's beard), and wild indigo. Thus, you might use the entire bottle of echinacea and half of each of the rest of the bottles. You now have your flu formula.

Start taking the above dose as soon as you suspect that you're getting the flu. You can take this formula during the acute phase, but don't continue for more than 3 or 4 weeks.

Garlic

Each day, take capsules providing a total of 10 milligrams of allicin. Garlic's therapeutic powers are widely accepted, including its ability to destroy viruses and help speed your recovery from flu. For this we can thank allicin, the principal active ingredient that's helped garlic earn its reputation as a natural antibiotic. The key to using garlic in capsules—which are easy to find, easy to take, and often odorless—is to do a little label reading, because you need to know how much allicin is in the capsule.

First, find capsules that are standardized for allicin content. "For flu, take 10 milligrams of allicin a day, or 4,000 micrograms a day of what's called total allicin potential," says Susan B. Kowalsky, N.D., a naturopathic physician in Norwich, Vermont. "This is all equal to about one clove, or 4,000 milligrams, of fresh garlic. Otherwise, follow the manufacturer's recommendations."

Chamomile and Peppermint

Drink two or more cups of tea a day. Part of the misery of influenza is a general sort of malaise that goes beyond the individual symptoms. You just feel rotten. As tired as you may be, though, you're far from relaxed. That's where chamomile-and-peppermint tea comes in.

Chamomile is soothing, and it has some ability to resist microbial invaders, says Dr. Bloom. "Peppermint is also relaxing, and it's soothing to the digestive system. If you're restless, irritable, and having stomach problems, this is something nice to sip."

There are no complicated procedures here. Simply steep dried chamomile flowers and peppermint leaves at a strength you feel comfortable with. Or you can buy packaged chamomile and peppermint tea and put the tea bags in the same cup. Drink plenty of it throughout the day, says Dr. Bloom. It's mild and tastes wonderful.

FOOD CRAVINGS

*R*ight now, you're probably wondering how all that food got to know you. Like the double-chocolate fudge cake nestled in the cupboard, the leftover lasagna in the back of the refrigerator, the roll of slice-and-bake cookies sitting in the freezer.

Those foods must know you. Why else would they all be calling your name?

Food cravings, that's why. Those overpowering urges that dissolve your willpower and shatter your diet. The things that turn your most noble intentions into a mad scramble for something filling.

Don't beat yourself up too much. It feels like a simple lack of willpower, but there's more to food cravings than that, says Fred Garcia, M.D., founder of Slim and Slimmer Medical Associates clinics in Newport Beach and Beverly Hills, California. If you want to blame food cravings on something other than yourself for a while, try society.

"We, as a society, are addicted to simple carbohydrates in food," he explains. Simple carbohydrates are foods that raise blood sugar quickly. This in turn causes your body to release various hormones that ultimately make you hanker for even more sweets. Complex carbohydrates do the opposite. They gradually release energy-providing sugars into the bloodstream, giving you a steady burn of energy.

The best thing you can do to control food cravings is adjust your diet, says Dr. Garcia. Get rid of the refined grains and sugars. Go for complex carbohydrates: whole grains and lots of vegetables and fruit. You've been told that pasta is great for you, but make sure it's the kind made with whole grains, not the refined kind. Look for spinach on the label rather than flour.

An attack of cravings will generally remind you how faithful you've been to watching what you put in your mouth. "My patients can almost always look back over the past few days and tell by their cravings if they've been eating well," says Willow Moore, N.D., D.C., a naturopathic physician and chiropractor at the Maryland Natural Medicine Center in Owings Mills.

While eating wisely is the most important weapon in the fight against food cravings, it's not the only one. Herbs can help, too. Here are some you should consider.

St. John's Wort

Take 300 milligrams of extract standardized to 0.3 percent hypericin twice a day for as long as needed. Your brain has an interesting relationship with food. When you succumb to the binge that food cravings demand, your brain releases compounds that make you feel happier and more content. They're called neurotransmitters and

Fast FACTS

Cause: Food cravings are preventable. A diet high in refined grains and sugars is almost certain to lead to cravings. Your body rapidly turns these foods into glucose, the sugar that runs through your bloodstream and provides energy. Because the sugar hits your system quickly, your body responds by trying to normalize the level by increasing insulin production. It tends to overcompensate, though, leaving you deprived of blood sugar. Then your body craves more carbohydrates to restore blood sugar levels.

Incidence: Anyone who eats poorly is prone to food cravings, as are people who drink a lot of caffeinated beverages. It's been estimated that well over half the population deals with food cravings on a regular basis.

When to see the doctor: The problem with food cravings is that they usually lead to weight problems and even obesity. If you are seriously overweight (30 percent over your ideal weight), you should see a doctor who specializes in weight control.

include natural compounds like serotonin and dopamine. This reaction was the reason that the prescription drug Fen-phen was so effective. It raised brains levels of these compounds and removed the cravings for food. Fen-phen was pulled from the market, though, due to dangerous side effects.

The good news is that the increasingly popular herb St. John's wort has similar properties without the nasty side effects, says Dr. Garcia. Just don't expect to pop a pill and see your cravings melt away. "St. John's wort takes about a month before it's effective," he says.

Licorice

Take one or two 300-milligram capsules twice daily. Licorice acts to keep your blood sugar levels stable, says Dr. Moore. That means fewer cravings.

The dosage above is for powdered root. If you come across the concentrated extract, steer clear. It can have unpleasant side effects in some people. Take the capsules for 4 to 6 weeks to see if it works for you.

Asian Ginseng

Take one 300-milligram capsule of extract standardized to 0.3 percent ginsenosides three times a day. Ginseng could easily be considered Asia's ultimate herb, says Dr. Moore. It has long been used in that part of the world as a treatment for many conditions and as an overall tonic. Asian ginseng, also called Chinese, Korean, or panax ginseng, seems to have many beneficial effects, but for food cravings, its ability to stabilize blood sugar swings is what's important to you. You can take it indefinitely.

Wild Yam

Women, once a day between the 15th and 25th day of your cycle, rub ¼ to ½ teaspoon of progesterone cream (derived from wild yam) into your abdomen, inner thighs, and neck. Many women experience more forceful cravings in the 2 weeks prior to their periods, when their hormones are in full swing, says Dr. Garcia. Progesterone cream is believed to help you through this time by restoring some hormone balance. Made from Mexican wild yam, progesterone cream is widely available at health food stores and some drugstores.

FOOD POISONING

*B*y golly, it smelled good, didn't it? Maybe it was a Polish sausage smothered in sauerkraut, onions, and mustard, purchased on a fragrant whim from a street vendor. Maybe it was a bowl of chili from a local hangout. Perhaps it was an egg salad sandwich that was in the refrigerator a little longer than you thought.

Whatever it was, it's not smelling good anymore. As a matter of fact, the mere thought of food makes your already cramped stomach lurch in indignation. You probably have diarrhea, stomach pain, vomiting, chills, and a fever from the offending food you ate 3 hours ago. Sometimes, food poisoning can cause a major headache, too, and an overall achy, flulike feeling.

The worst cases of food poisoning can hang on for a couple of weeks. Fortunately, that's the minority. Most of the time, they last only a day or two.

The first thing to do in cases of food poisoning is to be sure that you remain hydrated, says James S. Sensenig, N.D., distinguished visiting professor at the University of Bridgeport College of Naturopathic Medicine in Connecticut and founding president of the American Association of Naturopathic Physicians. You're losing a lot of fluids through both diarrhea and vomiting. Extreme dehydration can be life-threatening. If you cannot keep any food or fluids down for 12 hours, you need to be concerned about dehydration.

Dr. Sensenig suggests Gatorade or some other sports drink, which has the electrolytes and minerals that you're losing. If you can't bear the thought of running to the store for some, you can make do with a pinch of salt in a glass of water, he says. Whatever you choose to drink, sip it slowly. If you take too much at once, it's likely come right back up.

In addition to staying hydrated, try some of these herbs to help you get through this more quickly and with less pain.

Garlic

Eat two fresh cloves up to three times a day. Garlic, that kitchen staple, has many more uses than just flavoring your spaghetti, says Dr. Sensenig. Combating food poisoning is one of them. Garlic has powerful antibiotic and antimicrobial properties and goes right to work on the bugs that are making you sick.

To get the benefits of garlic, mash or chop two small to medium cloves. The taste will be strong, but you might be surprised at how well you can tolerate it, given your condition. You can mix the garlic with a glass of water to help it go down, or spread it on some crackers. "That masks the taste," says Dr. Sensenig. Take small bites. You can do this up to three times a day if your stomach can keep it down.

Lemon

Take ½ teaspoon of juice in 4 ounces of water as needed. Lemon juice acts in a twofold manner, says Dr. Sensenig. First, it increases stomach acidity, which makes an inhospitable environment for bacteria. Second, it flushes toxins from the bugs out of your liver and the rest of your system, reducing the symptoms of poisoning.

Sip the concoction slowly to keep your stomach from rejecting it. You can do this every hour as necessary.

Fast FACTS

Cause: Food poisoning happens when you ingest nasty bacteria that have taken root in your food. Bugs like salmonella and *Escherichia coli* proliferate when food hasn't been cooked or refrigerated properly or has been handled by someone with contaminated hands.

Incidence: The Centers for Disease Control and Prevention in Atlanta estimates that more than six million Americans come down with foodborne illnesses every year. Some cases can even result in death.

When to see the doctor: If a young child or elderly person has symptoms of food poisoning, you should head to a doctor right away. The same is true for someone who has an immune-system-related disorder. These groups of people are most susceptible to the deadly effects of food poisoning.

Even if you're a normally healthy adult, get to a doctor if your fever exceeds 100°F or if you have severe or persistent vomiting (meaning that you can't hold down any liquids) or diarrhea for most of a day. Likewise, seek medical attention if you see blood in your stool.

Miso

Drink 8 ounces of broth up to three times daily. Miso is a flavorful, fermented paste that you can get in the refrigerated section of most health food stores, says Yvonne Tyson, M.D., a physician in Long Beach, California, and a member of the American Holistic Health Association. It's made from soybeans or barley and has lots of sea salt in it. You want the kind made from barley. It has many digestive enzymes that can calm the stomach churning that you're experiencing.

To make the broth, boil some water, then let it stand for about 5 minutes to cool a little. Don't use the water while it's at boiling temperature because it will kill the active enzymes. Add about a teaspoon of miso paste to 8 ounces of water. (It will look a bit like curdled milk, so don't look at it.)

Sip it slowly. Since miso has a large amount of salt, you might want to consult your physician before using it if you're under treatment for high blood pressure, says Dr. Tyson.

Kudzu

Add 1 heaping tablespoon to warm water and sip slowly up to three times a day. Kudzu is a high-quality thickener with uses similar to those of cornstarch, says Dr. Tyson. It comes from a tuberous vegetable that is best harvested during the coldest time of the year.

You can find it at well-stocked grocery stores or health food stores. The starchy powder has beneficial effects on the inflamed lining of your digestive tract.

"It doesn't do much to get rid of the infection, but it reduces the cramping and other symptoms," says Dr. Tyson. "And, quite honestly, that's what people are most concerned with when they have food poisoning."

Ginger

Drink three cups of tea daily. Ginger can be one of your best allies against food poisoning, says Willow Moore, N.D., D.C., a naturopathic physician and chiropractor at the Maryland Natural Medicine Center in Owings Mills.

Ginger is chock-full of compounds that help infections and bacterial invasions. It boosts your immune response, aiding your body in getting rid of the bug. It also has strong anti-nausea compounds to keep your stomach down where it belongs.

Pick up the tea at any health food store or well-stocked supermarket and steep 1 teaspoon in hot water for about 10 minutes. Sip it slowly. You can also get ginger in capsules and powder, but stick with the tea for food poisoning. You need the fluids that come with it.

FOOT ODOR

A pair of feet has approximately 250,000 sweat glands, and they excrete as much as a half-pint of moisture each day. Seal up all that moisture inside a pair of shoes and socks, and you have the perfect breeding ground for bacteria and fungi, two guests that will stink up any party.

The first steps toward combating foot odor, says Beverly Yates, N.D., a naturopathic physician with the Natural Health Care Group in Portland, Oregon, and Seattle, are to own more than one pair of shoes and to rotate them regularly. Give each pair a chance to air out and dry out before you wear it again. This includes the shoes that you wear to work out.

Wearing clean socks each day is also vital. If your feet perspire heavily, change your socks two or three times a day as needed to keep your feet dry, and add powder or bentonite clay (a drying agent available at health food stores) to socks and shoes. Also, wash your feet once a day with soap and water, reminds Dr. Yates, and dry them thoroughly each time.

You can reduce the amount of sweat that accumulates on your feet, says John E. Hahn, N.D., D.P.M., a naturopathic doctor and podiatrist in Bend, Oregon, by cutting back on the many sources of caffeine in your diet, including cola drinks, coffee, and chocolate. He also prescribes reducing the amount of stress in your life.

While you're working on that, here are some herbal remedies that will help kill off the critters that are fouling your feet.

Goldenseal and Myrrh

Soak in a disinfecting herbal footbath. Goldenseal is one of the best antifungal and antibacterial herbs in the herbalists' arsenal, while myrrh fights not only bacteria but also inflammation. That matters in the case of foot odor, says Dr. Hahn, because the bacteria that cause it can actually eat into the surface of the skin.

Fast FACTS

Dr. Hahn recommends mixing a tablespoon each of goldenseal and myrrh tincture in $\frac{1}{2}$ quart of warm water and soaking your feet for 5 to 10 minutes. Do this once a week for recurrent foot odor and perspiration. The goldenseal may stain your skin yellow, Dr. Hahn says, but it's no cause for concern. The color wears off in 2 to 3 days.

Lavender and Tea Tree

Rub a mixture of these essential oils into your feet twice a day to kill foot bacteria. Lavender is among the most skin-friendly of all the healing herbs and can help soothe the tissues on your feet that have been irritated by invading bacteria. Meanwhile, the potent antifungal properties of tea tree oil will help wipe the offending critters off your podiatric map.

Dr. Hahn suggests mixing 1 teaspoon of tea tree essential oil with 3 teaspoons of lavender essential oil and rubbing the combination into your feet until it disappears, once in the morning and once at night. Use this rub every other day or every third day. Dr. Hahn cautions that in advanced cases of foot odor, bacteria sometimes cause tiny pits in the surface of the skin so that it seems soft and mushy or cracked. Using lavender oil may increase the mushiness.

Garlic

Take enough capsules to equal 7,500 micrograms of allicin a day in three divided doses. Allicin is the active ingredient in garlic, and it has potent antifungal properties. Garlic can make your body an inhospitable environment for the types of fungus that create foot odor, says Kathleen Janel, N.D., a naturopathic doctor with the Brattleboro Naturopathic Clinic in Vermont. As a bonus, oral garlic will boost your immune system, help regulate blood sugar, and lower blood cholesterol levels, Dr. Janel adds.

Since the amount of allicin in store-bought garlic capsules varies widely, she recommends that you read the label of the brand you buy and gauge the appropriate daily dosage by the amount of allicin listed there.

FORGETFULNESS

Sometimes, when a love affair goes sour or a day at work goes badly, forgetfulness can seem like a blessing.

Most of the time, though, we want to remember as much as we can, and many of us are frustrated that we seem to remember less than we'd like. The stressful pace of modern life all but guarantees that a growing number of details will slip through our mental sieves, while all the talk about Alzheimer's disease makes us squirm a little more each time it happens.

We worry about memory more than we should, according to Andrew Weil, M.D., director of the program in integrative medicine at the University of Arizona College of Medicine in Tucson and author of *8 Weeks to Optimum Health*. "The vast majority of people who think they are losing memory are not," he says. The secret of memory, he says, is paying attention, and the secret of attention is motivation. If our memories aren't what we think they should be, the reason could be that we simply don't care enough about recalling certain details to focus on remembering them.

"Try not to worry about your memory," Dr. Weil concludes. "The chances are good that nothing is wrong with it." He suggests watching your diet, exercising regularly, practicing stress reduction, taking antioxidant vitamins, and keeping your mind active.

If you'd like to take steps beyond that to make sure your memory is as strong as it can possibly be, an herbal remedy or two can help.

Ginkgo

Take 60 to 120 milligrams of standardized extract in capsule form twice a day. Ginkgo is one of the best-researched of all the medicinal herbs, and its ability to increase blood circulation to the brain—thereby enhancing memory—is well-documented. There is evidence that it helps enhance the function of the brain's synapses as well, says William Warnock, N.D., director of the Champlain Center for Natural Medicine in Shelburne, Vermont.

Ginkgo is almost always used for treating memory problems once they've already developed, Dr. Warnock says, although it can be used on an ongoing, preventive basis by taking 60 to 80 milligrams twice a day. He recommends taking ginkgo extract in capsule form that is standardized to 24 percent ginkgoflavoglycosides, the active ingredients.

Ginseng

Take 20 drops of tincture three times a day. Dr. Warnock recommends taking ginseng for memory problems for a very specific reason: It stimulates production of a hormone called DHEA by the adrenal glands. A decline in DHEA is thought to be one of the factors that contributes to aging, so theoretically, increasing DHEA production could help keep aging at bay.

One study found that DHEA supplements increased older women's sense of well-being—measured by soundness of sleep, joint comfort, mobility, and ability to cope—by an astonishing 84 percent. Men's sense of well-being increased by 67 percent.

In order to achieve the benefits of ginseng, Dr. Warnock recommends taking it on an ongoing basis. Take it for 6 weeks, then take a break for 2 weeks. Do this in a constant cycle to prevent your body from adapting to the ginseng and causing the herb to lose its effectiveness. Both the Asian and Siberian varieties stimulate the production of DHEA, he says.

Because ginseng is imported, it's difficult to be certain that it is correctly standardized. Look for a product that will give you approximately 10 to 15 milligrams of ginsenosides, the active ingredients, in a 20-drop dose. Dr. Warnock says that you should try as many different brands of ginseng as necessary to find the one that works well for you.

Ashwaganda

Take one 500-milligram capsule two or three times a day. Ashwaganda, which is often called the Indian ginseng, is a staple of Ayurveda, the ancient Indian system of medicine. According to C. Leigh Broadhurst, Ph.D., a nutrition consultant and herbal researcher based in Clovery, Maryland, it's a type of herb known as an adaptogen, meaning that it has a broad range of effects that help restore the body to normal function when it's out of balance in various ways. Among those restorative properties, she says, is an ability to enhance the function of the brain—hence its ability to improve memory. It's safe to take the suggested dose on an ongoing basis, Dr. Broadhurst says.

Gotu Kola

Take 2,000 milligrams in capsule form twice a day. Practitioners of Ayurveda in India regard gotu kola as an important rejuvenating herb, especially for nerve and brain cells. It works in part because it has anti-anxiety properties, according to Dr. Warnock, which help counter the negative effects of stress.

"Although the brain is infinitely more complicated than a computer, it has a similar tendency to freeze up if you ask it to do too many things at one time," he says. "Anxiety occupies the brain, and by reducing anxiety, you allow it to focus on other things."

Forget-Me-Not Formula

Smells go directly to the limbic system, one of the brain's key repositories of memories, which is why aromas can so often spur recollections of times past. Aromatherapist Victoria Edwards, owner of Leydet Aromatics in Fair Oaks, California, has designed an essential oil blend specifically to take advantage of that brain-memory connection. You can use the formula in an aromatherapy diffuser or simply put a drop or two on a handkerchief or cotton ball and take a sniff when you feel you need it.

5 drops ginger essential oil
10 drops lemon essential oil
5 drops peppermint essential oil

Combine the ginger, lemon, and peppermint oils in a clean glass dropper bottle and shake well.

Dr. Warnock recommends buying capsules of gotu kola that contain 40 percent asiaticoside, the active ingredient.

Rosemary

Drink three cups of tea a day. Rosemary's reputation as the herb of remembrance is well-deserved, says Dr. Broadhurst. Its rich antioxidant properties help prevent the breakdown of chemicals in the brain that are key to memory.

To make a good cup of rosemary tea, add 1½ tablespoons of the dried herb to about 8 ounces of boiling water. Cover and simmer for 5 minutes, then remove from the heat and let stand for 5 minutes. Strain it, if you choose, and drink. It is fine to drink this on a long-term basis. In fact, older people should use this tea regularly, since rosemary may help prevent or treat Alzheimer's disease and other related dementias.

Fast Facts

Cause: Some degree of memory loss is a normal part of aging. Exactly why that's so is uncertain, but it may be because of deterioration of the nervous system, the circulatory system, or other natural systems. A host of other factors can contribute to forgetfulness, including Alzheimer's disease, depression, alcohol abuse, hypothyroidism, tumors, stroke, multiple sclerosis, vitamin deficiencies, and Parkinson's disease.

Incidence: Because the possible causes of memory loss are so diverse, it can affect anyone, but it's far more common in people over 65.

When to see the doctor: An evaluation is advisable if you or those close to you notice consistent lapses in memory for which there seems to be no obvious cause.

Cypress

Use this essential oil as aromatherapy to enhance memory. Cypress is another herb that has traditional associations with memory, according to aromatherapist Victoria Edwards, owner of Leydet Aromatics in Fair Oaks, California. For centuries, it was planted around the graveyards of Europe, she says, to help visitors remember the souls buried there. Cypress has what Edwards describes as a bright, piercing smell that stimulates and clears the mind.

If you don't have a diffuser for essential oils, you can use cypress essential oil by simply putting a drop or two on a cotton ball or handkerchief and taking a sniff when you feel like it.

Ginger

Sniff a few drops of essential oil for mental stimulation. Ginger is Edwards's second favorite oil for forgetfulness, after cypress. "Ginger is spicy and warming," she says. "It heats up the cold corners of the mind."

Like other scents, ginger can be used with a diffuser, a cotton ball, or a handkerchief. Edwards cautions, however, that ginger is a heavy scent that can be overpowering if you overdo it. She recommends using no more than a few drops at a time.

Frankincense and Black Pepper

Use these essential oils to clear your mind for better memory. Frankincense is one of the most ancient of all scents to be used medicinally, says Edwards. Its capacity for stimulating memory is suggested by its widespread use in ancient religious ceremonies, she says, where it serves to remind the faithful aromatically of their connection to God.

Black pepper is another essential oil that is strong enough to dispel the distractions that dislodge the memories we'd like to keep. "It's very stimulating and energizing for the brain," Edwards says. "It will keep you awake and paying attention."

GINGIVITIS

*F*rom ancient Egypt to eighteenth-century France, whenever teeth rotted and fell from the mouth, people and their dentists blamed the toothworm. Coiled in the pulp of the tooth, this malevolent creature was said to gnaw its way free from the inside out, causing excruciating pain on its way.

Modern dentists know that the real toothworm—the underlying cause of tooth loss—is gingivitis, or inflammation of the gums. Typically, gingivitis is caused by a buildup of plaque, a sticky mixture of

In-the-Pink Gum Swab

This blend of herbs can help clear up a mild case of gingivitis in a matter of days, says Barry Sherr, a professional member of the American Herbalists Guild who practices in Danbury, Connecticut.

The myrrh, tea tree oil, goldenseal, and propolis contain substances that act as antiseptics, reduce inflammation, or kill off bacteria. The prickly ash helps oxygenate the gums, discouraging bacterial growth. The peppermint fights bad breath, a common result of gingivitis, and may also offer some relief from discomfort. Swab your gums liberally with the mixture two or three times a day. While most people notice improvement after a couple of days, it may take up to 2 weeks to see results. After your symptoms are gone, swab your gums once a week as a preventive measure.

- **1 part myrrh tincture**
- **1 part goldenseal tincture**
- **3 parts prickly ash tincture**
- **2 parts tea tree oil**
- **2 parts propolis tincture**
- **2 parts peppermint tincture**

Mix the myrrh, goldenseal, prickly ash, tea tree, propolis, and peppermint in a bottle and shake.

---

mucus, saliva, food particles, and bacteria, on the teeth and gums. The bacteria release toxins that damage the gums, leaving them red, puffy, and prone to bleeding.

If plaque isn't properly brushed and flossed away, gingivitis can lead to periodontitis, a major cause of tooth loss. In people susceptible to periodontitis who don't seek treatment, the gums can pull away from the teeth and the gaps fill with bacteria and fluid. Eventually, the bacteria destroy the gums, teeth, and bone. The teeth start to wobble in their sockets. The next thing you know, you're pricing dentures.

The best way to keep your gums in the pink is to brush and floss your teeth at least twice a day. Brushing scrubs plaque from the teeth, while flossing digs it out from between the teeth and gumline, says Roy Page, D.D.S., Ph.D., professor of periodontics in the school of dentistry at the University of Washington in Seattle. Another gum-saving tactic: Cut back on sugary snacks, which encourage plaque, says Dr. Page. Opt for more gum-healthy fare such as raw vegetables, plain yogurt, or cheese.

Along with proper oral hygiene, certain herbs can help prevent and treat gingivitis, says Ellen Kamhi, R.N., Ph.D., a professional member of the American Herbalists Guild (AHG), an herbalist in Oyster Bay, New York, and author of *The Natural Medicine Chest*. Some herbs act as powerful antiseptics, slowing the growth of microbial marauders. Others help soothe tender, swollen gums.

Echinacea

Combine 30 drops of tincture with a few ounces of water and rinse your mouth at bedtime. "I use echinacea for any condition that causes inflammation," says Ed Smith, a professional member of the AHG and founder of Herb Pharm in Williams, Oregon. Echinacea helps your immune system fight the bacteria and viruses that attack the body. It also helps heal existing infections.

Goldenseal

Rinse your mouth with a solution of 1 tablespoon of root powder, 1 teaspoon of baking soda, and a few ounces of water. Swish the rinse around for a minute or so, then spit it out. Use the rinse two or three times a day until your symptoms subside. If after 2 weeks, you don't notice any improvement, try another remedy. "Goldenseal is excellent for soothing inflamed gums," says Flora Parsa Stay, D.D.S., a dentist in Oxnard, California, and author of *The Complete Book of Dental Remedies*.

For convenience, look for goldenseal root power in capsule form, says Dr. Stay. Simply empty the capsule into the water-and-baking-soda mixture. Goldenseal contains hydrastine and berberine, sub-

Fast FACTS

Cause: Gingivitis comes from an overgrowth of plaque, the sticky film that you feel on your teeth in the morning. Plaque is teeming with bacteria, which produce toxins that can damage the gums. Another culprit is the typical American diet, which is low in fiber (a natural plaque scrubber) and high in plaque-promoting sugary and refined foods.

Incidence: Seventy-five percent of all Americans over 35 develop gingivitis at some point in their lives.

When to see the doctor: If your gums are red, tender, or swollen, or if they bleed when you brush your teeth, get to a dentist pronto. Also see a dentist if you have persistent bad breath, if your gums seem to be pulling away from your teeth, or if your teeth seem looser, with wider spacing.

---

stances that are thought to have a soothing effect on the mucous membranes that line the mouth and digestive system.

Myrrh

Mix 30 drops of tincture in a couple of ounces of water and rinse your mouth. Myrrh contains tannins, substances that reduce inflammation and promote the formation of a protective "seal" on the skin and the mucous membranes, says Smith.

Goldenseal, Myrrh, and Aloe

Combine myrrh and goldenseal powders with aloe gel and massage into your gums. This two-step treatment is definitely a before-bed remedy, notes Dr. Kamhi—but it works. "I know people who have saved their teeth using this treatment," she says.

You should use it for only 2 to 3 days during an actual infection, says Dr. Stay.

First, brush and floss your teeth. Pour a little baking soda into your palm. Wet your toothbrush with water, dip it in the baking soda, and brush your teeth. With the baking soda still in your mouth, take a healthy swig of hydrogen peroxide. Your mouth will foam—a by-product of a chemical process called oxygenation, which helps flush away bacteria. Spit everything out, then floss your teeth.

Next, pack your gums with an herbal paste. Combine equal amounts of goldenseal and myrrh powders. In the palm of your hand, mix ½ teaspoon of the combined powders with enough aloe gel to make a paste. Then, use your finger or a cotton swab to pack the paste onto your gums, using a slow, circular motion. Put extra paste on very sore areas. Leave it on overnight. "You may swallow some, but that's perfectly safe," says Dr. Kamhi.

Propolis

Mix 30 drops of tincture with a few ounces of water and rinse your mouth three to five times a day. Commonly known as bee glue, this sticky substance made by bees to fill the cracks in their hives "is extremely high in aromatic resins, essential oils, and flavonoids, all of which help reduce inflammation and kill viruses and bacteria," says Smith.

Rosemary, Thyme, Peppermint, and Myrrh

Use an herbal mouthwash three or four times a day. Mix six drops each of rosemary, thyme, and peppermint tinctures and two drops of myrrh tincture with ½ cup of freshly boiled water. Let it cool, then rinse your mouth, says Harwinder Matthu, a member of Britain's National Institute of Medical Herbalists in Exeter, England, and an herbalist in British Columbia. "These herbs contain high amounts of volatile oils, which reduce inflammation and kill microbes," she says. You should see results in a few days, so don't use this mouthwash for more than a month at a time.

GOUT

Gout has a long and distinguished hit list. Its many victims include King Henry VIII of England, Benjamin Franklin, poet John Milton, and a fifteenth-century Florentine ruler so badly afflicted that he was nicknamed Piero the Gouty.

If you're in the midst of a gout flare-up, though, being in good company may seem like cold comfort. Gout is actually a form of arthritis that starts when too much uric acid, one of the body's waste products, starts to collect in a joint—usually the big toe. Normally, this acid is excreted in urine, but when levels get too high, the excess can settle in your joints, forming needlelike crystals that cause swelling and pain. Although gout generally targets the toe or foot, it can affect other body parts, including the knee, hand, wrist, and even the ear.

You can keep uric acid in check by avoiding rich foods. Such foods tend to be high in purines, substances that turn to uric acid in the blood. Organ meats, aged cheeses, beer and aged wines, and brewer's yeast are chief offenders, says Jennifer Brett, N.D., a naturopathic doctor in Stratford, Connecticut.

While gout usually requires a doctor's attention, several herbs can ease the pain and help the body rid itself of gout-causing purines before they have a chance to build up and cause trouble.

Ginger

Treat tender joints with a compress. When gout flares up, boil 2 quarts of water. Remove from the heat and grate a 2-inch piece of fresh ginger into the water. Cover and steep for 5 to 10 minutes. While the tea is still hot, but not so hot that you can't put your hand in it, soak a washcloth, wring it out, and apply it to your tender joint. Leave the cloth on until the heat dissipates, then immediately apply another cloth soaked in ice water. Leave the cold cloth on for 3 to 4 minutes, then reapply the hot cloth. Continue to alternate for about 15 minutes. As you're applying the treatment, keep the lid on the pot as much as possible so the tea stays hot.

Apply this hot/cold treatment every day until the swelling subsides, says Roy Upton, vice president of the American Herbalists Guild (AHG) and executive director of American Herbal Pharmacopeia, an herbal education foundation based in Santa Cruz, California. When using this treatment, always begin by applying the hot compress and end by applying the cold.

Black Cherry

Take 1 tablespoon of juice three times a day. Black cherry juice, which is available in health food stores as a concentrate, can help your body get rid of excess purines. The concentrated juice is very sweet, but you can dilute it with 8 ounces of water, Dr. Brett says. It all depends on the extent of your sweet tooth. The above amount should be taken for acute gouty attacks until the pain subsides. For prevention, people generally take 1 tablespoon daily, she says.

Horsetail

Take 60 drops of tincture a day or three 400- to 500-milligram capsules three or four times a day, or drink three cups of tea daily. This mild diuretic also helps get rid of excess purines, Dr. Brett explains. Use the above dosages for an acute attack until the pain and swelling subside. To make horsetail tea, use 1 tablespoon of dried, loose herb for each cup of hot water. Steep for 10 to 20 minutes and strain before drinking.

To prevent attacks, take two or three 400- to 500-milligram capsules or 20 drops of tincture a day. If you're taking capsules, remember that freshness is extremely important, Dr. Brett says. Check the date information on the container before buying.

<h1>Fast FACTS</h1>

Causes: Gout occurs when high levels of uric acid build up in the blood, crystallize, and collect in the joints. Most people with gout produce normal levels of uric acid but excrete too little in the urine. A small percentage of gout-prone people overproduce uric acid.

Incidence: Although it commonly strikes men between the ages of 40 and 60, it can affect men as young as 25. In women, it can occur after menopause.

When to see the doctor: If you have sudden swelling and tenderness in a joint, don't assume that it's gout. See your doctor for a proper diagnosis. Even if you've had gout in the past, and your physician has prescribed medication to take during an attack, you should consult your physician whenever you have a flare-up.

Celery Seed

Drink a cup of tea once a day until pain and swelling subside. Celery seed is another cleansing herb, which means that it helps the body rid itself of wastes, including excess uric acid. Simply add 1 teaspoon of dried celery seed to 8 ounces of water and bring to a boil. Boil for 3 to 5 minutes, then steep for another 5 minutes. Dr. Brett doesn't recommend this as a preventive because of the taste. She also cautions that since you'd need copious amounts of the spice to get the benefit of one cup of tea, simply adding celery seed to food during cooking probably isn't a good idea for treating gout.

Nettle

Have three to four cups of tea per day. Another easy-to-find cleansing herb, nettle makes a good tea that's mildly herb-flavored and pleasant, says Betzy Bancroft, a professional member of the AHG and instructor at Herbal Therapeutics School of Botanical Medicine in Washington, New Jersey. It is rich in minerals and can be found in dried bulk form at most natural or organic markets. The herbalists' rule of thumb for how long to take a remedy is one month for every year that you've had a chronic problem, she says. "Generally, people should always keep using a remedy for at least a short while after they feel better."

To use as a tea, add 1 teaspoon of dried herb to 8 ounces of boiling water. Steep for 1 hour, then strain and drink. When shopping, look for nettle that is leafy rather than having a lot of stems.

Burdock

Take 20 to 30 drops of tincture in 1 to 8 ounces of water three or four times a day. Burdock is another herb that acts to gently cleanse the body and purify the blood. The root can be found in dried form, as capsules, or as a tincture, but the tincture is probably most effective, Bancroft says. Continue to take this herb for a short time after you feel better.

HANGOVER

*T*hey say that you can't buy alcohol, you can only rent it. If that's true, then a hangover must be like the landlord pounding on your door—with a sledgehammer.

A hangover headache is caused by lowered blood sugar, excessive blood vessel dilation, and the dehydration that occurs as the body attempts to rid itself of excess alcohol. There is some evidence that drinking dark-colored alcoholic drinks, such as red wine, is more apt to cause pain in your brain. These drinks contain congeners, chemicals that add color and flavor and may promote a headache, says Frederick G. Freitag, D.O., of the Diamond Headache Clinic in Chicago.

The only real cure for a hangover is time—the time your body needs to process the toxins out of your system. But to help your body—and your poor head—there are several herbal remedies that may ease hangover symptoms.

Ginkgo

Take two 80-milligram capsules twice a day for 2 days. Ginkgo is well-known for its ability to aid circulation and revitalize your

Fast FACTS

Cause: Alcohol is a natural diuretic, so it dehydrates you. Brain tissue is more sensitive to this dehydration than the rest of your body, hence the typical hangover headache. This type of headache is worse than run-of-the-mill tension pain because alcohol also dilates blood vessels and lowers blood sugar, causing metabolic disturbances.

Incidence: Anyone, regardless of gender, race, or age, who overindulges in alcohol may be hammered by a hangover.

When to see the doctor: A hangover isn't normally cause for medical attention, but there are exceptions. If you experience withdrawal reactions—hand tremors, anxiety, sweating, rapid pulse, insomnia, hallucinations, or seizures—or find yourself drinking more than intended, you should seek professional help.

body's systems, says Steven Margolis, M.D., an alternative family physician in Sterling Heights, Michigan. Look for ginkgo phytosome, which is absorbed better than other forms of the herb, he advises. And take it for 48 hours, even when you start feeling better, he recommends, to help prevent hangover symptoms from recurring.

Ginger

Drink ½ to 1 cup of tea. Ginger is a great soother for all types of nausea, even the kind brought about by overimbibing, says Rosemary Gladstar, an herbalist at the Sage Mountain herbal education center in East Barre, Vermont, and author of *Herbal Healing for Women*. To 1 cup of boiling water, add 1 teaspoon of dried ginger or 2 teaspoons of grated fresh ginger. Remove from the heat and steep, covered, for 10 minutes.

Dandelion and Burdock

Drink ¼ cup of tea every 30 to 45 minutes, for a total of 3 to 4 cups. If half a day goes by and you still feel woozy, try a tea made from dandelion root and burdock. Add ½ teaspoon of each herb to 1 cup of boiling water and steep, covered, for 10 minutes, Gladstar suggests. Dandelion root and burdock are liver-detoxifying herbs that can help your body purge itself a little better, she says.

Feverfew

Take three 80-milligram capsules three times a day. If you attend a party where the beer and wine are flowing, start this regimen during the party and repeat it the day after, suggests Terry Willard, Ph.D., a clinical herbalist, professional member of the American Herbalists Guild, and founder and president of Wild Rose College of Natural Healing in Calgary, Alberta. Feverfew capsules are also popular for treating migraine headaches.

Reishi

Take three 60-milligram capsules twice a day. You should take this herb the day after you've overindulged, suggests Dr. Willard. Reishi is a mushroom that helps the liver process alcohol. Some capsules are a combination of reishi and ginger—an even better hangover remedy.

Milk Thistle

Take three capsules three times a day. Milk thistle protects the liver from alcohol poisoning and is often an ingredient in a formula containing other herbs such as St. John's wort, says Dr. Willard. Take this herb during the time when you are drinking, then again the following day. Look for capsules with at least 120 milligrams of milk thistle.

HEADACHES

Life is full of simple truths. Telemarketers will call at the exact moment that you sit down to eat dinner. Kids will scowl when you serve brussels sprouts. And when you're in the throes of an end-of-the-day headache, the little arrows on the pill bottle will never line up.

Despite this fact, most people turn to over-the-counter pain relievers for headache relief. Although pills like aspirin and acetaminophen may help get rid of the pain within a half-hour or so after you take them, some herbal remedies can offer almost immediate relief. The anti-inflammatory, antispasmodic, analgesic, and relaxant actions of many herbs can quiet the steady ache of the average tension-type headache—the kind that affects 9 out of 10 of us.

So take the phone off the hook at dinnertime and ignore the kids' complaints. And instead of a tongue-twisting pharmaceutical concoction, try some soothing herbal remedies the next time your head hurts. You won't even have to line up any arrows.

Lavender and Peppermint

Gently massage the blended oils into your temples at the first sign of pain. Lavender or peppermint essential oil can be used singly to relieve a tension headache. When blended together, though, they are even more effective for a headache brought on by stress, says Connie Catellani, M.D., medical director of the Miro Center for Integrative Medicine in Evanston, Illinois.

"Lavender is known for its soothing effect on the nervous system, while peppermint is a mild analgesic and anti-inflammatory agent," says Dr. Catellani. In a German study of 41 people with tension headaches, a solution containing 10 percent peppermint essential oil and 90 percent alcohol was massaged into the foreheads and temples of participants. Researchers noted that it relieved pain as effectively

Old-Fashioned Headache Sack

In colonial times, settlers sniffed tiny sachets of aromatic herbs to ward off head pain. A farmer might stash one in his hat so he could take a whiff now and then as needed. This updated version of the headache sack from Phoebe Reeve, a professional member of the American Herbalists Guild and an herbalist in Winchester, Virginia, combines the healing aromatic properties of lavender with the principles of massage therapy. When you have a headache, lie down and place the sack across your eyes. The scent will soothe, while the weight of the grain will provide counterpressure against your eyes and face to help relieve the pain, says Reeve.

 1 **piece calico or plain muslin, 8" by 8"**
   About 1 cup rice or flaxseed
 3–5 **drops lavender essential oil**

Fold the fabric in half so that it forms a 4"-by-8" rectangle. Stitch the sides together, leaving a small opening. Place the rice or flaxseed in a small bowl, add the lavender oil, and mix. Fill the sack with the grain and stitch it shut.

If you prefer a different scent, rosemary, bergamot, peppermint, and sweet marjoram essential oils also have pain-relieving properties.

as the same treatment combined with a dose of 1,000 milligrams of acetaminophen. The relief was quick, too—in just 15 minutes, pain began to subside.

For your own quick relief, keep a bottle of headache oil on hand. To make it, mix 1 tablespoon of vegetable oil, 10 drops of lavender essential oil, 5 drops of peppermint essential oil, and the contents of a vitamin E capsule in an amber glass bottle. Shake well to mix completely. To use the oil, warm a few drops in your hands and gently apply it to your temples and just beyond your hairline. Slowly breathe in the soothing aroma of the oil from your cupped hands and relax.

Fast FACTS

Cause: Research has shown that many headaches involve a combination of painfully inflamed blood vessels and tight, aching muscles. Stress, poor posture, tiredness, and eyestrain can generate muscle tension in the head, neck, or shoulders that brings on pain. Caffeine, alcohol, drugs, food allergies, and low blood sugar can also trigger a headache.

Incidence: Headache is among the most common reasons for missing work or school. Nearly 90 percent of men and 95 percent of women have had at least one headache in the past year. Between 40 and 50 million people suffer from chronic or repeated headaches.

When to see the doctor: Call your doctor if you have three or more headaches a week, or if you must take a pain reliever every day or almost every day. If you have a sudden onset of severe head pain that's different from any headache you've previously experienced, you should see a doctor right away. If a headache seems to be steadily worsening or is accompanied by fever and a stiff neck, seek immediate medical attention. Headache that begins after a head injury and persists longer than a week also warrants a checkup. If your headache is accompanied by unexpected eye, ear, or nose problems; slurred speech; numbness or weakness; blackouts; or difficulty thinking and remembering, you need to see your doctor.

Skullcap, Lavender, Peppermint, and Chamomile

Drink a cup of tension-soothing tea at the first sign of pain. You can use these herbs individually or in a tea blend that will help relax tense muscles, says Phoebe Reeve, a professional member of the American Herbalists Guild and an herbalist in Winchester, Virginia. Skullcap and lavender are antispasmodics that relax the nervous system. Peppermint and chamomile are mild relaxants that also add a pleasant taste to the tea, she says.

To make an herbal tea, just follow this basic recipe. For dried herbs, use 1 teaspoon of either an individual herb or a mixture of equal parts of each herb for each cup of water. If you are using fresh herbs, add 1 tablespoon of fresh herb or herb blend. Put the herbs in a saucepan and pour the water over them, then cover the pan and steep for 20 minutes. "The volatile oils in these herbs help to relax you. That's why it's important to cover the pot as they steep so you don't lose the volatile or aromatic oils," says Reeve. You can add a little honey as sweetener or use a twist of lemon.

HEARTBURN

*D*espite its familiar name's association with the heart, heartburn's real medical name is pretty unromantic. It's gastro-esophageal reflux disease, or GERD. As you probably know from the feeling in your belly, it's marked by a burning, acidic feeling, caustic burps, and the occasional hiccup. Sometimes, you'll hear it called in-digestion or acid indigestion.

There are a few things that you can do before you try herbal reme-dies to cool the fire in your belly, says Robert Jay Rowen, M.D., a holistic physician at the Complementary Medicine Center in An-chorage, Alaska, and a pioneer in the effort to have alternative med-icine recognized in Alaska.

Number one, slow down. Cramming your food down during a 5-minute lunch break just doesn't cut it. Sure, life is speeding up all the time, but put on the brakes at mealtime. Eating too much food too quickly doesn't give your digestive system time to get in gear. Chew your food about 40 times before swallowing, says Dr. Rowen.

The second thing you can do is back off the coffee for a while. If you need caffeine, get it from tea, which is less caustic to your in-nards.

That said, botanicals can come to your aid when other methods fail. Here's how to gird yourself for GERD.

Ginger

Drink one cup of tea after meals. Ginger is a powerful stomach soother, says Dr. Rowen. Pick up the tea at any health food store or well-stocked supermarket. Steep for about 10 minutes, then sip it slowly.

You can also make tea from the root. Finely chop or grate 1 teaspoon of fresh ginger, put it in a mug, and fill the mug with boiling water. Cover the mug with a saucer and steep for 10 minutes. Let it cool slightly, then sip it slowly.

In a pinch, you can even make tea from the powdered ginger in your spice rack (a lot of the volatile oils are missing, though, so use the other methods if possible). Add ¼ to ½ teaspoon of ginger to 1 cup of boiling water. Steep for 10 minutes, let cool, and sip slowly.

Aloe

Take 1 to 3 teaspoons of juice each day after meals. Taking a small amount of aloe juice every day can help soothe a sour stomach, says Dr. Rowen. Make sure you buy fresh juice, though, not the kind made from concentrate. The concentrate contains fewer active ingredients. Aloe vera products are also available in health food stores. Follow the dosage instructions on the label, and refrigerate after opening. Be careful not to exceed the recommended dose, since aloe can be a powerful laxative in high amounts.

Licorice

Take one or two DGL lozenges after eating. Licorice root lozenges have compounds that put a damper on the fire down below, says Theresa MacLean, R.Ph., N.D., a naturopathic physician and pharmacist based in Berwick, Nova Scotia.

Deglycyrrhizinated licorice, or DGL, is a modified form that has none of the compounds in the regular root that can raise your blood

Fast FACTS

Cause: Excess, for the most part—too much fatty or spicy food, too much coffee or alcohol, or eating too quickly—is at the heart of heartburn. Being overweight or pregnant can be a factor, too, as the extra girth below pushes on your stomach, forcing acid up into the esophagus.

Incidence: Heartburn is almost as common as stomachs. About 7 percent of American adults have heartburn daily. That number jumps to around 14 percent weekly, and a whopping 40 percent of people have heartburn on a monthly basis.

When to see the doctor: If you have heartburn on a daily basis, make an appointment to rule out anything serious, such as an ulcer or esophageal cancer. Also, if your heartburn becomes more of a blaze than in the past, have it checked. Increased pain often signifies that something else is wrong.

---

pressure. If your blood pressure is normally fine, you can also use plain licorice tablets. "It's important to chew them slowly to mix it with saliva," points out Dr. MacLean. That puts more of the active ingredients to work.

Marshmallow

Take 10 to 40 drops of tincture a day. Marshmallow root is a traditional cure for indigestion that is very appropriate even today, says Dr. MacLean. Yes, marshmallow does grow in marshes. Yes, candied marshmallow root was the precursor of the marshmallows we roast over fires today. Don't bother eating the commercial ones, though. They don't contain actual marshmallow root anymore.

When you're buying the tincture, look for one that is made with 1 part root to 5 parts of whatever fluid extract it's in. At any lower proportion, it's not as effective. Mix the tincture in a small glass of water and sip it slowly.

Swedish Bitters

Take 1 teaspoon or one capsule before meals. Swedish bitters is a strong-smelling liquid that is said to have been formulated by a Swedish doctor named Samst, who died at the age of 104—from a horseback riding accident. Bitters in general are herbs that prompt the digestive system into action, says Tim Hagney, N.D., a naturopathic physician in Anchorage, Alaska.

"Instead of the food just sitting in your stomach and backing up, bitters help your body digest it," he explains. You can also get Swedish bitters in capsule form.

Gentian

Drink one cup of tea 10 to 15 minutes before meals. If you prefer your bitters in tea form, gentian is for you, says Dr. Hagney. The mechanism at work here is the same as with Swedish bitters. To make the tea, place 1 teaspoon of grated gentian root in a pan with 1 cup of water, cover, and bring to a boil. Simmer for about 10 minutes, then strain.

HEMORRHOIDS

*O*nce upon a time, when the Philistines met the Israelites on the battlefield, they got more than they bargained for. Although they defeated the Israelites, they literally got it in the end.

After the Philistines won the battle described in the Book of Samuel, they celebrated by taking the ark of the covenant, a sacred chest representing the presence of God among the Israelites. Little did they know how much this displeased God. Their celebrations were cut short when the heavy hand of the Lord smote them all with hemorrhoids.

Perhaps you can empathize. Sometimes, hemorrhoids can feel as if a great power has taken hold of your hinder parts. There's pain when you pass stool, and often you find bright red blood in the toilet. In the worst cases, bleeding can continue slowly throughout the day.

Hemorrhoids occur when the many veins in the rectum become stretched, swollen, and inflamed. Basically, they're like the varicose veins that you see on people's legs, except that they're in a far more sensitive spot. And the rich supply of nerves around the rectum lets you know clearly that they're there. In some cases, such as with large or chronic hemorrhoids, conventional medical intervention may include removing them surgically. Naturally oriented doctors are more inclined to help people avoid hemorrhoids in the first place.

Sometimes known as the grapes of wrath due to their appearance and the discomfort they bring, hemorrhoids are almost entirely preventable, says Samuel D. Benjamin, M.D., director of the University Center for Complementary and Alternative Medicine at the State University of New York at Stony Brook and medical director of Mariposa Botanicals, an herbal producer in New York City.

Yours were most likely a result of a low-fiber diet and a low intake of water, which led to a state of chronic constipation, says Brenda Snowman, M.D., a physician in Cleveland, Tennessee. Lack of exercise also contributes because physical activity tends to keep matter moving through the intestines. A bowel full of dense, hard, dry stool puts tremendous pressure on the veins in the rectum. From that come hemorrhoids.

There are a few herbal products that can help you turn the grapes of wrath into the raisins of moderate displeasure.

Psyllium

Take 3 grams daily. Psyllium, sold under brand names such as Metamucil, is your number one ally in the fight against hemorrhoids, says

Cause: Hemorrhoids are almost always self-inflicted. A diet low in fiber can often cause chronic constipation, which results in lots of pressure on the delicate veins surrounding the rectum. They become inflamed and protrude and often bleed.

    Pregnant women often get hemorrhoids, too. The weight of the baby, plus the fact that pregnant women are often constipated, leads to the condition.

Incidence: More than 75 percent of people in the United States get hemorrhoids at some point in their lives. They are a particular problem for people over 50.

When to see the doctor: If home remedies simply don't work for your hemorrhoids, or the hemorrhoids worsen over a period of several weeks, get yourself to the doctor. There are simple outpatient procedures that can get rid of the worst cases. While it's common to see bright red blood on the toilet paper or on stool when you have a hemorrhoid, it is best to have any rectal bleeding evaluated by your doctor.

Dr. Snowman. Psyllium is a high-fiber supplement made from plant husks that is widely available at drugstores and health food stores.

Psyllium adds bulk to your digestive system, bulk that you're probably missing in your regular diet. Bulking agents like psyllium keep stool moving freely through your digestive tract. The dosage above is for psyllium husks. Some manufacturers use the whole seed, which has less fiber. Check the package for directions.

"Psyllium can backfire on people who don't increase their water intake," says Dr. Snowman. The bulking agent can quickly turn into a bowel obstruction if you aren't properly hydrated. She likens it to making cement. Be sure to drink at least eight 8-ounce glasses of water a day.

Witch Hazel

Apply as needed. Witch hazel is a popular herbal product. That's because it works on things like hemorrhoids, says Dr. Snowman. It is an astringent, which means that it constricts swollen blood vessels like your hemorrhoids. It rarely causes skin irritation, but if it does, stop using it.

You can also avoid some of the pain of wiping tender tissues after a bowel movement if you dampen a wad of toilet paper with witch hazel and gently use it to clean yourself.

Comfrey

Apply topical balm as needed. Comfrey is rich in allantoin, which is an anti-inflammatory agent and promotes healing, says Connie Catellani, M.D., medical director of the Miro Center for Integrative Medicine in Evanston, Illinois. Comfrey also contains mucilage, which soothes the irritation associated with hemorrhoids.

Look for a topical balm made with comfrey, she suggests. Alternatively, you can moisten powdered comfrey with a little bit of vegetable oil and apply it with a cotton ball or your clean fingers. Leave it on until the next time you bathe.

HIGH BLOOD PRESSURE

*H*igh blood pressure is a stealthy enemy. You can't see it, you can't feel it, and in most cases, you can't even pin down what's causing it. What you can do, though, is take advantage of some very effective and problem-free herbs to help get that pressure down to healthy levels.

That's important, because high blood pressure can kill. Not directly, mind you, but if you're eager for a heart attack or stroke, having high blood pressure is a good way to start.

Simply put, too much pressure on your arteries as blood circulates through them means that your heart's working harder than it should to pump blood and oxygen. Over time, that takes its toll on your heart as well as your arteries, and the next thing you know, your risk for serious heart disease—among other things—has skyrocketed.

How high is too high? Well, a blood pressure test gives you two numbers. The first number, the systolic (top) reading, is a measurement of blood pressure while your heart is pumping. The second, the diastolic (bottom) number, measures the pressure between beats. Any reading higher than 140/90 indicates high blood pressure, according to the American Heart Association, and needs attention.

Because high blood pressure (more formally known as hypertension) is so risky, conventional medicine offers a smorgasbord of pharmaceutical wonders to bring it down. The problem is that all of these drugs can have potentially nasty side effects. Hence, standard and alternative medicine agree on at least one point: When it comes to lowering your blood pressure, lifestyle changes take precedence over drugs.

"Most conventional physicians won't just jump in and prescribe blood pressure pills, because of the side effects," says George Milowe, M.D., a holistic physician in Saratoga Springs, New York. "But they will encourage you to lose weight, to eat healthier, to be more active physically, and to take up yoga or meditation."

Minerals also matter in controlling blood pressure, Dr. Milowe says. Most of us take in too much salt, not enough magnesium, and usually (though not always) the right amounts of calcium and potassium. "Supplementing with magnesium can be very helpful," he says. Take 1,000 milligrams daily in divided doses, or less if it produces diarrhea, but be sure to talk to your doctor before taking supplements.

Dr. Milowe also recommends enriching your diet with more omega-3 fatty acids, which are heart-healthy nutrients with an anti-hypertensive effect. You can get them from fish, shellfish, and flaxseed.

What it all comes down to is that drugs may lower your high blood pressure quickly, but a healthier lifestyle—helped along by the following herbs—may do it *permanently*.

Garlic

Take four to six 600-milligram capsules or tablets a day in divided doses. Sometimes, there's a thin line between heart-healthy foods and heart-healthy herbs. You'll find garlic on both sides of that line. "Garlic is a good example of something that's common in the diet and also helpful as a botanical medicine," Dr. Milowe says. "Studies have shown that it actually lowers blood pressure."

If your blood pressure is at an acceptable level and you want to keep it that way, eat a clove a day—preferably raw—alone or as flavoring in some other dish. That will definitely help, says Robert Rountree, M.D., a holistic physician at the Helios Health Center in Boulder, Colorado. "If you already have high blood pressure, though, you need something more potent," he says.

Get that potency by swallowing garlic capsules or tablets daily. Although that sounds like a simple suggestion, things can get a little confusing, because what's actually in those tablets or capsules depends on a wide array of processing methods. And the array of arguments about which process is best is just as wide.

Dr. Rountree recommends cutting through the controversy by finding a garlic product that's standardized for allicin, the beneficial natural constituent of garlic. It may be in the form of substances that convert to allicin in the body, so you'll measure your dose in "allicin potential." Dr. Rountree suggests taking capsules that provide 8,000 micrograms of allicin potential daily. You'll probably need to keep taking the above dosage for at least a month before seeing results. It's safe to take garlic indefinitely.

Hawthorn

Take two 500-milligram capsules or 1 teaspoon of tincture three times a day. The leaves, berries, and flowers of the hawthorn tree get standing ovations for their cardiovascular health benefits. Does that include helping to lower elevated blood pressure? You bet.

"Hawthorn is one of the most commonly used herbs for hypertension," says Ian Bier, N.D., Ph.D., a naturopathic physician, licensed acupuncturist, and natural medicine researcher in Portsmouth, New Hampshire. "It's very powerful yet very gentle. It takes a while, but it works."

Actually, hawthorn works a lot like conventionally prescribed medications, but it does so naturally and without side effects.

For high blood pressure, look for hawthorn standardized for a specific flavonoid (a natural plant nutrient) known as vitexin, Dr. Rountree says. The liquid extract of hawthorn in tincture form is not as potent as capsules, he says, but if you prefer that route, put a teaspoon in some water and drink it three times a day.

If you've been diagnosed with high blood pressure or other cardiovascular condition, you should not take hawthorn regularly for more than a few weeks without medical supervision. You should also have your blood pressure checked at least every 2 weeks. When it starts to come down, take one 500-milligram capsule or $\frac{1}{2}$ teaspoon of tincture three times a day, then reduce it to twice a day.

Reishi

Take 2,000 to 4,000 milligrams daily in capsule form. There's an all-star lineup of oriental mushrooms that natural and holistic physicians prescribe for lots of things. The best one for high blood pressure is reishi. "I recommend reishi a lot for blood pressure, both as a tonic (long-term preventive) and a medicinal," Dr. Rountree says. "It's a direct blood pressure reducer, it's very safe, and it has all kinds of other benefits, too."

You can get reishi in capsules at health food stores or by mail order. Dr. Rountree suggests finding them in concentrations that are strong enough to let you take 2 to 4 grams (2,000 to 4,000 milligrams) daily without having to swallow too many capsules. It's safe to take this dose forever.

Fast Facts

Cause: Sometimes, high blood pressure results from another condition, such as a kidney problem, a heart defect, a central nervous system disorder, or even an environmental factor such as lead exposure. Ninety percent of the time, however, the cause is unknown. It can be related to genetics, but often it can be linked to lifestyle factors such as poor diet, lack of exercise, or unmanaged stress.

Incidence: Blacks, the middle-aged, and the elderly are more prone to high blood pressure. People who are obese or drink heavily and women who take oral contraceptives are also at higher risk.

When to see the doctor: You should have your blood pressure checked by a doctor or other health professional at least once every 2 years. If it's higher than 140/90, your doctor will probably want to monitor it more often.

Motherwort

Take two to three droppers of tincture a day. Traditional Chinese Medicine uses the flowering herb motherwort extensively for controlling blood pressure. "It has a calming effect and also directly lowers blood pressure," Dr. Rountree says.

Motherwort is easily found in health food stores. The dose above is typical, according to Dr. Rountree, and it is safe for you to take on an ongoing basis. You can mix it with a glass of water or drink it straight.

Ginkgo and Hawthorn

Take a teaspoon of this tincture combination three times a day. Ginkgo is best-known as a brain herb, but it has cardiovascular benefits as well, including mild blood pressure–lowering effects. "Ginkgo dilates the peripheral vessels, and anything that does that will automatically bring the pressure down by giving the blood more room to move through," Dr. Bier says. "I would definitely throw it into a formula with hawthorn."

Dr. Bier recommends making your own formula from the tinctures, using twice as much hawthorn as ginkgo. Just buy a 1-ounce bottle of ginkgo and a 2-ounce bottle of hawthorn and pour the two together. Take the resulting formula mixed in a little water.

HIGH CHOLESTEROL

*Y*ou're either part of the solution or part of the problem.

If you're old enough to remember that stirring (if simplistic) call to action from the 1960s, you're old enough to be concerned about how much cholesterol is camped out in your arteries.

Indeed, a majority of adult Americans have at least borderline high cholesterol, and the levels rise with age. Rising along with those levels is your risk of heart attack, stroke, kidney disease, and other unpleasantries.

Turn that old slogan around, however, and you'll find some encouraging news for your cholesterol count: What's not part of the problem is part of the solution. You eat cholesterol and saturated fat when you eat animal products (the problem) but not when you eat plant foods (part of the solution). And when those plants are certain medicinal herbs, they can actually lower your cholesterol levels.

Thus, you get the most out of herbal remedies when you use them in tandem with good, healthy, cholesterol-lowering food choices. That advice holds true even with conventional cholesterol-lowering pharmaceutical drugs such as symvastatin (Zocor) or pravastatin (Pravachol). "It all comes down to diet," says George Milowe, M.D., a holistic physician in Saratoga Springs, New York.

It also comes down to saturated fats, which raise cholesterol levels even more than cholesterol consumed directly from meat and dairy products. Again, animal foods are the guiltiest suppliers of saturated fats, but there's a Benedict Arnold in the plant kingdom, too. When it comes to saturated fats, some vegetable oils could also be part of the problem, so besides cutting down on meat and dairy products, use vegetable oils with more monounsaturated fat (such as canola and olive oil), says Dr. Milowe.

Dr. Milowe also suggests that you help your herbal remedies by supplementing with antioxidants such as vitamins C and E, since cholesterol is even more harmful when it's oxidized. And, he says, you should eat more fish, flaxseed, and nuts. Not only can they substitute for meat, they also supply omega-3 fatty acids, which help protect blood vessel walls from the bad things that too much cholesterol does. "It's really a matter of getting back to basics," Dr. Milowe says. "Try to eat pure, simple, whole foods like fruits, nuts, seeds, and especially vegetables."

For the record, cholesterol is a victim of character assassination. We've all heard plenty about good cholesterol (HDL) and its evil twin (LDL). The truth is, though, that there's nothing inherently bad about either kind of cholesterol. In fact, your body makes its own cholesterol in just the right amounts to protect cell walls and build your sex hormones, among other things. Nothing bad about that, is there?

"The problems come when you have too much cholesterol circulating," Dr. Milowe says. "Then you have oxidized cholesterol damaging cells and artery walls, which can lead to arteriosclerosis (hardening of the arteries), one risk factor for a heart attack." The following herbs can help keep that from happening.

Garlic

Eat a clove or more a day, or take two to four 300- to 400-milligram capsules daily. Since HDL cholesterol routes excess cholesterol out of your body, it's good to increase it relative to LDL cholesterol. Garlic does just that, according to Ralph T. Golan, M.D., a holistic general practitioner in Seattle and author of *Optimal Wellness: Where Mainstream and Alternative Medicine Meet.* What's more, he says, there are plenty of studies showing that regular garlic consumption lowers overall levels of cholesterol in your bloodstream, which is exactly what you want.

So how do you get garlic's goodness into your body?

"Just eat it," Dr. Golan says. "For cardiovascular benefits, raw or cooked garlic seems to work quite well."

That's a pretty good piece of dietary news, since it means that the garlic-rich spaghetti sauce you love so much is as pleasing to your cardiovascular system as it is to your tastebuds. "But only if you eat spaghetti 5 days a week," points out Ian Bier, N.D., Ph.D., a naturopathic physician, licensed acupuncturist, and natural medicine researcher in Portsmouth, New Hampshire. "For garlic to work best in the long term, try to eat a clove or more a day, or as close to that as you can."

Now, working that much garlic into your daily diet may present something of a culinary challenge, especially if you're not a big fan of its taste. No problem. The simplest way to take garlic is to swallow capsules of powdered extract, which are easy to find at health food stores, drugstores, and even a lot of supermarkets. In fact, the only difficulty is the confusing variety of preparations available.

Your best bet, according to Robert Rountree, M.D., a holistic physician at the Helios Health Center in Boulder, Colorado, is to look for a product whose label promises 4,000 micrograms of allicin potential per capsule. (Garlic's botanical name is *Allium sativum*, and allicin is its principal active constituent.)

Taking any herbal remedies for high cholesterol is a long-term affair, so continue with your two daily garlic capsules for at least several months. "Pushing cholesterol down takes time," Dr. Bier says. "Check your cholesterol level again in 6 weeks if you really want, but be prepared to give it 6 months."

Guggul

Take three 500-milligram capsules daily with meals. Its name sounds like baby talk, but the small guggul tree from India yields a gummy resin that lowers LDL cholesterol, raises HDL cholesterol, and reduces overall cholesterol. "I've seen it dramatically lower cholesterol," Dr. Golan says. "I've had patients whose cholesterol levels have come down as much as 20 percent with guggul."

Also called gugulipid (which sounds even more like baby talk), the powdered extract is available in capsule form and usually standard-

Fast FACTS

Cause: Genetics can be a factor, especially for those with extremely high cholesterol levels, but far and away the main cause is the modern industrialized world's dietary imbalance in favor of meat and dairy products, which are rich in cholesterol and saturated fat.

Incidence: According to the American Heart Association, nearly 100 million American adults have cholesterol counts higher than the borderline-high cutoff point of 200 (meaning 200 milligrams of total cholesterol per deciliter of blood). That's more than half of the adult population. About 20 percent of adults exceed the 240 mark, which is considered high, with nothing borderline about it. Women on average have lower total cholesterol levels than men until the age of menopause, when the trend reverses.

When to see the doctor: Heart disease is silent until it's fairly well along, so it's important to have your cholesterol checked and have it checked early. Having a doctor monitor your risk factors is key to preventing heart disease.

---

ized for an active constituent called guggulsterone. At the dosage above, you should get a daily total of 75 milligrams of guggulsterone. Once you are able to optimize your cholesterol through diet, exercise, and other lifestyle changes, you don't need to continue taking guggul, says Dr. Golan.

Hawthorn

Take 2,000 milligrams daily in capsule form or 1 teaspoon of tincture two to four times a day. Hawthorn's the best herb there is for your heart, which is too often the victim when cholesterol accumulates in your bloodstream. That by itself is enough reason to take hawthorn if you have high cholesterol. But here's another one: "There's also some research that shows that hawthorn lowers cholesterol," Dr. Milowe says.

Hawthorn is best when it's standardized for a flavonoid called vitexin. If you prefer the liquid extract, Dr. Milowe suggests a 1:5 (1 part hawthorn to 5 parts alcohol) tincture.

You can take hawthorn indefinitely, but if you have any type of cardiovascular condition, talk to your physician before starting, advises Dr. Milowe.

Dandelion

Take 1 teaspoon of tincture three times a day. Natural healers often concentrate on the connection between blood cholesterol and your liver.

"A neglected liver can really elevate cholesterol," says Pamela Sky Jeanne, R.N., N.D., a naturopathic family physician in Gresham, Oregon. "Your digestive system may not be eliminating the cholesterol, or your liver may be overproducing it."

That's where dandelion root can help. Although there's no direct evidence linking dandelion to reduced cholesterol levels, there's no doubt that it's a great herb for your liver, according to naturopathic doctors. It's easy to find, but make sure the tincture is made from the root, says Dr. Jeanne. Use the bottle's dropper to fill a teaspoon, put the tincture in a small amount of water, and drink it down. It's best to take dandelion for about 2 months and then stop for about 2 weeks, says Dr. Jeanne. You can then take it for another 2 months and continue cycling until your cholesterol is lowered.

HIVES

*T*he pale red swellings typical of hives (or urticaria, to give them their official name) show up in clusters on any part of the body and, like a freak snowstorm in May, usually disappear without a trace after a few hours.

Hobbs's Hives Helper

Fourth-generation herbalist and botanist Christopher Hobbs, of Santa Cruz, California, has his patients make an infusion of dried herbs to treat hives. According to Hobbs, who is also a professional member of the American Herbalists Guild, a licensed acupuncturist, and author of Handmade Medicines: Simple Recipes for Herbal Health, *the herbs in this formula are astringent, soothing, and healing.*

To make a compress, wrap about ¼ cup of wet herbs in a piece of muslin and apply it to the hives for 10 to 15 minutes. Soak the compress in the tea and reapply it, then repeat the whole process once more. Repeat for two or three sessions daily as needed. If the rash is hot and itchy, says Hobbs, blend several drops of peppermint essential oil into the herbs before applying the compress to your skin. Between sessions of using the compress, apply some St. John's wort infused oil to which a few drops of peppermint essential oil have been added.

- ⅞ **cup calendula flowers**
- ⅝ **cup witch hazel bark**
- ½ **cup gotu kola leaves**
- ½ **cup white oak bark**
- 10 **cups water**

Grind the calendula, witch hazel, gotu kola, and white oak. Place them in a large saucepan with the water and simmer, covered, for about 20 minutes. Remove from the heat and let cool before using.

Hives can be as small as kernels of corn or several inches across, and sometimes they band together to form one large swelling. They can burn. They can sting. But what they do best is itch. And itch. And itch.

What makes those bumps appear (and itch!) is blood plasma seeping out of tiny blood vessels in the skin, a reaction that's triggered by the release of a chemical called histamine. This histamine release may occur as a result of an allergic reaction to a certain food (nuts, chocolate, fish, tomatoes, eggs, fresh berries, and milk are all potential allergens) or a medication. Emotional stress or a simple infection like a cold can also be to blame. Often, though, the root cause remains a mystery.

Diet is certainly one of the most common causes. But as dermatologist Nia Terezakis, M.D., clinical professor of dermatology at Tulane University School of Medicine and Louisiana State University School of Medicine, both in New Orleans, points out, "You can run the bills up into the thousands of dollars doing tests, but that's not likely to cure your hives." She counsels her patients to avoid anything packaged, prepared, or canned and to stick to fresh vegetables and meats without hormones.

Identifying the triggering factor is the best treatment of all, but because that can be such a challenge, doctors often prescribe antihistamines in the meantime to deal with the symptoms. In severe cases, oral steroids are sometimes used, although there are many adverse effects associated with their long-term use. Other simple remedies that help alleviate the itching are cool compresses and soaking baths.

On the herbal front, there are several plants that have antihistaminic or anti-itching properties that can be very effective. Naturopathic doctors also often prescribe supplemental bioflavonoids and vitamin C to reduce the inflammation.

If itchy hives have you wanting to jump out of your skin, try some of these natural herbal remedies. You'll probably have some of them handy in your pantry.

Oats

Soak in a lukewarm oatmeal bath to soothe the itch until you feel relaxed. You don't want to take a hot bath, says Thomas Kruzel, N.D., former president of the American Association of Naturopathic Physicians, who practices in Portland, Oregon, because it can be irritating to the skin. "I recommend what we call a neutral bath, just a degree or two over body temperature." Adding oatmeal has an immediately soothing effect, says Dr. Kruzel.

Put 2 cups of oatmeal, the type called old-fashioned (any brand is fine), in a white sock and let the water from the faucet run through it into the tub. Between baths, you can get some relief by putting a

Fast FACTS

Cause: Hives are caused by a chemical called histamine that makes blood plasma leak out of small blood vessels in the skin. Often, the release of histamine is caused by an allergic reaction to a particular food or medication. Physical factors such as a fever and exercise can also bring on a bout of hives. Often it's impossible to figure out why hives happen.

Incidence: Hives are extremely common. Ten to 20 percent of the population will have at least one outbreak in their lifetimes.

When to see the doctor: If your hives don't go away on their own within a few hours, or if you start to have trouble breathing or notice swelling around your lips, see your doctor or go to the emergency room immediately.

cup of oatmeal in a sock or piece of muslin, wetting it, and dabbing it on your skin. Let it dry without rinsing it off so that the emollients in the oats can form a natural, protective barrier on your skin.

Another option is to pick up a colloidal oatmeal product like Aveeno, which is available in health food stores and some drugstores. You can add this oatmeal powder and oil mixture directly to the bathwater according to the label instructions.

Lavender

Smooth a thin layer of essential oil onto acute hives as needed. Lavender oil helps soothe prickly, irritated skin because of its calming effect on the nervous system, says Christopher Robbins, a member of Britain's National Institute of Medical Herbalists who practices herbal medicine in Ross-on-Wye, Herefordshire, England, and has written several books, including *The Natural Pharmacy*. Buy the essential oil and apply it directly to the hives.

Tarragon, Basil, Chamomile, Fennel, and Oregano

For chronic hives, make a strong tea and drink a cup two or three times a day. Some herbs, such as the ones that go into this tea, have natural antihistaminic properties that make them useful for treating hives. This remedy, says Dr. Kruzel, is best for hives that are a persistent problem, because its effects build up over time.

Put 1 tablespoon of each dried herb in a canning jar. Boil 5 cups of water and pour it over the herbs. Put the jar in the refrigerator, leaving the herbs in the tea to strengthen the infusion. Two or three times a day, pour some tea into a cup, heat it, and drink. If you're trying to prevent an outbreak, drink a cup once a day with a meal. If you develop digestive problems, cut back until the side effects subside.

Nettle

Take two 300-milligram capsules three times a day for 7 days. Nettle is another herb that acts as a natural antihistamine. You could follow the example of the ancient yogis, who made a stew out of the herb, but it tastes like bitter gruel, according to William Wulsin, N.D., who has a naturopathic family practice in Seattle. "The capsules are much more palatable," he says. Discontinue this treatment after 7 days if you do not see any improvement.

Green Tea

Drink a cup twice a day. Compounds called catechins that are found in green tea are powerful antioxidants, says Tammy Alex, N.D., a naturopathic doctor based in Guilford, Connecticut. If you tend to get hives often, green tea can be helpful for stabilizing the cell membranes and preventing breakouts. Add 1 tablespoon of tea to 1 cup of boiling water, steep for 10 minutes, and drink. Not only is it safe to drink green tea long-term, it's a good idea because it has many health benefits, says Dr. Alex.

INCONTINENCE

*I*f you're too embarrassed to discuss incontinence with your doctor, you're not alone. In a national survey, women ranked talking to their doctors about incontinence higher on the embarrassment scale than problems with birth control, family planning, or menopause. Only problems with sexual performance ranked higher. In fact, doctors estimate that nearly half of the 15 million people who are affected by incontinence choose to suffer in silence rather than seek treatment.

"Fear of having an accident can be so acute that people with bladder problems may voluntarily restrict their lives, giving up outings and social activities," says Andrew Weil, M.D., director of the program in integrative medicine at the University of Arizona College of Medicine in Tucson and author of *8 Weeks to Optimum Health*. "Yet, I assure my patients that urinary incontinence is treatable 90 percent of the time," he says.

The herbs listed here will promote healing and toning of the muscle and nerve tissue of the kidneys, bladder, and urethra. You won't see improvement in a day or even a week, but you should begin to notice a better sense of control in about a month.

Horsetail

Drink one cup of tea daily, or take 10 to 12 drops of alcohol-free extract twice a day for a month. Also called bottlebrush, horsetail is an abrasive plant that was once used to polish metal and wood. The primitive perennial contains large amounts of silica, which helps support the regeneration of connective tissue. If you have stress incontinence due to weak muscle tone, a daily dose of silica-rich horsetail tea combined with a regimen of Kegel exercises can help restore muscle tone in your urinary tract, says Lynn Newman, a professional member of the American Herbalists Guild and a medical herbalist in

Glen Head, New York. To do Kegels, you simply clench and unclench the pelvic muscles that control urine flow,

Since a large proportion of its silica content is water soluble, take horsetail as a tea. Bring 1 cup of water to a boil, remove it from the heat, and add ½ teaspoon of dried herb. Steep for 15 to 20 minutes, then strain. Since horsetail can irritate the digestive tract if used daily for more than 6 weeks, Newman recommends the following monthly routine: Drink a cup of tea every day for a month, take a week off, then resume taking the tea for another month.

If you take horsetail as an extract, says Newman, add each dose to 1 cup of water and adhere to the same monthly pattern as with the tea.

To get the maximum benefit from the herb, your daily routine should also include three sets of Kegel exercises. Start with 10 contractions per set and work up to 30.

Hawthorn

Take ¼ teaspoon of solid extract three times a day. Used primarily for heart and circulatory disorders, a daily dose of hawthorn can also promote healing of the muscles, ligaments, and nerve tissue of the urinary tract, says Erik Von Kiel, M.D., D.O., a holistic physician in Allentown, Pennsylvania. The concentrated extract is a tarlike syrup. You can lick it off a spoon or make tea by adding ¼ teaspoon to 1 cup of warm water. Let the mixture stand for 10 minutes before drinking. You can also use a tea bag instead of the extract.

Known as a symbol of hope in the Middle Ages, hawthorn is a powerful antioxidant whose main medicinal benefit comes from its high bioflavonoid content. Although you may see some improvement after taking it regularly for a week, typically it may be 1 to 3 months before you notice more bladder control. You can use the same dose daily or every other day for a year or longer, says Dr. Von Kiel.

Corn Silk and Agrimony

Every day, drink three cups of tea. An overactive, irritated bladder can send you running to the bathroom. Corn silk and agrimony work together to soothe the irritation, says Claudia Wingo, R.N., a medical

Fast FACTS

Cause: Bladder infections, constipation, and some medications, such as diuretics, pain relievers, sedatives, cold remedies, and medicines for depression and high blood pressure, can all cause temporary, reversible loss of control. Childbirth may stretch muscles or damage nerve tissue, interfering with normal urination. In postmenopausal women, incontinence may result from thinning of the tissues in the urinary tract and the sagging of the pelvic floor as estrogen levels drop.

Incidence: More than 15 million people—nearly 85 percent of them women—in the United States have some form of urinary incontinence. Female stress incontinence, which results from strain on the bladder caused by coughing or sneezing, is the most common type, accounting for about 75 percent of cases seen by doctors. Although incidence increases with age, loss of bladder control is not an inevitable part of aging.

When to see the doctor: You need to call your doctor if you experience an abrupt loss of bladder control. It can indicate a serious disease or disorder such as cancer, diabetes, stroke, Parkinson's disease, multiple sclerosis, or, in men, an enlarged prostate gland.

herbalist in College Park, Maryland, and a member of the National Herbalists Association of Australia.

As a treatment for incontinence when bladder irritation is the cause, agrimony works best in combination with corn silk. Known for its diuretic properties, corn silk may seem like an herb to avoid if you want to regain control of your bladder. Actually, the nourishing tea made from the stamens of this everyday vegetable contains mucilage that helps soothe the walls of the urinary tract, explains Silena Heron, N.D., adjunct professor at Southwest College of Naturopathic Medicine and Health Sciences in Tempe, Arizona, and vice president of the Botanical Medicine Academy.

Finding good-quality corn silk can be a challenge. It's often simpler just to use your own, says Dr. Heron. Buy organic corn on the cob and save the silk as you husk the corn. Trim away any brown or dried-up areas. Chop it and use it in salads or dry it in a food dehydrator or on a ventilated rack. The silk tastes like fresh corn.

To make sure that you always have a supply of ready-to-drink tea on hand, make it at night before you go to bed, says Wingo. Place 1 heaping tablespoon of a blend of equal parts dried corn silk and agrimony in a 1-quart jar. Cover the herbs with boiling water and steep overnight. "You'll have a nice, strong tea the next day," she says. You can use this remedy daily for up to a year.

Kava Kava

Take 30 drops of tincture with water three times a day. While it may be better-known for its power to induce a calm, euphoric state of mind, kava is a valuable herb to help settle an irritable bladder, says Wingo. As you age, your bladder can become overactive, causing contractions that are too strong to control; this is called urge incontinence. You feel an overwhelming urge to urinate but can't get to the bathroom before your bladder releases the urine. Taking kava can help quiet and soothe the bladder and the pressing urge to urinate. But don't take it before going to bed, she advises, as it can increase urination through the night.

INFERTILITY IN MEN

*R*eproduction should be easy, but it's not. Here are the facts: It's estimated that roughly 15 percent of couples in the United States have some sort of problem with fertility, and the problem resides with the male partner in about one-third of the cases.

A man can be infertile for a number of reasons: His sperm count may be low, the sperm may be misshapen, or they may simply be lousy swimmers, unable to make it all the way to their destination.

Experts continue to debate whether sperm counts worldwide may be dropping. We do know that in a Finnish study, the percentage of men with normal sperm counts dropped from 56 percent in 1981 to 27 percent 10 years later. A more recent study shows a steady rate of decline in sperm counts for North America and Europe, with inconclusive results for non-Western countries. If you're among those concerned about this problem, read on.

Certain steps will help increase your chances of conceiving. If you smoke, quit now, because nicotine damages sperm in a number of ways. Make sure that you're getting enough vitamin C and E, two antioxidants that have been shown to help sperm, says John J. Mulcahy, M.D., professor of urology at Indiana University Medical Center in Bloomington. And although experts disagree, it may help to ditch your tight jeans and switch to more loose-fitting cotton trousers that allow air to circulate. Jeans aren't very porous, says Dr. Mulcahy, and they trap body heat in the groin, possibly increasing the internal temperature and harming sperm motility and production.

Herbs can also play a role in successful conception. You should discuss the pros and cons of your proposed fertility regimen with a qualified practitioner, and in most cases, you'll want to discontinue this particular herbal regimen once your partner has conceived. But here are some male fertility boosters that experts recommend.

Pygeum

Take a capsule containing 100 to 200 milligrams each day. This African tree bark extract is a common treatment for enlarged prostate, as it's known to help relieve some urinary symptoms. However, pygeum also causes an increase in prostate secretions, improving the composition of semen and the odds for conception, says Steven Rissman, N.D., a naturopathic physician at American WholeHealth in Cherry Creek, Colorado.

Fast Facts

Cause: Male infertility can be traced to sperm production mishaps. Either not enough sperm are produced, the sperm aren't shaped correctly, or they don't swim well enough. A common reason for these defects is a varicocele, a vein malfunction located near the testicle that drives up the testicular temperature and harms sperm. Environmental and health factors also play a role.

Incidence: It's estimated that roughly 5 percent of men in the United States have some problems with fertility.

When to see the doctor: If you and your partner have been trying to conceive for a year without success, see a fertility specialist.

Ginger

Take two capsules totaling 1,000 milligrams a day. Ginger has been shown to enhance sperm count and motility, says Steven Margolis, M.D., an alternative family physician in Sterling Heights, Michigan. "Take the ginger along with a 500-milligram dose of vitamin C," he says. Vitamin C is an antioxidant that has a protective effect on sperm, and coupled with ginger, it packs a serious pro-fertility punch.

Flaxseed

Take 1 tablespoon of oil every day. This oil can be found in the refrigerated or frozen foods section of health food stores. Why is it important for fertility? Most other oils and shortenings are extremely high in omega-6 and omega-9 fatty acids, which are fairly toxic to male reproductive function, says Dr. Margolis. So much so, in fact, that a compound from cottonseed oil, which is frequently used to cook potato chips and corn chips, is being investigated for possible use in a male birth control pill, he adds.

Flaxseed oil, on the other hand, is one of the best vegetable sources of omega-3 fatty acids, associated with heart health and gland function. Research in Germany has indicated that supplementation with flaxseed oil improves circulation throughout the body, increases thyroid function, and enables the body to produce more sex hormones that are beneficial to fertility, Dr. Margolis says.

Asian Ginseng

Take 100- to 200-milligram capsules that provide a total of 15 milligrams of ginsenosides daily. Asian ginseng, also called panax, Chinese, or Korean ginseng, is a traditional Chinese virility tonic. In a number of animal studies, it has been shown to increase testosterone, testicle size, and sperm formation. It's commonly available. "Check the label so you know the amount of ginsenosides in each capsule," says Dr. Rissman.

Siberian Ginseng

Take capsules containing 100 to 200 milligrams three times a day. This form of ginseng also appears to have fertility benefits. "It's been shown to increase testosterone and sperm counts," says Dr. Rissman. An animal study confirmed this and showed that boosting sperm counts in such a manner also strengthened reproductive capacity. Siberian ginseng is not considered to be as effective as Asian ginseng, but they can be taken together without side effects. If you take the combination product, your total daily dose should be 100 to 200 milligrams, says Dr. Rissman.

Ashwaganda

Take capsules containing 250 milligrams twice a day. This Indian herb dates back 500 years as a fertility treatment, says Dr. Margolis. It has a positive effect throughout the reproductive system, stimulating hormone production and improving the composition of semen.

INFERTILITY IN WOMEN

*B*abies require loads of energy and tons of time from the mothers who love them. Because of that, there's a cosmic logic in Mother Nature's decree that babies are less likely to come along the older a woman gets. In fact, beyond age 35, conception rates for women fall significantly. But how do we explain the situation when a young woman—even one with ample energy and more than enough time on her hands—has trouble conceiving? We call it infertility.

Forty percent of the time, the issue of infertility can be narrowed down to the female half of the equation. For three out of four infertile women, there are procedures and prescription drugs that can solve the problem. There remains a group of women, however, who will be told that they have "unexplained" infertility. For them, even expensive, uncomfortable treatments can't help.

With your doctor's supervision, the following herbal remedies can be another step to take in your quest for a family. If you've tried other treatments without success, herbs may be just the thing to make a gentle miracle possible.

Chasteberry

Take 175 milligrams in capsule form once a day or 40 drops of tincture each morning until your periods are regular. A common cause of infertility in women is a problem called anovulation, which happens when an ovary doesn't release a monthly egg as it should. Signs of anovulation include a lack of periods or periods that are unpredictable. Getting your menstrual cycle back on track is the first step toward making ovulation—and conception—possible, says Mercedes Cameron, M.D., family practitioner at The Woman's Place at St. Mary's Hospital in Grand Junction, Colorado. This herb has hor-

Fast FACTS

Cause: Infertility in women can be caused by many factors. Age, sexually transmitted diseases, smoking, certain drugs, environmental toxins, and extremely low body fat can all contribute to making conception difficult or impossible.

In addition, reproductive system disorders (including uterine fibroids or cysts), lack of ovulation, and too much or too little of certain hormones will prevent pregnancy.

Incidence: Between 10 and 20 percent of married couples in America are infertile, including five million women.

When to see the doctor: Most couples conceive within 6 months when having regular, unprotected sex. If you have been trying to conceive for at least that long with no success, a visit to your obstetrician/gynecologist is in order. She can examine you to be sure there isn't a physical problem that may be preventing conception.

If you are over age 35 and haven't conceived after a year of trying, seek out a doctor who specializes in infertility. You'll need her supervision to try herbs or other medical treatments to help you conceive.

---

monelike actions that have a proven balancing effect on menstrual irregularities.

Progesterone is a female hormone that is normally balanced by another hormone, estrogen. While some herbs have estrogen-like effects in the body, chasteberry is similar to progesterone, says Dr. Cameron. Since anovulation may cause a lack of progesterone that results in irregular periods, the extra hormonelike action provided by chasteberry can be just enough to set things right. Whichever form of chasteberry you take, you'll have to take it for 3 to 6 months, until your periods become regular.

Once your periods are fairly regular again, Dr. Cameron recommends stopping the chasteberry *before* you attempt to become pregnant. "My feelings about herbs and pregnancy are the same as for prescription medicine," she says. "None is best, especially for the first trimester."

Red Clover, Nettle, Catnip, and Partridgeberry

Drink two cups of this tea daily until conception. Herbal tea is a time-honored way to assist fertility, says Dr. Cameron. The herbs in this particular recipe have effects that can help conception occur naturally.

Red clover has estrogen-like effects, nettle helps restore proper reproductive functioning, catnip has a relaxing effect, and partridgeberry (also known as squaw vine) is a tonic herb that has additional hormone-balancing actions.

Mix equal parts of the dried herbs together in a bowl. For each cup of tea that you're making, put 1 rounded tablespoon of the mixture into a teapot. Add 1 cup of boiling water per serving, cover, and steep for 5 to 10 minutes (depending on the strength you prefer). Pour the tea through a strainer into a mug.

When you become pregnant, you should stop drinking this tea. While it's probably completely safe, says Dr. Cameron, there's no reason to use these herbs once infertility has been overcome.

INFLAMMATORY BOWEL DISEASE

*I*nflammatory bowel disease (IBD) consists mostly of three disorders, Crohn's disease, ulcerative colitis, and gastritis, which is really just a general term for inflammation of the gastrointestinal tract. Beyond that, you'd be surprised how little experts know about these conditions. It's a mystery, for example, why some people get it and some don't, although you'll find more theories about IBD than about JFK's assassination.

The differences between the two major types of IBD are largely matters of location and how deeply the inflammation penetrates the bowel wall. Ulcerative colitis remains mostly in the colon, while Crohn's can strike any part of the intestine. In either case, part of the digestive tract is inflamed and possibly scarred by ulcers and abscesses. IBD symptoms—diarrhea up to 10 to 20 times a day, bloody stool, abdominal pain, fever, and even eye problems—are no picnic either.

The most common conventional course of action is to hit IBD with rounds of corticosteroids, powerful hormones that help reduce the inflammation and rebuild the tissue that's being destroyed in your digestive tract. Antibiotics and immune system–suppressing drugs may also be used.

As you can imagine, complex rounds of powerful pharmaceuticals bring with them some undesirable side effects, such as osteoporosis, cataracts, high blood pressure, mood changes, and even a change in the way your body stores fat, resulting in a swollen-looking face and torso.

That's where herbs can play a significant role, says Zoltan P. Rona, M.D., a Toronto physician, former president of the Canadian Holistic Medical Association, and author of *The Joy of Health*. The herbs used to treat IBD are far less toxic than these drugs and often work with considerable success, he says. Here are several doctors' top herbal remedies.

Cat's Claw

Take 300 milligrams in capsule form twice a day with meals until symptoms subside. Cat's claw has been used since ancient times by the native population of Peru to treat a variety of conditions, says Mark J. S. Miller, Ph.D., professor of pediatrics and physiology at Albany Medical College in New York. And when Dr. Miller and a colleague began testing cat's claw, they found its folk use justified.

Cat's claw is a powerful antioxidant, and that's good news for you because mounting evidence shows that oxidants play a role in chronic gut inflammations like IBD. The herb is also an anti-inflammatory, effectively taking the *I* out of IBD.

"It's really good for that," says Dr. Miller. "Impressively so. And we've never seen the side effects associated with steroids." To get maximum benefits from cat's claw, it's important to know how it was manufactured, he adds.

The dosage above is for cat's claw that's been atomized, or ground exceptionally fine. If the herb has only been pulverized, a less-refined form, you'll need to increase the dosage to 1,500 milligrams twice daily with meals until symptoms subside, says Dr. Miller. The reason for this is that with the cruder form, fewer of the active compounds are digested.

How do you tell the difference? It's easy. It won't say on the label which method was used, but when you get home, break open a capsule and pour the powdered herb into a glass of water. If most of it settles to the bottom without dissolving, it was pulverized, so you should take the higher dose.

Licorice

Take one or two chewable tablets of DGL four to six times daily until symptoms subside. Licorice contains flavonoids that have the ability to reduce intestinal inflammation, says Dr. Rona. DGL (deglycyrrhizinated licorice) is a modified form of licorice root that contains no glycyrrhizin, a compound that can raise blood pressure and deplete potassium stores in the body. DGL chewable tablets have no such side effects, and they're a relatively pleasant way to get the medicine down.

Quercetin

Take 500 to 1,000 milligrams in capsule form 15 to 30 minutes before meals as a preventive measure. The last time you cooked up a couple of onions, you probably threw away the parchmentlike skins. Little did you know that you were tossing out a highly effective treatment for IBD.

Onion skins are high in a compound called quercetin. But have no fear, says Dr. Rona, you don't have to choke down crispy skins to get the benefits of the compound. Simply pick some up in capsule form at a health food store.

Many people with IBD feel worse right after they eat because their bodies sometimes release histamines in response to the food

Fast FACTS

Cause: No one is sure what causes inflammatory bowel disease. There may be a genetic link, as it sometimes runs in families, and environment may also play a role. Other theories include food allergies, bacterial and viral infections, and low-fiber diets.

Incidence: Fewer than 1 percent of the population has IBD. That number is even less in the developing world, where it is virtually unheard of. For reasons that aren't clear, Crohn's disease, one type of IBD, was on the rise for a while in Western society, but it has stabilized in recent years.

When to see the doctor: If you have any of the forms of IBD, you should be under the regular care of a doctor. Because some forms of the disease can lead to bowel cancer, it needs to be monitored closely. If a major change, such as increased blood in your stool, fever, or severe pain, occurs between your regular appointments, see your doctor as soon as possible.

---

traveling through their guts, similar to an allergic reaction. Quercetin helps prevent that histamine release by stabilizing cell membranes.

Slippery Elm

Eat this as a porridge up to three times a day until symptoms subside. Slippery elm has compounds that soothe the intestinal tract, says Carolyn DeMarco, M.D., a physician in Winlaw, British Columbia, and a member of the advisory board of Dominion Herbal College in Burnaby.

To get the gut-mellowing effects of slippery elm, mix 1 to 2 teaspoons of the powder with enough warm water or milk to give it the consistency of porridge, says Dr. DeMarco.

Robert's Formula

Take according to package directions. According to legend, a sailor named Robert began using plants recommended to him by various herbalists in each of the ports he visited. Eventually, the individual herbs were combined into the present-day mixture called Robert's Formula.

There are slight variations among manufacturers, says Dr. DeMarco. Ideally, you should look for a product that contains marshmallow root, slippery elm, echinacea, geranium, goldenseal, and pokeroot. Follow the dosage instructions on the brand you buy. This grab bag of herbs attacks IBD from numerous angles. Pokeroot, for example, helps heal the lining of your bowel, while echinacea boosts immunity.

Ginger

Take two to four 500-milligram capsules four to six times a day until symptoms subside. Ginger contains zingibain, a special kind of enzyme that chemically breaks down proteins. Some meat tenderizers work because of this type of enzyme.

No, you're not a T-bone in need of tenderizing, but zingibain can help because it has anti-inflammatory properties. This, says Dr. Rona, makes it ideal for IBD. Ginger also cuts down on the nausea that sometimes strikes those with IBD, and it's good for promoting an appetite. That's beneficial because people with IBD are prone to weight loss.

INSECT BITES AND STINGS

*W*hen you consider that there are more species of insects—almost a million that we know about—than of any other animal in the world, it's not surprising that once in a while, they invade our space and get a little more cozy with us than we'd like.

When an insect alights on your exposed skin, he'll either settle in for a tasty snack or jab you with his stinger and beat a swift re-treat. Mosquitoes, fleas, biting flies, and midges are the biters out to suck our blood, and it's the saliva they inject into our skin while feeding that causes all that nasty itching, redness, and swelling.

Stingers sting out of self-defense, not a hearty appetite, but if you cross paths with a honeybee, a velvet ant, a hornet, or a wasp, it can feel like an all-out attack. The piercing pain of an insect sting usually disappears quickly, but the redness and swelling can stick around for quite a while.

Honeybees, by the way, are the only stinging insects that leave stingers in their victims. To remove one, don't use tweezers—that will push more venom into the sting. Instead, use something flat and hard such as a butter knife or credit card. Carefully brush the knife or card across the sting with the edge against your skin. This should safely remove the stinger.

Here are a few herbs to quell the itch or sting of an insect assault, plus a few that will make you seem less appetizing to those biting bugs.

Aloe

Dab on gel as needed to stop the itch. "Aloe vera is one of the best anti-itch medicines you can find," says Eric A. Weiss, M.D., assistant professor and associate director of emergency medicine at Stanford University Medical Center and founder of Adventure Medical Kits, an Oakland, California–based company that makes first-aid kits that include both conventional and herbal remedies. "I like it because it's been studied medically as well as appearing through the ages in folklore," he says. "It's been found to be very effective, with no known side effects."

You can find pure aloe gel on the shelves of health food stores. Alternatively, you can grow your own plant on the kitchen windowsill. Simply pull off one of the spiky leaves and squeeze out the thick gel.

Witch Hazel

Apply a paste of witch hazel and baking soda, leave it on for about 10 minutes, then rinse. Witch hazel is a wonderful anti-inflammatory that can soothe the itchies, says William Dvorine, M.D., former chief of dermatology at St. Agnes Hospital in Baltimore and author of *The Dermatologist's Guide to Home Skin Treatment*. Take a tablespoon of baking soda and add enough witch hazel to make a paste. You may reapply it every few hours until the itch is gone.

St. John's Wort

Make a paste with bentonite clay and St. John's wort oil and smear it on a bee sting to draw out the venom. You can find bentonite clay at many health food stores. Mix a couple of drops of St. John's wort into the clay to make the paste, says Whitney Miller, N.D., a naturopathic doctor who has a family practice in New London and Colchester, Connecticut. The strong drawing action will help suck the venom right out of the sting, giving you welcome relief. Because of its anti-inflammatory properties, the St. John's wort oil will help alleviate some of the pain. Leave it on until the pain is gone.

Papaya

Slap a slice of fresh papaya on a sting, or make a paste with meat tenderizer containing papain. "If I could find fresh papaya, that's what I'd use," says Mark Stengler, N.D., a naturopathic doctor in Oceanside, California, and author of *The Natural Physician: Your Health Guide to Common Ailments*. If you don't have fresh papaya, a paste of meat tenderizer (the kind that contains papain) and water can also effectively neutralize the venom. Leave either the papaya or meat tenderizer on the sting for about an hour.

Garlic

Crush a clove and apply it directly to the bite. "If garlic bulbs were sold in the drugstore, they would be marketed as broad-spectrum antibacterial agents," says Dr. Stengler. This pantry staple has both antibacterial and antiviral properties, making it one of the most useful (and most readily available) herbs around. According to Dr. Stengler, the oil in garlic helps relieve the pain right away.

He also recommends garlic as an insect repellent. "If you start eating garlic a couple of weeks before you go on a camping trip, you'll have it in your system, and it will start to come through your skin, repelling mosquitoes, ticks, and other insects." Of course, you may repel your friends, too, but if that's the price you have to pay for being bug-free, perhaps it's worth it. Rubbing raw garlic on your skin will do the trick, too.

Lavender

Put a drop of pure essential oil on the sting. "I found out by accident that lavender works well," says Christopher Robbins, a member of Britain's National Institute of Medical Herbalists who practices herbal medicine in Ross-on-Wye, Herefordshire, England, and has written several books, including *The Natural Pharmacy*.

A colleague's small daughter had been stung on the face by a wasp and was screaming so loud that no one could hear themselves think. Robbins grabbed a vial of lavender oil and put a drop on the sting. Two minutes later, the child stopped screaming.

Robbins isn't sure why the remedy worked so rapidly. "I have a hunch that it could have been neutralizing the alkaline venom, but we also know it's a very good nervine," he says. "It may have just calmed the nerve endings."

Most essential oils will irritate the skin if used undiluted. For spot treatment, lavender oil is an exception to the rule, says Mindy Green, a founder and professional member of the American Herbalists Guild, director of educational services at the Herb Research Foundation in Boulder, Colorado, and co-author of *Aromatherapy: A Complete Guide to the Healing Art*. However, Green cautions, "Don't use it undiluted on large areas such as your entire back or the whole body."

Peppermint

Stop the itch with a bit of peppermint toothpaste. Peppermint oil is a great bite soother, but it has to be the right amount. On its own, the oil is too powerful to use on human skin. Use mint toothpaste instead, says Cathryn Flanagan, N.D., a naturopathic physician in Old

Saybrook, Connecticut. "If you're out camping and that's all you have at your disposal, it's a good choice because of the peppermint oils in it," she says. "The nongel kind works better because it's already in a paste and has the action to draw irritants from the bite." Keep the paste on until it dries.

Lemon

Scratch that itch with half a lemon. However much people tell you not to scratch, sometimes you just have to. The problem is that people often get secondary infections from scratching their bites with dirty fingers, says clinical herbalist 7Song, a professional member of the American Herbalists Guild and director of the Northeast School of Botanical Medicine in Ithaca, New York. "What I do is cut a lemon in half and scratch with the soft, pulpy side of it," he says. The logic? The acid in the lemon soothes the itch a little, and you're much less likely to rupture the bite.

California Poppy

Take two droppers of tincture right after you've been stung and one dropper every 2 hours for the rest of the day. 7Song recommends taking small amounts of California poppy, an herb that's well-known as a mild sedative, to relax frayed nerves. "It'll bring you down a little from the trauma and help you breathe again," he says. The dosage depends on body type. If you're tall or heavy, start with two droppers. Otherwise, one should be sufficient.

Onion

Cut a slice of white onion and tape it onto a sting for 1 hour. An old folk remedy, onion is still recommended by herbalists, although there's little consensus on why or how it works. "It's very cooling and moist, and it also has a drawing action," says Dr. Stengler. Don't mash the onion, he says; just cut a nice slice and tape it onto the sting. Be sure to remove the stinger first.

Fast FACTS

Cause: Insect bites happen when a mosquito, flea, biting fly, or midge inserts its mouth parts into your skin and removes a drop of blood. The saliva that's injected while the bug is enjoying his dinner is what causes the itching, redness, and swelling. Stings are the result of a bee, wasp, or ant injecting a poison into your skin with its stinger, causing sharp pain followed by swelling and redness.

Incidence: With nearly a million different species populating the world, insects are everywhere, and unless you seal yourself off from nature completely, being bitten or stung is just part of life's rich tapestry.

When to see the doctor: Some people experience severe allergic reactions when they're stung by a bee. If you find that you're having trouble breathing, notice that your lips and throat are swelling, or experience faintness, confusion, a rapid heartbeat, or hives after a sting, seek emergency care immediately. If your allergic reaction is less severe, with symptoms of nausea, intestinal cramps, diarrhea, or a swelling larger than 2 inches in diameter at the site, call your family doctor.

Most spider bites are harmless, but if there's excessive swelling at the site or you have breathing problems, seek care immediately. Insect bites rarely require professional treatment, but you should call your doctor if a bitten area of skin becomes excessively red, swollen, warm, and tender, or if your temperature rises above 101°F. This could indicate an infection.

Eucalyptus and Lemon

Add 1 part lemon-scented essential oil to 4 parts white vinegar and use as a repellent as needed. Most recipes for herbal insect repellents have a list of ingredients as long as your forearm. Jeanne Rose, San Francisco aroma herbalist and author of *The World of Aromatherapy*, has a much simpler solution—lemon-scented eucalyptus essential oil. One of the reasons Rose likes to use this oil instead of the commercial citronella-based repellents is that she says it has a much more pleasant odor and contains more of the mosquito repellent components citronellol and citronellal.

Mix up the repellent in a plastic spray bottle, using 10 drops of oil for every 4 ounces of water, and be sure to shake it well before spraying it on your body. Reapply it as often as needed, depending on how much you sweat, says Rose.

INSOMNIA

$\mathcal{T}$he great mezzo-soprano Marilyn Horne recommends reading an opera score if you can't sleep. "It will bore you to death," she says.

Of course, there's no need to resort to measures quite that drastic. While an inability to get to sleep, or to stay asleep, can be related to problems with physical or mental health, insomnia is more frequently a temporary inconvenience brought on by stress, extreme temperature, or noise.

For people who experience occasional sleepless nights, herbs are an option. Certain roots, flowers, and leaves are gentle alternatives to over-the-counter or prescription medications that often leave grogginess in their wake. In particular, the four herbs recommended here have repeatedly been shown to be effective in folk use, and they have been scrutinized for safety by scientific review.

Valerian

Take ½ to 1 teaspoon (1 to 3 milliliters) of tincture 1 hour before bedtime. Valerian root is a classic herbal insomnia remedy that really works. In some ways, it does the job better than prescription or over-the-counter sleep aids.

Herbal Sleepytime Pillow

Using tiny, hand-made pillows stuffed with sleep-inducing herbs is a time-honored path to dreamland. And they work well for everyone, including children and the elderly, says Phoebe Reeve, a professional member of the American Herbalists Guild and an herbalist in Winchester, Virginia. "It's something that's beautiful and natural, and that in itself is soothing," she says. "Plus, the scent is physiologically and psychologically soporific." That means that the fragrance is relaxing for body and soul.

If you can't find all of these dried herbs, any combination or even just one can help you sleep better. The pillow is not meant to cradle your whole head when you sleep; instead, just place it near your nose when you lie down. "It's also something nice to hold onto while you sleep," says Reeve.

- **Cotton fabric such as muslin**
- **I tablespoon lavender**
- **I tablespoon chamomile**
- **I tablespoon hops**
- **I tablespoon mugwort**
- **I tablespoon rose**

Cut two small rectangles of the same size from the piece of fabric (Reeve recommends 4" by 4", but you can make yours a bit bigger if you prefer). Sew the right sides of the fabric together on three sides, then turn the pieces inside-out.

Mix the lavender, chamomile, hops, mugwort, and rose together. Use the mixture to stuff the pillow, then sew it shut.

To reactivate the scent of the herbs, sprinkle vodka or any odorless grain alcohol on the pillow and let it dry. Your pillow should remain effective for about a year, when you can refill it with a new batch of herbs.

"Most people do fine with it and don't experience any hangover effect the next day," says Connie Catellani, M.D., medical director of the Miro Center for Integrative Medicine in Evanston, Illinois. And, unlike prescription sleeping pills, valerian has virtually no addictive qualities.

Valerian is particularly helpful for the kind of sleeplessness that comes from watching the clock, says Dr. Catellani. If it seems that there just isn't enough time in your day to get a good night's sleep, valerian makes a good choice.

To avoid the awful taste of valerian tea, try a tincture. Tinctures are more concentrated than tea and tend to work faster than capsules. "Some people even put the drops under their tongues so the herb can be absorbed without having to go through the gastrointestinal tract," says Dr. Catellani.

Start small. You may find that just ½ teaspoon of tincture is enough to send you off to dreamland. On the other hand, should you need to increase the dose, 1 teaspoon is also a safe amount to take. It's okay to take valerian every day on a long-term basis, says Dr. Catellani, but she recommends that you take it only periodically, when you need extra help to fall asleep.

Passionflower

One hour before bedtime, take 4,000 to 8,000 milligrams of dried passionflower in single-herb capsules, or take a combination formula according to package directions. Passionflower, with its exotic-looking blooms, makes a strikingly beautiful houseplant. When dried and crushed and included in an herbal sleep formula, it also does an excellent job of alleviating nervous restlessness.

"Passionflower is often found in combination with valerian root," says Dr. Catellani. It's a safe combination that may work better than either herb alone. "They seem to enhance each other's effects, making the remedy more likely to work." It's okay to take these herbs on an ongoing basis, she says. Since you'll probably find capsules of passionflower in doses of less than 1,000 milligrams, you can expect to take a goodly number to get the effective amount.

Kava Kava

Take the equivalent (in capsules or tincture) of 60 to 120 milligrams of kavalactones 1 hour before bed. Kava kava's special at-

Fast FACTS

Cause: Short-term insomnia can be caused by stress, noise, hot or cold temperatures, jet lag, or the side effects of some medicines. Chronic sleeplessness may be due to depression or underlying physical problems such as kidney disease, heart failure, arthritis, asthma, sleep apnea, or restless legs syndrome. Caffeine or alcohol abuse can also contribute to an inability to sleep.

Incidence: Insomnia is a problem for people of all ages and both genders, although it seems to be more common in the elderly and in women. Estimates indicate that approximately 10 percent of American adults experience chronic insomnia. Prescription sleeping pills are used by 4 percent of the population yearly.

When to see the doctor: If lack of sleep is causing daytime sleepiness and impaired performance, see your doctor for an evaluation.

---

traction is its muscle-relaxant properties, which make it helpful for someone with muscle tension or pain who is seeking some restful sleep.

Kava also counters anxiety, another common cause of lost sleep. "Most people can judge for themselves what's keeping them awake," says Dr. Catellani. "If you're anxious and your mind is racing, use kava."

Instead of the above dose, says Dr. Catellani, you can simply follow the recommendations on the label of the specific formula you purchase. In either case, take it an hour before bed to give the herb time to take effect. As with the other herbs recommended here, kava is safe to use daily, but herbal sleep aids should not replace your efforts to find a natural way to unwind.

Chamomile

Drink one cup of tea before bed. A rarely mentioned cause of insomnia is indigestion. If you're having trouble sleeping because of something you ate, or if your stomach hurts because something's eating you, chamomile's antispasmodic action makes it a worthy cure.

"Chamomile is a stomach-soothing remedy," says Dr. Catellani. "It can work for insomnia if your stomach is in knots from what you had for dinner or even if stress is giving you a stomachache."

Tea is probably the most pleasant way to take chamomile (it has a delicious, applelike flavor). You can find chamomile in single-cup tea bags at just about any grocery store. Or buy the pretty yellow dried chamomile flowers in bulk and brew your own. Use 1 rounded tablespoon of herb and cover with 1 cup of boiling water to make one serving. Steep for 10 minutes, then pour through a tea strainer or mesh sieve into a mug.

Chamomile is so safe and mild that you can feel free to use it to wash down any other sleep-inducing herbs that you might choose to take, and you can take it indefinitely without a break, says Dr. Catellani.

INTERMITTENT CLAUDICATION

*I*f you walk or run for any distance and develop cramping, aching, tiredness, or discomfort in one or more of the muscles of your legs, you may have intermittent claudication.

This condition is caused by too little blood flow to a muscle, usually the result of narrowing in an artery that normally supplies blood and oxygen to the leg. Other arteries nearby try to compensate by redirecting blood around the narrowed or blocked artery, but the appearance of symptoms signals that these smaller vessels aren't adequate to do the job that the bigger artery could do in its prime. Less blood flow means that less oxygen is supplied to the legs, causing pain and weakness during walking. Usually a few minutes of rest provides temporary relief, but it does nothing to get at the root causes of the condition.

Conventional remedies include stopping smoking, controlling high blood pressure, limiting dietary fat and cholesterol, and keeping a tight lid on your blood sugar if you have diabetes. Doctors also recommend as a treatment the very thing that causes pain—walking.

The key is to walk for 35 to 45 minutes a day, stopping briefly if you have discomfort, then continuing when it subsides, says Robert Di-Bianco, M.D., associate clinical professor of medicine at Georgetown University School of Medicine in Washington, D.C., and director of cardiology research at the risk factor and heart failure clinics at Washington Adventist Hospital in Takoma Park, Maryland. This training can make a dramatic improvement for some patients, rivaling the benefits of medication in many cases. In addition, new medications have been developed and are being used to help this very common problem.

Good hygiene to prevent infection or skin breakdown is important. Try to keep your feet clean, apply moisturizing lotion or baby oil to prevent cracking or dryness, and wear comfortable shoes and socks. Try not to impair circulation with tight garters, support stockings, or socks with tight elastic tops, says Dr. DiBianco.

Vitamins can also be useful in treating intermittent claudication, says Timothy Birdsall, N.D., director of naturopathic medicine at Midwestern Regional Medical Center in Zion, Illinois. He recommends taking 800 international units of vitamin E a day and 500 milligrams of inositol hexaniacinate (a special form of niacin) three times a day until your symptoms subside. These vitamins help increase circulation and blood flow, Dr. Birdsall says. If treatment is needed for longer than 3 months, you should be monitored by a physician experienced in nutritional medicine, he adds. Excess amounts of vitamin E have been associated with increased risk of hemorrhagic stroke.

These herbs can also help.

Fast Facts

Cause: As you age, fatty deposits may accumulate on the interior walls of arteries. This can cause narrowing of the arteries in the legs and reduced blood flow that leads to pain and swelling.

Incidence: Those at highest risk are smokers, men, women beyond menopause, people over age 60, and those with high blood pressure or high cholesterol. People who are overweight, sedentary, or have diabetes or a family history of atherosclerosis at an early age are also susceptible.

When to see the doctor: Any time you have leg pain and swelling, see your doctor to determine the cause. Also, if you develop sores on your legs that don't heal, consult your doctor right away.

Ginkgo

Take standardized tablets or capsules according to the manufacturer's directions. "We usually think of ginkgo for the brain, but it's really excellent for overall circulation," says herbalist Mindy Green, a founder and professional member of the American Herbalists Guild (AHG), director of educational services at the Herb Research Foundation in Boulder, Colorado, and co-author of *Aromatherapy: A Complete Guide to the Healing Art*.

Indeed, at least 13 studies have been done on ginkgo's ability to help people with intermittent claudication. Germany's Commission E, which evaluates herbs for safety and effectiveness, concluded that in four of these studies, the increase in pain-free walking distance was statistically significant and clinically relevant.

Garlic

Take two capsules two or three times a day for 2 to 6 months after you no longer have symptoms. While it's not entirely clear why, garlic does seem to help increase circulation throughout the body, says Terry Willard, Ph.D., a clinical herbalist, professional member of the AHG, and founder and president of Wild Rose College of Natural Healing in Calgary, Alberta. Capsules are the easiest—and least smelly—way to get garlic.

Onion

Take an average daily dose of 1.5 ounces of fresh onion or 20 grams of dried onion. Like garlic, onion can help prevent age-related narrowing of the arteries, says Varro E. Tyler, Ph.D., Sc.D., distinguished professor emeritus of pharmacognosy at Purdue University in West Lafayette, Indiana, and co-author of *Tyler's Honest Herbal*. Onion is said, among other things, to contain properties that keep your blood from clotting and causing the blockages that lead to intermittent claudication pain.

IRRITABILITY

*I*f you haven't been acting irritable lately, you may be in the minority.

"Irritability is endemic," says psychiatrist James Gordon, M.D., director of the Mind/Body Center in Washington, D.C., and author of *Manifesto for a New Medicine*. "It's a condition of our times."

There are lots of reasons for that: too many people, too little space, too much stuff to do in too little time—the whole litany of modern woes. Indeed, one of the reasons that irritability is so commonplace today is that there is any number of things—physical, psychological, and spiritual—that can set it off.

"You find yourself unable to tolerate the sorts of things you usually take in stride—the toast being burned in the morning, the driver

Victoria's Anti-Ballistic Formula

It's always a good idea to stop irritability before it goes too far. Toward that end, aromatherapist Victoria Edwards, owner of Leydet Aromatics in Fair Oaks, California, devised the following blend of essential oils. You can use a diffuser or simply sprinkle a few drops on a tissue or handkerchief. Take it out and sniff the fragrance whenever an irritable impulse looms.

5 drops lavender
2 drops Roman chamomile
4 drops ylang ylang

Mix the lavender, chamomile, and ylang ylang in a small, dark glass bottle and shake.

in front of you not moving the second the light turns green. Usually, it's things over which we have no control," says Timothy Birdsall, N.D., director of naturopathic medicine at Midwestern Regional Medical Center in Zion, Illinois. "Underlying that, very frequently, is an elevated sense of anxiety, almost always related to something completely different from the annoyance that happens to be irritating you at any given moment. You're not irritable about your toast being burned or the driver in front of you; you're irritable because you're anxious about your job, your family, your finances, your relationships—your life."

The best first step toward dealing with irritability, in Dr. Gordon's opinion, is to gain some perspective on its causes by learning to meditate. Meditation won't make the traffic jam or your annoying boss disappear, but it will allow you to contemplate them more calmly and perhaps even with humor. He also recommends taking steps to stabilize your blood sugar levels by cutting down on sugar and caffeine and by eating regular meals that include protein.

Another key element to consider in the area of general physical maintenance, says Dr. Gordon, is a daily multivitamin/mineral supplement. Deficiencies of vitamin C and B vitamins, in particular, and of magnesium can contribute to irritability, he says.

Exercise can also help. "Take out some of that irritability and aggressiveness in the gym and get the positive effect of some endorphins pumping through you," suggests Thomas Kruzel, N.D., former president of the American Association of Naturopathic Physicians, who practices in Portland, Oregon. Whatever the specific source or sources of the problem, though, herbs can be a part of the solution.

Kava Kava

Take 400 to 600 milligrams in capsule form with meals three times a day. When irritability is a by-product of anxiety, which it often is, kava kava can bring relief, says Dr. Birdsall. That's because it helps your central nervous system deal more efficiently with stress. Kava shouldn't be used indefinitely, though. Two to 4 weeks is a reasonable period to be on it, Dr. Birdsall believes.

He recommends looking for kava products that are standardized to 30 percent kavalactones, the active ingredients. Taking it with meals will help your body absorb the herb, he says.

Asian Ginseng

Take capsules totaling 75 to 150 milligrams twice a day. Stress is often a major contributor to irritability, Dr. Birdsall points out, and ginseng is an excellent tonic to help the body cope with stress. As one of the adaptogenic herbs, ginseng helps the body adapt in numerous ways to stresses in the environment—including burnt toast and inattentive drivers.

Look for extracts standardized to provide at least 20 percent ginsenosides, Dr. Birdsall says. Start with the lower dosage and increase to the higher amount if necessary. Siberian ginseng will provide the same irritability-beating benefits as the Asian form (also called Chinese, Korean, or panax ginseng), he adds. Take the same dose in extracts that are standardized to at least 0.5 percent eleutherosides. You can take either type for 4 to 12 weeks.

Chamomile

Drink a cup of tea a half-hour before bedtime as needed. "People are usually irritable because their nervous systems are overstimulated, and chamomile is very good for soothing that," says Dr. Kruzel. To brew a cup, simply put 1 tablespoon of dried chamomile in a wire tea ball, place it in a teacup, and pour 1 cup of boiling water over it. Steep for 5 to 10 minutes and drink.

Romaine Lettuce and Nutmeg

Drink a cup of soothing broth three times a day. Is the gypsy life stressful? Apparently so, because gypsies developed an excellent folk remedy for chilling out, according to Dr. Gordon. It could hardly be simpler to make: Finely chop a head of Romaine lettuce, put it in a pan with 3 pints of water, and boil until the liquid is reduced to 1½ pints. Add a dash of nutmeg for an extra tranquilizing effect, Dr. Gordon says. Use this remedy for a few weeks during periods of stress or occasionally if you are having trouble sleeping. It's not a substitute for addressing a stressful condition or meditating, but it certainly can help.

IRRITABLE BOWEL SYNDROME

*T*aking the bus. Standing in line for a movie. Searching through a crowded mall. Being caught in a traffic jam.

To most people, these are just parts of everyday life. Inconvenient, sure. Fear-inspiring? Not usually—unless you happen to have irritable bowel syndrome (IBS).

People with IBS never know when the rumbling in their intestines will turn into a full-fledged attack of diarrhea. At times like these, having access to a nearby toilet is critical. Along with bouts of the runs, those with IBS battle cramps and gas pain. And when diarrhea's not a problem, it just may be replaced by constipation.

Irritable bowel syndrome doesn't frustrate only those who have to live with it. It also frustrates those who try to treat it.

"Part of the problem is that we don't truly understand what causes it," says Robert J. Hilsden, M.D., a gastroenterologist and research fellow in the department of internal medicine at the University of Calgary in Alberta.

Added to that is the fact that conventional medicine has a poor track record in treating the disorder. It's estimated that more than half of IBS patients fail to respond to the normally prescribed rounds of antispasmodic drugs and tranquilizers, says Zoltan P. Rona, M.D., a Toronto physician, former president of the Canadian Holistic Medical Association, and author of *The Joy of Health*.

If you fall into that category, or if you just want to try a more natural approach, these herbal remedies may be well worth your time. Use them until your symptoms subside.

Peppermint

Take two 250-milligram enteric-coated capsules of oil twice a day. Peppermint oil can have multiple effects on IBS, says Dr. Rona. Its primary function is antispasmodic, to cut down on those incapacitating cramps. As a bonus, it reduces the production of gas, leaving you less bloated.

Make sure you take only the enteric-coated capsules, otherwise the oil will break down in your stomach before it has a chance to hit your intestines. The coating protects the oil on the ride through stomach acid.

Ginger

Drink four to six cups of tea daily. Ginger has a long history of use for digestive problems, says Dr. Rona. It's also good for the nausea that can accompany IBS. The prepared tea bags are available at almost any health food store or herbal apothecary. You should brew the tea moderately so that it doesn't have a strong spicy or sharp taste.

Chamomile and Catnip

Drink one cup of tea three times a day. This tea blend is soothing for people with IBS, says Connie Catellani, M.D., medical director of the Miro Center for Integrative Medicine in Evanston, Illinois. Blend 1 level teaspoon of dried catnip and 1 rounded teaspoon of chamomile and steep for 10 minutes in 1 cup of water.

Fast FACTS

Cause: There are many theories but little proven about the causes of irritable-bowel syndrome. Food allergies, psychological disorders, parasite infestations, and bacterial imbalances are among the theories discussed.

Incidence: IBS has been estimated to account for 50 percent of all referrals to gastroenterologists, doctors who specialize in gut disorders. Other estimates have placed the number of people experiencing IBS symptoms at 15 percent of the population.

When to see the doctor: If you experience abdominal pain so severe that it prevents you from walking, notice blood in your stool, or experience unintentional weight loss, make an appointment with a physician.

Evening Primrose

Take two 500-milligram capsules of oil daily. This remedy is especially helpful for women, says Mary Jane Minkin, M.D., an obstetrician/gynecologist in New Haven, Connecticut, because many women experience an increase in IBS symptoms as their periods approach. Menstrual hormones sometimes have the unfortunate effect of causing intestinal contractions and diarrhea.

British researchers have found that evening primrose oil is loaded with gamma-linolenic acid, a fatty substance that can soothe those symptoms. "It works for many women," says Dr. Minkin. "At least 50 to 60 percent of the women I treat with it see improvement." Although her practice deals exclusively with women, Dr. Minkin sees no reason why men wouldn't have similar success with evening primrose oil.

Flaxseed

Take some gel once or twice a day. Flaxseed contains many of the minerals that your body loses with the diarrhea that accompanies IBS. Unfortunately, those lost minerals also play a pivotal role in keeping IBS symptoms at bay. Flaxseed gel not only soothes the gut but also helps replace those depleted minerals, says Carolyn DeMarco, M.D., a physician in Winlaw, British Columbia, and a member of the advisory board of Dominion Herbal College in Burnaby.

Here's how to make the gel: To ½ cup of flaxseed, add 2 cups of boiling water. Stir, cover, and let stand at room temperature overnight. The next day, strain the mixture through cheesecloth. Toss away the seeds, and what you'll have left is a white, gel-like substance. It's bitter, so you may want to mix it with juice to improve the taste. Take the whole amount once a day, or twice a day during bad bouts.

"It's really very effective," says Dr. DeMarco. "Almost everyone who uses it sees improvement."

JET LAG

No matter how fast you travel, your body can't escape jet lag. In fact, as you're fast-forwarded into a new time zone, your brain needs time to catch up and readjust the orchestra of rhythms that regulate sleep schedules, body temperature, hormone release, and many other functions. Fly east, and you'll probably have trouble getting to sleep at the new bedtime (even though you feel bone-tired). Head west, and you may find yourself waking up before the birds.

This interruption of your daily rhythms can also cause headaches, difficulty concentrating, indigestion, and bowel irregularities. Whether you travel for business or pleasure, herbs can help your body handle the stress of travel and adjust more quickly, says Orest Pelechaty, O.M.D., a doctor of oriental medicine, professional member of the American Herbalists Guild, and founder of the ALOHA (Aware of Life Options and Healing Arts) Holistic Health Clinic in Short Hills, New Jersey. "When using herbs to fend off a case of jet lag, your treatment should begin before you even leave home," he advises.

Siberian Ginseng

Two weeks before your trip, start taking two 400-milligram capsules of powdered root twice a day. You can minimize the effects of jet lag by enhancing your body's resistance to stress, says Dr. Pelechaty. Also called eleuthero, Siberian ginseng is an invigorating tonic that can offset fatigue and boost your stamina. Although the herb has been studied since the 1950s, science hasn't determined exactly how it improves stamina. It's completely safe to use as a long-term therapy—before, during, and after your trip—but you shouldn't take it indefinitely, says Dr. Pelechaty.

American Ginseng

Take 500 milligrams of standardized extract once or twice a day for 2 weeks prior to departure. Like its distant cousin, Siberian ginseng, American ginseng increases tolerance to stress of all kinds— and air travel is full of its own peculiar stresses. The kind you feel while standing in line for an hour waiting to check in at the airport or sitting immobilized in a coach class seat that was designed to comfortably accommodate a 10-year-old. To contend with breathing dry cabin air that's full of other people's germs—a very real stress on your immune system—you may want to try American ginseng.

Dehydration contributes to jet lag. That's why you're always advised to fill up with water, not alcohol or caffeinated beverages, during the flight. In Chinese herbal medicine, American ginseng is believed to have a moistening effect on the body, explains Dr. Pelechaty. Taking this type of ginseng may help your tissues stay hydrated during long hours in the desert-dry cabin air.

"Use either of these herbs throughout your travels as long-term support so your body has more resiliency in meeting the demands of stress," says Dr. Pelechaty. "But they shouldn't be taken indefinitely, so if you feel better with these remedies, check with an herbalist about further beneficial use," he adds.

Green Tea

Perk up with a cup of strong tea. The first rule in re-establishing sleep patterns is to stay awake until nightfall in your new locale. Depending on how long it's steeped, one cup of green tea contains between 40 and 100 milligrams of caffeine—up to the amount in one cup of coffee. That should help you stay up if you need to, says Dr. Pelechaty.

Chamomile, Linden, Passionflower, Valerian, or Hops

Slip into sleep with any of these herbal sedatives. When you have jet lag, over-the-counter sleep aids can do more harm than good. While they do put you to sleep, they can leave you with a hangover effect in the morning, say experts. Herbs, which have been safely used for thousands of years to induce sleep, don't usually have this effect.

From the mildly relaxing properties of chamomile to the sleeping-pill strength of valerian, Mother Nature has created a wide range of plants to lure Mr. Sandman. But it's important to find the plant that suits your particular constitution before you leave on your trip. Start with chamomile, advises Dr. Pelechaty. "If one tea bag isn't strong enough, try two. On the other hand, if you're someone who can't turn off your brain, try passionflower," he says.

Many of the herbs used as sleep aids, such as chamomile and linden, have traditionally been consumed in the form of teas. About an hour before bedtime, brew a cup by bringing 8 ounces of water to a boil. Remove from the heat and stir in 1 heaping teaspoon of dried herb. Cover and steep for 10 minutes, then strain

Fast FACTS

Cause: At the base of your brain are small cells that control body temperature, sleep and wakefulness, and a variety of hormone changes. Scientists refer to the workings of this built-in body clock as circadian rhythm. Long-distance travel, which typically involves more than 4 hours' time difference, interrupts this rhythm, making you feel tired, irritable, and out-of-sorts.

Incidence: Jet lag is the most common problem that people experience with their circadian rhythms. People who travel regularly for business tend to be more prone to it. Generally, symptoms are worse the older you are and the more time zones you cross, and traveling east is associated with more severe symptoms than traveling west. Even if your feet never leave the ground, you may experience a mild form of jet lag twice a year when we make the time changes for daylight saving time.

When to see the doctor: If your job requires frequent travel or shift work, talk to a doctor who is familiar with this kind of problem about long-term strategies to minimize the health effects of chronic disruptions in your daily schedule.

out the herb. Even the simple ritual of steeping the tea and breathing in the warm steam from the cup will help promote sleep.

Chamomile and linden are gentle and safe for long-term relaxation. Passionflower is stronger and best used for about 1 week at a time. Valerian and hops teas should used to induce sleep only while you have jet lag, advises Dr. Pelechaty.

Ginger

To ease digestive distress, take two 500-milligram capsules of powdered ginger, 30 drops of tincture, or two slices of peeled raw root as needed. Eating a four-course dinner when your tummy says it's time for a bowl of cornflakes can give you a case of jet lag—induced indigestion, or worse. Whether taken as a tea or eaten fresh, ginger will soothe indigestion and gas and also act as a mild stimulant for weary travelers. For nausea, you can use the capsules or tincture, suggests Dr. Pelechaty. To use fresh root, cut it into slices about the size and thickness of a quarter.

"This is a plant that gives us many gifts," he says. "It's not a cup of coffee, but ginger's ability to stimulate your circulation can also make you feel more awake and alert."

Ylang Ylang, Lavender, and Frankincense

Dab a drop of each essential oil on a tissue and breathe in. Jane Buckle, R.N., of Hunter, New York, author of *Clinical Aromatherapy in Nursing*, jets back and forth between her homes in England and America. She uses this formula to sleep peacefully upon arrival.

"Pop the tissue under your pillow and get your zzzs," advises Buckle. As you breathe in the aromas, the scent of ylang ylang will ease nervous tension, true lavender will relieve insomnia, and frankincense will soothe your spirit.

Rosemary, Basil, Eucalyptus, and Peppermint

Put this blend on a handkerchief and breathe in each time your eyelids start to close. If you need to be at your best upon arrival in a new time zone, Buckle suggests an energizing blend of the essential oils of rosemary, a nervous system stimulant; basil, which overcomes mental fatigue; eucalyptus, an energy enhancer; and peppermint, which counters mental fogginess.

Dab a drop of each oil on a handkerchief. Not only will this invigorating blend wake you up, it may also help you fight off any germs that you may have breathed in during your hours on the flight. "The essential oils of lavender and peppermint have a definite antimicrobial effect in the sinuses," says Dr. Pelechaty.

Jock Itch

You don't have to be a jock to get jock itch, but it helps. Running around all day while chasing a football or shooting hoops can make your groin area nice and sweaty. Fungus—the cause of this annoying complaint—just loves moisture and warmth.

"There are two or three species of fungus that cause 99 percent of cases," says Scott Norton, M.D., chief of dermatology at the R. W. Bliss Army Health Center in Fort Huachuca, Arizona, and assistant professor of medicine at the University of Hawaii in Honolulu. "They're all closely related to each other and can also cause athlete's foot and ringworm." There are two things that you want to do when you have jock itch, says Dr. Norton: Clear the fungus and get rid of that irritating rash and the itch that goes with it.

The herbal pharmacy has its share of antifungal plants. In fact, says Dr. Norton, in the tropics, where fungal infections are nearly ubiquitous, antifungal medicines are among the most common natural medicines. Tea tree oil, native to Australia, is high on the list, and several other herbs that are readily available in the United States have similar actions.

Jock itch lends itself well to self-treatment. Keeping the skin clean and dry, says Dr. Norton, is the first step in healing the condition and avoiding future outbreaks. Here are the herbs that can help.

Tea Tree and Calendula

Mix tea tree oil with calendula cream and apply a thin layer to the area two to four times a day. "Tea tree oil is wonderful," says Christopher Robbins, a member of Britain's National Institute of Medical Herbalists who practices herbal medicine in Ross-on-Wye, Herefordshire, England, and has written several books, including *The Natural Pharmacy*. "It's cheap and easily available, and it's a wonderful antiseptic and antifungal."

Scientific studies have confirmed that the Australian aborigines who brewed the leaves of this shrublike tree 2 centuries ago for medicinal purposes were on the right track. Although its antifungal properties are not in dispute, however, tea tree oil can irritate sensitive skin.

"The groin has more delicate tissue than your foot, so it's wise to proceed with caution," says June Riedlinger, Pharm.D., assistant professor of clinical pharmacy at Massachusetts College of Pharmacy and Health Sciences in Boston.

To play it safe, try a drop on unaffected skin in the same area. Leave it for 10 to 15 minutes. If it's not irritated, itchy, or red, you're in business. Adding the oil to calendula cream dilutes it, making irritation even less likely, says Robbins. To 2 tablespoons of calendula cream, add 10 drops or ½ milliliter of tea tree essential oil.

This combination is a winner, says Robbins, because the little bit of oil in the cream keeps sweat and other moisture from aggravating the skin. Also, it's a good way of holding the essential oil in place without having a large concentration of it. "The two together are brilliant," he concludes.

Although twice-daily applications should be sufficient, if you are prone to being hot and sweaty or live in a hot climate, Robbins recommends upping the frequency to three or four times a day to treat jock itch.

Calendula and Comfrey

Apply a thin layer of cream twice a day. Calendula (or pot marigold) is a useful antifungal and an anti-inflammatory. Thomas Kruzel, N.D., former president of the American Association of Naturopathic Physicians, who practices in Portland, Oregon, has his patients start treatment by pouring 3 percent hydrogen peroxide over the area the first time, then washing with soap and water and drying off thoroughly. "Usually, after that, there are no more organisms there, and what I want to do is build the skin's protective layer up," he says.

The cream that Dr. Kruzel recommends includes comfrey and calendula in a base of olive oil and beeswax. Look for it at health food stores; if you have no luck there, you can order it from one of the many mail-order or Internet herbal catalogs. Apply the salve before turning in for the night and after your morning shower. It should help you heal within a week or so, he says.

Fast FACTS

Cause: Jock itch is caused by a fungal infection, which in turn is nurtured by a warm, moist environment.

Incidence: About one of every five Americans will have a fungal infection at some time in their lives. Jock itch often occurs in men who wear athletic support.

When to see the doctor: If your jock itch refuses to clear up within a couple of weeks, or if it keeps coming back, make an appointment with your doctor.

Goldenseal

Dust some powder on the affected area twice a day. David Richard Decatur, M.D., who runs the Decatur Medical Center, a holistic health facility in Indianapolis, says that he's had success in treating jock itch with goldenseal. Goldenseal powder is anti-inflammatory and antibacterial, and it helps to keep the groin area dry, which hastens healing.

Usnea

Make some powder and dust it over the area twice a day. "You can put this in your underwear and keep on going," says Beverly Yates, N.D., a naturopathic physician with the Natural Health Care Group in Portland, Oregon, and Seattle.

Buy this antifungal herb loose, she advises, and grind it to a powder in your kitchen blender. Every day for 2 months, dust some on the groin area whenever you change your underwear. "If you're naturally sweaty or do activities that cause a lot of perspiration, this will really help to treat your jock itch," says Dr. Yates. Usnea (also known as old man's beard) may be difficult to find, but it's worth looking for.

Apple Cider Vinegar

Dab the area once a day. This may sting a little, warns Tammy Alex, N.D., a naturopathic doctor based in Guilford, Connecticut, but it really works well for jock itch. Before applying anything topically, she says, it's a good idea to gently scrape the area with something with a dull edge, such as a butter knife or a credit card, to remove any scaly skin. It's safe to use this remedy until the fungus heals.

KIDNEY STONES

*P*icture something about the size of a sesame seed trying to pass through a tube as thin as a strand of spaghetti. Now imagine the smooth seed sprouting jagged spurs and becoming lodged in the tube.

That's what happens in a typical kidney stone attack, says Jean L. Fourcroy, M.D., Ph.D., editor of the *Women in Urology* newsletter and past president of the American Medical Women's Association and the National Council on Women's Health.

Bits of undissolved minerals can lie dormant in the kidneys for years without causing the slightest twinge. When one of the nasty little nuggets is finally evicted, your first clue is intense pain. As the jagged stone makes its way inch by agonizing inch through the ureter—the tube that passes urine from the kidneys to the bladder—dozens of needlelike protrusions slowly rake through the soft tissue, generating pain that radiates from your upper back to your lower abdomen and groin.

Stones can range from the size of a tiny speck of sand to—ouch—that of a dime or marble. Generally, though, as long as it's smaller than a pea—and 80 percent of stones are—doctors will let your body pass the stone on its own. When stones are larger than 8 to 10 millimeters, however, they are usually too large to be passed. Often, they remain in the kidneys, where they can become infected.

People who have had one bout with kidney stones are more likely to develop them again. But you don't have to accept this as an inevitable date with future agony. There's a lot you can do to prevent another attack. First, though, be sure to find out from your doctor what kinds of kidney stones you have or are prone to, since different types of stones are treated differently. The preventive measures and remedies suggested here are meant to deal mainly with the most common type of stones—those formed from calcium phosphate or calcium oxalate.

First, drink a lot of water. In the ongoing Nurses' Health Study, Harvard researchers reported that women who drank 11 full 8-ounce glasses of fluid per day were 38 percent less likely to form stones than those who drank about 6 glasses. Increased fluid dilutes the compounds that form the deposits, says Silena Heron, N.D., adjunct professor at Southwest College of Naturopathic Medicine and Health Sciences in Tempe, Arizona, and vice president of the Botanical Medicine Academy. Another good thing to drink is lemonade, which has been shown to help prevent the formation of mineral compounds that lead to kidney stones.

Supplementing your diet with vitamin B_6, calcium citrate, and magnesium citrate can also help retard stone growth, says Dr. Heron. She generally recommends 250 milligrams of vitamin B_6 daily, 500 milligrams of calcium citrate three times daily with meals, and a magnesium citrate supplement that provides roughly 150 milligrams of elemental magnesium twice a day. You should take this amount of vitamin B_6 only under medical supervision, however.

Your doctor may also advise you to avoid the foods that increase the level of oxalate (the stone-forming mineral) in your urine—namely spinach and other leafy vegetables, chocolate, tea, nuts, strawberries, rhubarb, and wheat bran. For best results when attempting to treat or prevent kidney stones, Dr. Heron recommends that you consult a naturopathic physician. Self-treating with these preventive measures or the natural remedies that follow without the advice of a medical doctor is not advisable, she says. Kidney stones can be serious business.

If, despite your best efforts, your kidneys churn out another stone, natural therapies, used with medical supervision, can help facilitate the painful process of passage.

Dandelion or Goldenrod

During the acute phase of an attack, steadily drink tea made from either herb to help expel the stone. To pass the stone as quickly as possible, doctors recommend drinking copious amounts of water. Instead of plain water, Dr. Heron recommends dandelion leaf tea. Dandelion and other diuretic herbs increase urine output by stimulating blood circulation through the kidneys. This action helps flush the stone from your system faster. Unlike diuretic drugs, which can deplete the body of potassium, dandelion leaf is one of the best plant sources of this crucial mineral. A cup of cooked dandelion greens contains as much potassium as a small banana.

If you can't find dandelion leaf tea in your local health food store, you can substitute goldenrod tea, suggests Dr. Heron. Along with its diuretic properties, goldenrod helps repair the inflammation caused by the passage of the stone.

To make either tea, add 2 teaspoons of dried herb to 1 cup of boiling water and steep for 15 minutes.

Marshmallow or Corn Silk

To help protect and repair tissues in the urinary tract, drink one cup of tea three times a day before meals. Your urinary tract is lined with mucous membranes to protect it from irritation and inflammation. As a kidney stone passes through, it strips away this protective layer. You can help replace it by drinking tea made from marshmallow root or corn silk, says Orest Pelechaty, O.M.D., a doctor of oriental medicine, professional member of the American Herbalists Guild, and founder of the ALOHA (Aware of Life Options and Healing Arts) Holistic Health Clinic in Short Hills, New Jersey. The slimy texture of the tea helps by assisting the mucous membranes.

Marshmallow is a good source of mucilage—large sugar molecules that produce a sticky, jellylike mass when they soak up water. The silica content of corn silk will aid in the repair of the urinary tract tissues.

Fast FACTS

Cause: In people who develop kidney stones, excess mineral matter in the urine stays in the kidneys, eventually forming a full-fledged stone. Calcium stones often run in families because the tendency to absorb too much calcium is hereditary. Irritable bowel syndrome, Crohn's disease, or eating a diet high in oxalic acid (found in spinach and other leafy vegetables, chocolate, tea, nuts, strawberries, rhubarb, and wheat bran) can cause kidney stones.

Incidence: For unknown reasons, the incidence of kidney stones has been rising steadily in the United States for the past 20 years. Roughly 10 percent of Americans will develop a kidney stone in their lifetimes. They are most common in white men between 20 and 40 years old, but over the past 10 years, they've become increasingly common in women. Although no one knows why, kidney stones are more prevalent in the southern United States, an area some doctors refer to as the Stone Belt.

When to see the doctor: Contact your doctor if you develop symptoms of kidney stones, which include pain that radiates from the upper back to the lower abdomen and groin, frequent urination, pus and blood in the urine, and sometimes chills and fever.

It's probably easier to find good-quality marshmallow than corn silk, says Dr. Heron. "Corn silk is one herb that is best used in fresh form, and it should be carefully collected so that you're using only the green or yellowish parts. Most commercially available corn silk is of a low quality," she says. To collect your own, buy organic corn on the cob and keep the silk as you husk the ears. Trim away any dried-up or brown pieces of silk.

To make the most soothing tea from marshmallow root, simmer the herb for several minutes in a pan of water. "Use 2 ounces of herb to 1 quart of water and boil for 5 to 10 minutes," says Dr. Pelechaty. "Corn silk is best steeped using 1 ounce of material to 1 pint of water," he continues. "Let it stand and cool for 5 minutes so it thickens."

Gravel Root

To soften a stone, take 30 drops of tincture three times a day. As its name implies, gravel root has been used traditionally for treating urinary "gravel." It helps prevent the formation of kidney stones and may help dissolve existing ones, says Dr. Pelechaty. It also helps relax the ureter, allowing a stone to pass more easily. Long-term use may be required. It is best to consult a professional herbalist or trained holistic physician to match the treatment to the individual.

Cranberry

To discourage calcium stones from forming again, drink 16 ounces of juice every day. Preliminary research suggests that cranberry juice may help reduce the amount of calcium in the urine, says Amy Howell, Ph.D., a researcher for the Blueberry and Cranberry Research Center of Rutgers University in Chatsworth, New Jersey. In a study of people with calcium-containing kidney stones, cranberry was shown to reduce the amount of ionized calcium in the urine by 50 percent. Less calcium in the urine means that there may be less risk of forming new stones. Cranberry juice also has a very cleansing effect on the urinary tract.

Saw Palmetto

Take two 160-milligram capsules of extract daily or ½ teaspoon of tincture three times a day for as long as needed. Known for its benefits in treating prostate problems, saw palmetto relaxes the ureter, making it easier for both men and women to pass kidney stones.

"Saw palmetto is also believed to reduce the pressure on the neck of the bladder," says Dr. Heron. She feels it's key because of its general tonic effect on the entire urinary tract. For preventive purposes, take the same dosage as recommended above, she says.

LARYNGITIS

You don't have to be a rock star or political candidate to get laryngitis. Those are just the cases we hear the most about, because one symptom of laryngitis—inflammation of the larynx, or voice box—is hoarseness or even complete loss of voice. Next thing you know, concerts are postponed or campaign stops canceled.

Just spend enough time drinking and smoking while shouting nonstop encouragement to your favorite team on the tube, though, and you can get laryngitis, too. Alcohol, tobacco, and overuse of the voice are major causes of chronic laryngitis.

On the other hand, acute laryngitis, which can come and go very quickly, is usually the result of a viral infection, and there are lots of herbal remedies to help you deal with it. The first thing you should do, to put it bluntly, is shut up. Resting your voice (a more polite way of saying it) is key to recovery. You can help things along by inhaling steam, getting bed rest, steering clear of irritating agents such as smoke and alcohol, and avoiding immune depressors such as caffeine and sugar, suggests Connie Catellani, M.D., medical director of the Miro Center for Integrative Medicine in Evanston, Illinois.

The conventional medical approach might include pain relievers and antibiotics. Natural medicine enlists herbal remedies such as those that follow.

Goldenseal and Cayenne

Gargle five times a day with this herbal solution. "This is a high-powered, hard-punching remedy for when you really have to get well fast," says Willow Moore, N.D., D.C., a naturopathic physician and chiropractor at the Maryland Natural Medicine Center in Owings Mills. "I've had people use it who didn't even have a voice, their laryngitis was so bad. And within 24 hours, they turned around."

Such results come at a price, though. Goldenseal is one of the more bitter herbs in the plant kingdom, and as we all know, cayenne pepper is hot, hot, hot. Buy the two herbs in dry, powdered form—the cayenne can come right off your spice rack, Dr. Moore says—and put ¼ teaspoon of each in ½ cup of water. Take a mouthful, swirl it around a few times, tilt your head back, and gargle deeply. "You really want to coat the back of your throat with the goldenseal and cayenne pepper," she says.

You'll probably need to do several wash-and-gargles to finish up the ½ cup. Repeat the whole process five times a day for just a day or two.

Echinacea

Take 20 to 60 drops of tincture every 2 hours. Echinacea is one of the best herbs there is to help the body fight the infection that causes the inflammation of laryngitis, says Dr. Moore.

This native American plant is often combined with other herbs (such as goldenseal) in an immune-stimulating formula. But it's also powerful on its own, especially when you use it at high doses at the very beginning of an infection.

Jill Stansbury, N.D., chair of the botanical medicine department at the National College of Naturopathic Medicine in Portland, Oregon, and author of *Herbs for Health and Healing*, recommends using the tinctured root, available in 1- or 2-ounce bottles at health food stores or by mail order. Start with anywhere from 20 to 60 drops (that should be one to two droppers), then reduce the dosage daily as symptoms subside.

Collinsonia

Take 20 drops of tincture three or four times a day. *Collinsonia* is herbal terminology for a plant called stone root. It's not a big anti-in-

Fast Facts

Cause: Chronic laryngitis is caused by direct irritation of the larynx, often from smoking, drinking alcohol, or talking a lot. Acute laryngitis is usually the result of a viral or bacterial infection, either in the larynx itself or as part of a more general upper respiratory infection.

Incidence: Exposure to certain viruses or bacteria can lead to acute laryngitis, which can also be an unwelcome follow-up to other infections, such as tonsillitis, bronchitis, or flu. Smokers, drinkers, and those who use their voices a lot are more prone to chronic laryngitis.

When to see the doctor: Laryngitis shouldn't linger. If things aren't getting better after 4 to 5 days, consult your doctor.

fective herb like echinacea or goldenseal, but it's great for laryngitis because it actually helps reduce the tissue inflammation, thus relieving the "-itis" part of laryngitis.

"Collinsonia helps with the hoarseness or a raspy voice and with swelling in the larynx, especially the vocal cords," says Dr. Stansbury.

You can find the tinctured root of collinsonia in 1-ounce dropper bottles in health food stores or by mail order. Reduce the dose after a day or two and gradually taper off to nothing within a week.

Sage, Rosemary, and Thyme

Do three consecutive gargles with this tea blend, and repeat often. Gargling with astringent herbs such as sage, thyme, and rosemary is a super sore throat soother that you can use for laryngitis as well.

Dr. Moore recommends mixing equal parts of dried sage, thyme, and rosemary leaves to make a tea blend. Steep 1 heaping tablespoon of the blend in 1 cup of boiling water for 10 to 20 minutes, let it cool until it's comfortably warm, then strain. Take a mouthful of tea and gargle for 30 seconds, then repeat two more times. You don't have to swallow, but you should try to gargle while the tea is still warm. You can make several cups of tea at a time, then refrigerate it in a jar with a tight-fitting lid so you can reheat it to use throughout the day. As your symptoms improve, you can gargle less often.

LOW IMMUNITY

*I*f you find yourself constantly coming down with whatever bug is going around, you have two choices: One, curse your luck, or two, strengthen your immune system.

The first is quicker, but it won't help you stay healthy. The second will.

That's because an underachieving immune system is like an undermanned fort. There just aren't enough troops to keep the invaders from taking over. When your immune system is functioning properly, it takes advantage of your body's miraculous ability to recognize "self" (that would be you) from "non-self" (that would be viruses, bacteria, yeast, and so on). When the "non-selfs" are present—which is all the time—the immune system deploys an elite force of chemical weapons to keep the invaders at bay.

A weakened immune system isn't always up to the task. "A lot of people today have chronically low-performance immune systems," says George Milowe, M.D., a holistic physician in Saratoga Springs, New York. "That makes them susceptible to all kinds of infections—not just colds and flu but also urinary tract and gastrointestinal infections."

Lifestyle and environment factors have plenty to do with low immunity. According to natural and holistic medical experts, any combination of pollution, poor diet, inadequate vitamin or mineral intake, bad sleep habits, stress, smoking, and countless other toxins can wear down your immune system. In short, your body spends so much time resisting the effects of these harmful elements that by the time a real cold comes along, your immunity army has already been decimated.

Herbal medicine can help strengthen your immune system in two ways. First, when you do get sick, you should use natural methods to help your body heal (rather than zapping the disease with drugs), says David McLeod, an herbalist and acupuncturist and president of the National Herbalists Association of Australia in Sydney. That way, "once you get better using natural medicine, the next time you get a cold, you'll probably get better in half the time," he says. "It's a process of training your body to get better itself." Second, there are herbs that you can take tonically—that is, as strengtheners—over the long haul to improve your immune system. Think of it as enhancing your military preparedness during peacetime.

Astragalus

Drink one to two cups of tea a day, or take ½ to ¾ teaspoon of tincture two or three times a day or 1,500 milligrams in capsule form three times a day. Astragalus is everything you could possibly ask for in a long-term immune booster. It's from China, but it's well-known and readily available in the West. And for good reason. Rich in polysaccharides, astragalus increases the activity of lots of different kinds of immune system cells, including macrophages, T-lymphocytes, and natural killer cells.

"Its best use is for chronic low immunity," says Susan B. Kowalsky, N.D., a naturopathic physician in Norwich, Vermont.

Astragalus works right in the bone marrow, where your immune cells are manufactured. "It takes months to really be effective," says Chanchal Cabrera, a member of Britain's National Institute of Medical Herbalists, a professional member of the American Herbalists Guild,

ADVENTURES IN HERBALISM

A METHODIST'S MEDICINE

*M*any of the medicinal herbs that we now take for granted we first learned about from Native Americans. Indeed, Europeans who arrived on these shores were often impressed with the natural healing skills of the native tribes. One of these was the English minister John Wesley, founder of Methodism, who spent some time early in his career as a missionary in Georgia.

Wesley eventually wrote his own volume of herbal and other home remedies, called *Primitive Physic, An Easy and Natural Way of Curing Most Diseases*, that was first published in 1747. Written largely for poor people who couldn't afford doctors or apothecary drugs, the hugely popular book was filled with the sorts of herbal cures and preventive methods that have been used for centuries, both before and since.

A wave of similar collections of home remedies hit the English market during Wesley's era because of widespread mistrust of the standard medical practices of the day, which were not only expensive but were also often painful and not very effective.

Sound familiar?

and an herbalist in Vancouver. "This is not an herb to take just when you feel a sniffle. It is taken day in and day out for chronic immune weakness, so if you always seem to have a cold during the winter, start taking it in September."

You have lots of options for taking your astragalus. If you can handle a strong medicinal tea, buy plenty of loose astragalus root in cut-and-sifted form, either at a Chinese herb store or a well-supplied health food store. Since it's a root, you'll need to decoct it, which simply means that you put 2 tablespoons of the herb into 1 pint of cold water, bring it to a boil, then immediately lower the heat and let it simmer for 10 minutes. Cabrera recommends one to two cups a day.

A little honey is okay as a sweetener in your astragalus tea, but avoid refined sugars, because they deplete immunity. Besides, tea made from astragalus root is pretty neutral-tasting, according to Cabrera.

If you just don't like the tea, however, you can try astragalus tincture—that is, an alcohol-based liquid extract. You'll usually find it in 1- or 2-ounce bottles, with an herb-to-alcohol ratio of 1:5. You can dilute it in a little water or fruit juice to help it go down.

A third option is powdered astragalus root in capsules, which, like the tincture, is easily found at health food stores.

Ginseng

Take 200 milligrams of standardized extract in capsule form one to five times a day. Ginseng is one of the world's more famous tonic herbs. It's also a super long-term immune booster.

Buy either American or Asian (also called panax, Chinese, or Korean) ginseng. There are many different versions on the market, from the whole root to chewing gum, but your best bet, according to Dr. Kowalsky, is to buy capsules. Read labels to make sure the ones you buy are standardized for their ginsenoside content.

Dr. Kowalsky recommends taking ginseng standardized for 5 percent ginsenosides. "It's best to start off with low doses between meals and gradually work up," she says. "Use it cyclically, 3 weeks on and 2 weeks off."

Shiitake

Take one or two 300-milligram capsules three times a day for 3 to 6 months. The Chinese mushroom called shiitake (shee-tah-kay) is,

Fast Facts

Cause: The exact cause of low immunity is not fully known, but prominent factors include lifestyle (poor diet, smoking, and so forth), environment (toxins and pollution), and genetics.

Incidence: There are no precise numbers, but natural practitioners agree that low immunity is becoming increasingly common. Some holistic practitioners consider it a syndrome of modern times, blaming it on the growing amount of chemicals in our food, the air, the water, the workplace, and the home.

When to see the doctor: Getting sick once or twice a year is normal. If you have a healthy immune system, you're ill for 3 to 4 days, at most (although the lingering symptoms of a cold, such as a runny or stuffy nose, may last a week or so, and some flu symptoms, such as a persistent cough and fatigue, may last for up to a month).

If you get sick more than twice a year, and you feel no better at all after a few days, it's likely that you have an immunity problem. See your doctor for an evaluation.

---

like astragalus, high in immune-stimulating polysaccharides, according to Mary Bove, N.D., a naturopathic physician at the Brattleboro Naturopathic Clinic in Vermont and a member of Britain's National Institute of Medical Herbalists. What's more, it tastes good and makes an excellent immune-boosting soup.

A more practical way to benefit from shiitake over the long term is to use it in capsule form. "Sometimes they include maitake (my-tah-kay) mushroom powder, which is also immune-stimulating," says Dr. Bove.

Reishi

Take one or two capsules three times a day. A third type of mushroom that helps you overcome low immunity is called reishi (ray-shee).

"Reishi is highly esteemed in the Orient," says Jill Stansbury, N.D., chair of the botanical medicine department at the National College of Naturopathic Medicine in Portland, Oregon, and author of *Herbs for Health and Healing*. "It's considered good for your overall vital energy as well as your immune function." You can find encapsulated reishi powder fairly easily in health food stores. Follow the label instructions carefully, she adds.

Garlic

Eat one clove a day, or take the equivalent in capsule form. The allicin in garlic is a well-known wonder worker for acute infections. In small daily doses, garlic is also a great long-term general immunity enhancer. If your immunity isn't what it should be, Dr. Kowalsky suggests working garlic into your daily routine at the rate of one clove a day. If you want to get your daily dose in capsule form, read the label to be sure that the product you're using provides 10 milligrams of allicin a day.

Low Sex Drive

*A*ccording to many television shows these days, the only time people *aren't* having sex is when they're saving lives in a hospital or arguing before the Supreme Court. Yet, in the real world, not only are we not having sex all the time, we're also not always in the mood. That's normal.

If you find that you almost never want to have sex, however, even when you have access to a willing partner, it might be worth wondering if you have a low sex drive, says Steven Margolis, M.D., an alternative family physician in Sterling Heights, Michigan.

"Low sex drive can be caused by a large number of physical and psychological factors," says Dr. Margolis. Common reasons include stress, depression, fatigue, interpersonal conflicts between partners, certain prescription drugs, and low testosterone levels in men.

The first step is to talk about it with your partner. After that, check with your doctor to see if there's a medical reason that your libido has dropped. Find a way to take some time off from stress, either with a workout routine (which will help you look and feel better about yourself—not a bad way to increase desire) or some other stress-management technique. And if relationship conflicts appear to be at the root of the problem, it might be a good idea for the two of you to visit a counselor or sex therapist, Dr. Margolis suggests.

That said, daily herbal supplementation can play a role in restoring your desire, and some folks continue to take the herbs below even after their sexual spark has been restored. Dr. Margolis okays them for long-term use, noting that some of them have other benefits, such as increased energy. Here's the best of what experts have to offer.

Tribulus

Take one 250-milligram capsule each day. This little-known herb from Eastern Europe shows exciting potential as a treatment for low sex drive in men, says Dr. Margolis. It works primarily by stimulating the body's natural production of testosterone, and it appears to increase sexual desire and maximize blood flow to the penis.

Damiana

Take 2 to 4 milliliters of tincture, or drink one cup of tea daily. Damiana leaves appear to benefit mainly the female libido, says Dr. Margolis, but the herb can have benefits for both sexes.

Fast FACTS

Cause: Common reasons for a reduced or inhibited sex drive include stress, depression, fatigue, interpersonal conflicts between partners, certain prescription drugs, and low testosterone levels in men.

Incidence: One study found that roughly 30 percent of women and 15 percent of men consider themselves uninterested in sex over extended periods of time.

When to see the doctor: If your reduced sex drive seems to be a permanent condition (that is, it has lasted for several months, even in circumstances that you would normally respond to) and appears to be taking a toll on your relationship, it's time to visit an expert.

For one thing, it appears to be a mild antidepressant, which would be helpful for both women and men if the lack of sex drive has an emotional component, says Steven Rissman, N.D., a naturopathic physician at American WholeHealth in Cherry Creek, Colorado. In addition, experts speculate that damiana causes mild inflammation of the urethra, thus increasing penile sensitivity for men.

Dang Gui

Take capsules containing 300 milligrams daily. In the Far East, this Chinese herb (also known as dong quai) has a variety of different uses, including revitalizing the sexual organs. It's the closest herbal equivalent to estrogen that you'll find, says Dr. Margolis, which makes it particularly suited to charging up the female sex drive. It's his top choice for women.

Muira Puama

Take a 300-milligram tablet once a day. Also known as potency wood, this herb is derived from a tropical Brazilian plant and has a long history in South America as a male libido booster. In a study done at the Institute of Sexology in Paris, 62 percent of male subjects with low sex drive reported improvement after taking muira puama daily for 2 weeks. "It's very effective," Dr. Margolis says, "and there are no side effects."

MACULAR DEGENERATION

*W*hen you're young, there's a tendency to believe that you see everything perfectly clearly. As you age, you begin to understand how limited your vision can be. This is called wisdom.

As your mental vision becomes more acute, however, your physical vision is likely to go downhill. Macular degeneration is among the most serious of those potential vision problems, but according to Alice Laule, M.D., who practices holistic medicine and ophthalmology in Harrison, Arkansas, several readily available herbs can help prevent onset of the disease and even retard its development once it has started.

The macula is a part of the retina, located on the back portion of the eye, that allows you to see fine details clearly. With age, it can deteriorate. Exactly why this happens is unknown, but vitamin deficiencies, a breakdown of blood circulation to the eye, and excessive exposure to ultraviolet light are among the suspected causes.

If you develop macular degeneration, your vision is likely to become blurry, straight lines may seem slightly wavy, or you may see a dark or empty area in the center of your field of vision. Usually, the loss of vision is gradual, but in about 10 percent of cases, it can be rapid and severe.

There is at present no known cure for macular degeneration, but a growing body of research suggests that a healthy diet rich in vitamins can help prevent it. "If you take a good multivitamin and eat sensibly, you'll probably greatly reduce your chances of getting severe macular degeneration," Dr. Laule says. "People in the early stages of the disease should take an extra-potency multivitamin that gives them more than the recommended daily requirement of all the minerals and vitamins, especially zinc and magnesium." What's more, these supplements should be high in antioxidants, chemicals that are important for nourishing the eyes and eliminating harmful substances that can cause damage.

A good diet for the eyes, Dr. Laule adds, includes lots of green, leafy vegetables, such as spinach, turnip greens, chard, kale, romaine lettuce, cilantro, and parsley. These provide antioxidant substances called lutein and zeaxanthin, which have been shown to be particularly effective at warding off macular degeneration. Wearing good sunglasses that filter out ultraviolet sunlight also protects your eyes.

If you're in the early stages of macular degeneration or you want to keep it from developing, give these herbal remedies a try.

Ginkgo

Take 60 to 80 milligrams in capsule form or 15 drops of tincture in 1 cup of cold water twice a day. One of the best ways to avoid deterioration of the tissues in your eyes is to maintain the health of the blood vessels and capillaries that supply them, says Dr. Laule. Several studies have shown that ginkgo does exactly that. It also helps thin out the platelets in the blood that can sludge up circulation.

If you're taking the tincture, Dr. Laule warns that the taste isn't great, so you may want to dilute it. Instead of putting 15 drops in 1 cup of water, you can add them to a glass or two. "Some people would rather drink a little bit of really bad-tasting stuff, and others would rather drink a lot of moderately bad-tasting stuff," she says. "It doesn't matter, just so you get it down."

Morning and evening doses, before or after meals, are fine for both capsules and tincture. You can take this herb on an ongoing basis, she says.

Bilberry

Take 100 milligrams a day. Bilberry, which has been described as the European version of the blueberry, is well-known there for its eye-saving properties. During World War II, British pilots were given bilberry jam to improve their night vision, according to Andrew Weil, M.D., director of the program in integrative medicine at the University of Arizona College of Medicine in Tucson and author of *8 Weeks to Optimum Health*.

European studies indicate that the dark purple pigment in bilberry—found in greater amounts than in our native blueberry—contains a potent form of antioxidants called bioflavonoids. These are thought to improve the circulation of blood through the eye. Dr. Laule says that bilberry is safe to take long-term.

Grape Seed

Take a 50-milligram capsule of extract twice a day. The pip, or seed, of the grape, is an especially rich source of flavonoids, according to Dr. Laule. Health food stores often sell this in an antioxidant mixture containing vitamin C. Since antioxidant vitamins are considered vital for maintaining vision, that makes a potent eye-saving combination. You can take this on an ongoing basis.

Pine

Take a daily supplement of bark extract, following instructions on the bottle. Pine bark contains proanthocyanidin, one of

Fast FACTS

Cause: Macular degeneration is a condition of aging in which the macula, the central part of the retina in the back of the eye, begins to deteriorate. Exactly why this occurs is unknown, but heredity, a breakdown of circulation in the eyes, vitamin deficiencies, and exposure to sunlight are thought to be some of the contributing factors.

Incidence: More than 13 million Americans have experienced at least some symptoms of macular degeneration, making it the leading cause of vision loss among older people. While early warning signs can appear in people in their thirties, this is rare. Symptoms usually don't begin until people are in their sixties.

When to see the doctor: During a thorough eye examination, an ophthalmologist will normally check for macular degeneration. Be sure to see an ophthalmologist if you notice any deterioration in your vision, especially blurring, distortion, or a blind spot in the center of your vision field.

the same potent bioflavonoids in grape seeds, says Dr. Weil. The product is often sold in health food stores under the brand name Pycnogenol.

Clove

Drink one to three cups of tea a day. To make a vision-protecting tea, pour 8 ounces of boiling water over 2 teaspoons of whole cloves and a piece of cinnamon stick, if desired, for extra flavor. Steep for a few minutes, then strain the tea and enjoy it while it's hot.

"I would recommend three cups a day for the short term, but if you intend to use it for more than 4 to 6 months, stick to one or two cups a day," says C. Leigh Broadhurst, Ph.D., an herbal researcher and nutrition consultant based in Clovery, Maryland.

The oil in cloves is a powerful antioxidant, according to James A. Duke, Ph.D., an herbalist and ethnobotanist in Fulton, Maryland, and author of *The Green Pharmacy*. Studies have shown that it helps prevent the breakdown of important chemicals that help keep the retina healthy.

MENOPAUSAL PROBLEMS

*M*enopause is kind of like puberty, only in reverse. That means that it isn't a disease or an illness. It is, however, a transitional time of unpredictable hormone levels and often uncomfortable symptoms.

The body changes associated with menopause are caused by sudden drops in estrogen levels. Many parts of the female body—the breasts, vagina, vulva, and ovaries in particular, but also the skin, bones, and heart—depend on estrogen to function normally, says Larry Kincheloe, M.D., chairman of the department of obstetrics and gynecology at the Central Oklahoma Medical Group in Oklahoma City. When estrogen levels falter and fall, symptoms abound.

The most common and probably most annoying side effect of dwindling estrogen is hot flashes. These waves of uncontrollable body heat seem to be the cause of other menopausal problems, such as insomnia and mood swings. Low estrogen also leads the usually soft, moist vaginal tissues to become thinner and drier, making sex uncomfortable for some women. More seriously, hormone changes due to menopause also increase a woman's risk for heart disease, osteoporosis, and maybe even Alzheimer's disease.

Not all women experience discomfort during menopause. For those who do, there are three basic paths to choose from. Some women go it alone—what's often referred to as suffering in silence. Millions of others take hormone replacement therapy (HRT), prescription medication that's designed to replace the body's hormones. HRT reduces the chances of developing a menopause-related health problem while also helping with hot flashes and other symptoms. Yet another group of women is now opting to try the new and "natural" over-the-counter remedies containing herbs that mimic estrogen as HRT does, only in a milder way. But there's an even better method for managing menopause.

An approach that Dr. Kincheloe uses frequently with his patients is to prescribe the lowest dose of synthetic hormones necessary to lower the risk of the more life-threatening menopause-related problems. On top of that, he recommends certain herbs to help with other symptoms, which could be called lifestyle-threatening. "The dose of hormones needed to protect the heart and bones may not be enough to prevent hot flashes or vaginal dryness. That's where herbs can help," he says.

If you're currently taking HRT and would like to reduce your dose, the herbs that follow are the ones to discuss with your doctor. For women who may be just sensing the first twinges of premenopause symptoms, the same herbs can help harmonize fluctuating hormones and make the transition to full menopause easier.

Sage

Drink one to three cups of tea, or take 3 to 15 drops of tincture three times a day. The common, everyday sage found in herb gardens and used in cooking is a good choice for checking the profuse perspiration that can come with hot flashes, says Matthew Wood, a member of the American Herbalists Guild in Minnetrista, Minnesota, and author of *The Book of Herbal Wisdom*.

Interestingly, even as sage helps dry out perspiration, it has a re-moistening effect on the rest of the body. When menopause brings hot flashes plus a lack of vaginal lubrication, sage can be a savior. "It's considered a little bit of an anti-aging remedy because of its ability to relubricate internal tissues," says Wood.

Perimenopausal Relief Tincture Tonic

This combination of herb tinctures can help stabilize symptoms that occur during perimenopause, the 5 to 10 years before menstruation actually stops. Take this mixture to regulate off-kilter menstrual cycles or just to cool the occasional hot flash, says Virginia Frazer, N.D., a naturopathic physician and licensed midwife in Kennewick, Washington.

Use a dosing syringe (available at drugstores) to accurately measure your doses. Take 5 milliliters of the blend two or three times a day, depending on the severity of your symptoms, says Dr. Frazer. Tinctures tend to have a strong taste, so to make your herbal combo easier to swallow, add the measured amount to a half-glass of water, tea, or juice.

- **4 ounces black cohosh**
- **2 ounces partridgeberry**
- **2 ounces motherwort**
- **I ounce chasteberry**
- **I ounce wild yam**

Pour the black cohosh, partridgeberry, motherwort, chasteberry, and wild yam into a glass mixing bowl and set the empty bottles aside. Stir gently to blend, then use a small funnel to carefully rebottle your custom combination.

Make a fragrant sage tea by pouring 1 cup of boiling water over 1 to 2 teaspoons of dried herb. Cover and steep for 5 to 10 minutes, then strain into a mug. To take sage in tincture form, simply add the drops to $\frac{1}{2}$ cup of water or tea.

Red Clover

Take two capsules three times daily and drink tea throughout the day. When it comes to naturally balancing estrogen loss, herbal con-

Fast Facts

Cause: Menopause is the end of a woman's reproductive years and typically occurs between the ages of 42 and 58. It's marked by the permanent cessation of menstrual cycles. The wide variety of symptoms associated with menopause is caused by flagging levels of estrogen, the chief female hormone.

While menopause usually happens naturally, it can also be artificially induced through surgical removal of the ovaries or uterus, as with hysterectomy. Bothersome symptoms are much more common in women who have gone through surgical menopause than in those who have a natural menopause.

Incidence: While there are no precise figures, most women experience some menopause symptoms.

When to see the doctor: Menopause is a natural transition, not a disease. While some symptoms of menopause seem merely annoying, others can be life-threatening. If a woman has a family history of osteoporosis, heart disease, stroke, colon cancer, or Alzheimer's disease, menopause may be best managed with some form of hormone replacement. All women, regardless of symptoms or history, should discuss their options with a gynecologist.

---

stituents known as phytoestrogens can be a big help, says Dr. Kincheloe. While they are not exact substitutes for the body's true hormones, phytoestrogens do have similar effects. Often, their mild action is just enough to reverse troubling menopause symptoms that are due to too little estrogen.

Red clover is an herb that's high in multiple types of phytoestrogens as well as isoflavones, the beneficial, naturally occurring chemicals that are also found in soy foods. In fact, the little globe-shaped clover flower is so potent that an extract is now sold over the counter as a menopause-targeted formula called Promensil.

You can look for red clover capsules with a dosage range between 370 and 435 milligrams per capsule at health food stores.

While you're taking the capsules, you can also drink red clover tea. For one serving, pour 1 cup of boiling water over 1 to 2 teaspoons of dried herb. Cover and steep for 5 minutes, then strain into a mug.

It's fine to drink as much of this tea as you like. The amount of phytoestrogens in red clover is small compared to the levels of hormones that your body produced every month in preparation for pregnancy or menstruation, says Dr. Kincheloe. "You're not going to overdose on these phytoestrogens."

Black Cohosh

Take ½ to 1 milliliter of tincture two to four times daily. Like red clover, black cohosh contains natural phytoestrogens. "It's a classic American herb widely used by menopausal women in Europe," according to master herbalist Susun Weed of Woodstock, New York, author of *Menopausal Years: The Wise Woman Way*.

Native American people used black cohosh first for female health complaints, and German physicians have been recommending it since the 1940s for hormone disturbances.

One study involving 110 women at the University of Gottingen in Germany showed that black cohosh can stop hot flashes before they start. The women were split into two groups. One was given two tablets a day of a standardized black cohosh extract, while the other took placebos (inactive look-alikes).

After just 2 months, blood levels of luteinizing hormone (LH) were found to be much lower in the women who took black cohosh than in those who didn't. LH is what's known as a vasodilator. It opens up blood vessels, sending waves of heat out to the skin. In menopause, sharp rises in LH lead to the feeling that you are suddenly standing in front of an open furnace. Naturally lowering levels of LH with black cohosh can keep hot flashes at bay.

Take the herb in tincture form. Add your dose to a half-glass of water or tea two to four times a day for 6 weeks, says Weed, then take a month off. After that, you may repeat the cycle if you wish.

MENSTRUAL CRAMPS

*C*all it the Arnold Schwarzenegger of the female anatomy: the uterus. Suspended in the abdomen, this pear-shaped powerhouse is one of the strongest muscles in a woman's body.

Of course, if you're prone to menstrual cramps, you're reminded monthly of just how strong the viselike grip of its dense, muscular layers can be.

What makes the uterus tense up once a month like a body builder bench-pressing a few hundred pounds? In a word, hormones. Not the estrogen and progesterone that orchestrate the menstrual cycle in the first place, but another type called prostaglandins, which control inflammation and body temperature. Released during menstruation, prostaglandins help your uterus contract by prompting blood vessels to tighten. The decrease in blood flow causes the uterine muscle to cramp, making you feel pain in your lower abdomen.

Whether they last a few hours or a few days, the searing pain of menstrual cramps can disrupt your everyday life with dismal regularity. While conventional medications like ibuprofen can successfully help you manage the pain, they do nothing to decrease the incidence of menstrual cramps. The herbal remedies recommended here offer a different approach. They can regulate hormones so that cramps become less of a problem in the long run.

Black Cohosh and Blue Cohosh

During the last 2 weeks of your menstrual cycle, take 15 drops of each tincture three times a day. To make your own cramp-relief formula, mix equal parts of these antispasmodic and anti-inflammatory herbs, suggests Beverly Yates, N.D., a naturopathic physician with the

ADVENTURES IN HERBALISM

A REVOLUTION IN A YAM

*M*any of the drugs that we take for granted today are based on chemical compounds originally found in plants. Aspirin, a chemical version of the salicin found in willow, is probably the most famous. A less well known example is the birth control pill.

According to Barbara Griggs, an herbal historian in London and author of *Green Pharmacy*, chemists in the 1930s and 1940s became intrigued by the possibility of using sex hormones to effect changes in the reproductive cycles of men and women. The problem was finding an affordable source of animal hormones to use as a base for producing a pharmaceutical version. One researcher had to use a whole ton of bull testicles to get less than 300 milligrams of the male sex hormone testosterone.

The problem was solved by Russell E. Marker, an "unpredictable genius" then working at Pennsylvania State College (now Pennsylvania State University) in University Park. Marker was convinced that he could find the hormone model he needed in plants—an idea that was greeted by his peers as absurd. Undeterred, Marker persevered, and eventually he discovered in the Mexican yam the chemical constituents he needed to artificially produce the female sex hormone progesterone.

When Marker announced his discovery, no one believed him, so he quit his job and moved to Mexico City. There, in a tiny rented cottage, he set up a lab, acquired a supply of yams, and began pumping out progesterone. "The Pill" eventually became economically feasible, and the sexual revolution was on its way.

Natural Health Care Group in Portland, Oregon, and Seattle. Viewed as a fortifier of the female reproductive system in Native American medicine, black and blue cohosh contain volatile oils and plant-based hormones that tone the uterine muscle, soothe menstrual cramps, and ease hormone-related headaches.

"I see these herbs as a team. If you suffer from severe cramps, they may not be a 'magic bullet' cure, but you'll likely notice that your cramps become less of a problem," says Dr. Yates.

Cramp Bark or Black Haw and Ginger

Take ½ teaspoon of tincture in hot water twice a day, or drink ½ cup of tea every 3 hours. As its name implies, cramp bark's primary use is to relieve cramps. It works as both an antispasmodic and a sedative to relax the uterus, explains Joel Evans, M.D., a holistic physician and founder and director of the Center for Women's Health in Darien, Connecticut.

A Native American remedy, cramp bark comes from a shrubby tree that grows in North America and Europe. The bark is peeled off in the spring and summer while the plant is flowering. The herb can also be applied externally to relieve muscle tension.

Black haw, which is often used interchangeably with cramp bark, has antispasmodic properties that are thought to be more specific to the uterus. One of the active substances in the root is scopoletine, a strong uterine sedative.

To make tea from either herb, slowly simmer 4 tablespoons of root with 1 tablespoon of grated fresh ginger in 1 quart of water for 20 minutes, then strain. Ginger improves the flavor, is a mild antispasmodic, and helps boost circulation so that you will feel relief faster, says Dr. Evans.

Valerian

If cramps tend to keep you awake, take 40 drops of tincture in a small glass of warm water about an hour before bedtime. Although you may be more familiar with its use as a sleep aid, valerian has been used since the Middle Ages to relieve menstrual cramps. It combines well with cramp bark, says Gayle Eversole, Ph.D., a certified nurse practitioner and a professional member of the American Herbalists Guild (AHG) in Everett, Washington.

If necessary, you can repeat the dose once during the night, but don't take it any later than 4:00 A.M., or you may not wake up on time. If you need daytime relief, you can take 15 to 30 drops of tincture one to three times a day. "Since valerian is somewhat sedating, I wouldn't take it during the day unless cramping is severe," Dr. Eversole advises.

Evening Primrose

Take 3 to 6 grams of oil a day with meals. When cramp-inducing hormones are released during your menstrual period, evening prim-

Fast FACTS

Cause: Hormonelike compounds called prostaglandins that are released during menstruation cause the blood vessels in the uterus to constrict, decreasing blood flow to the area. The uterine muscle then tenses up like a tight fist. This process helps the uterus expel the menstrual flow. Women who have excessive levels of prostaglandins experience monthly occurrences of tenderness and pain.

Incidence: Women tend to develop menstrual cramps from 1 to 2 years after their first menstrual periods. In a study of 265 women ages 17 to 19, 60 percent reported at least one episode of severe pain during their periods, while 13 percent reported severe pain more than half the time. By age 25, cramps usually begin to dissipate, and they may disappear altogether following childbirth.

When to see the doctor: Call your physician if you have pain at an abnormal time in your cycle or if it is severe or lasts longer than 2 to 3 days.

---

rose oil can help counteract their effects, notes Paula Ceh, Pharm.D., assistant professor of pharmacy at Butler University College of Pharmacy and Health Sciences in Indianapolis. Evening primrose oil stimulates production of a good group of prostaglandins—the kind that discourage pain and inflammation.

Dang Gui

To relax the uterus, drink one cup of tea a day, or take ½ teaspoon of tincture in a glass of water up to four times a day 2 weeks before your period. Respected in Chinese medicine as an herb that works well for women's complaints, dang gui (also known as dong quai) regulates the menstrual cycle and eases premenstrual cramping and pain, says Dr. Yates. It functions as a uterine tonic.

A cousin to the parsley plant, dang gui is the most widely used traditional medicine in China. Its slightly sweet-tasting root normalizes irregular uterine contractions and improves blood flow to the uterus. To make a cramp-preventive tea, place 1 teaspoon of root in hot water, cover the pan or mug to preserve the volatile oils, and steep. Strain out the herb before drinking.

There's a hitch, however. You shouldn't use dang gui during menstruation, as it can stimulate bleeding, warns Dr. Evans. Stop taking it a week before your period begins, then resume once your menstrual flow ends. Women who are prone to heavy menstrual bleeding should not use this herb at all.

Raspberry

Drink one cup of tea two or three times day. A daily cup of this pleasant-tasting tea will help relax uterine muscles, says Dr. Evans. For centuries, raspberry leaf has been valued as a nutritive tonic for the female reproductive tract. Midwives still advise pregnant women to drink raspberry tea to tone and prepare the uterus for giving birth.

To make a day's supply, place 1 heaping tablespoon of dried leaves in a quart jar. Fill the jar with just-boiled water, steep for at least 10 minutes, and strain. Store the tea in the refrigerator.

Lavender, Marjoram, Chamomile, Geranium, and Ginger

Massage this blend of cramp-relieving oils onto your hips, abdomen, and lower back two or three times a day. Essential oils can help ease the pain of menstrual cramps through their anti-inflammatory action, says Mindy Green, a founder and professional member of the AHG and director of educational services at the Herb Research Foundation in Boulder, Colorado, in her book *Aromatherapy: A Complete Guide to the Healing Art*. "For best results, start using it a few days before symptoms are expected," she advises.

In the book, Green suggests mixing 4 drops of lavender essential oil, 3 drops each of marjoram, chamomile, and geranium essential oils, 1 drop of ginger oil, and 1 ounce of a carrier oil in a dark glass bottle.

Menstrual
Irregularities

*T*he clockwork regularity of the 28-day menstrual cycle is something of a myth. If you're getting your period every 23 days or every 35 days, you don't have a menstrual irregularity. In fact, you're probably perfectly fine.

Anything between 21 and 36 days is considered normal or regular, explains Joel Evans, M.D., a holistic physician and founder and director of the Women's Health Center in Darien, Connecticut. A bout with the flu, too much exercise, travel, or stress can cause your cycle to fluctuate from month to month. It's also normal for your cycles to become somewhat irregular as you approach menopause, when hormone levels begin to diminish.

"There are two kinds of irregularities," says Beverly Yates, N.D., a naturopathic physician with the Natural Health Care Group in Portland, Oregon, and Seattle. "There are women who are regularly irregular, and there are others with cycles that are sort of free-wheeling. It just shows up whenever it wants to show up. This could be a sign that the body's intricate dance of signals is jumbled."

How do you know if your cycles are truly irregular and in need of fixing? If your periods are more than 6 weeks or less than 3 weeks apart and don't seem to follow a regular pattern, a hormone imbalance may be the problem. The herbs listed here can help restore normal hormone levels and regulate your cycle.

Chasteberry

Take one or two 225-milligram capsules standardized for 0.5 percent agnuside every day. "The single best herb for regulating the menstrual cycle is chasteberry," says Robert Rountree, M.D., a holistic physician at the Helios Health Center in Boulder, Colorado. When taken regularly, chasteberry (also called vitex), regulates the timing of the menstrual cycle by acting on the pituitary gland, which in turn releases the hormones that regulate ovarian function.

Recommended for a number of menstrual disorders by Germany's Commission E, which evaluates herbs for safety and effectiveness, chasteberry is now approved as a common treatment for menstrual irregularity. If you want to use the herb in a less medicinal way, grind the dried fruits and sprinkle them on your food for a peppery flavor.

Don't take chasteberry during the week that you're menstruating, advises Dr. Yates. Constant use of the herb could cause hormone changes that make your period disappear altogether.

Black Cohosh

Drink two to four droppers of tincture in a little water or tea three times a day, or take two capsules of standardized extract daily. Among Native Americans, black cohosh was a widely used folk remedy for menstrual irregularities. Like chasteberry, it has a balancing effect on female hormone production.

"Black cohosh works by acting as a mild estrogen," says Dr. Yates. If your estrogen levels are too low, plant estrogens in the root, called isoflavones, pick up the slack and help regulate your cycle. Research indicates that black cohosh contains three compounds that affect the behavior of estrogen.

Dang Gui

Take ½ teaspoon of alcohol-based tincture in a glass of water up to four times a day. In China, dang gui (also known as dong quai) is widely prescribed for abnormal menstruation. The phytoestrogens in this member of the carrot family help regulate and balance the menstrual cycle, especially if your periods are scanty, says Dr. Yates.

Dang gui's slightly sweet-tasting root can normalize irregular

Fast Facts

Cause: The most frequent cause of irregular menstrual cycles is a hormone imbalance that interferes with estrogen and progesterone production. Occasionally, irregular periods can be related to stress, anxiety, crash dieting, or any of a variety of serious systemic diseases, including kidney and thyroid disorders.

Incidence: Irregular periods are most common at the beginning and end of a woman's reproductive years. Younger women tend to have longer cycles—about 32 days for those in their twenties—while women over 35 may have cycles shorter than 28 days.

When to see the doctor: If your cycle is consistently shorter than 21 days or longer than 36 days, you should see a doctor to determine the cause.

---

uterine contractions and improve blood flow to the uterus. Since it can stimulate bleeding, it's best to stop taking it a week before your period begins and resume once your menstrual flow ends, says Dr. Yates. Women who are prone to heavy menstrual bleeding should not use dang gui at all. Be especially cautious if you have uterine fibroids or endometriosis, as anything that might promote uterine bleeding could aggravate these conditions.

Red Clover and Raspberry

Drink a cup of tea made with equal parts of these herbs every day. A daily cup of this pleasant-tasting tea will support your reproductive system and help correct nutritional deficiencies that may be interfering with hormone activity, says Dr. Yates. For centuries, raspberry leaf has been valued as a tonic for the female reproductive tract. It contains concentrations of a compound called fragarine, which, in combination with several other plant constituents, serves to tone and relax the pelvic and uterine muscles. It is a rich source of many vitamins and minerals and is particularly high in calcium, iron, phosphorus, potassium, and vitamins B, C, and E. The astringent properties of the herb make it a good remedy for excessive menstruation.

Like black cohosh, red clover is rich in hormonelike substances that can help regulate your own estrogen levels.

To make a cup, pour 1 cup of just-boiled water over 1 tablespoon of dried red clover flowers and raspberry leaves and steep for 10 to 15 minutes. Drink it warm or at room temperature.

MIGRAINE

When workers in munitions plants around the end of the nineteenth century were plagued by blinding headaches, they discovered that the word *trigger* had a double meaning in their line of work. The cause of their headaches—nitrate, a common ingredient in gunpowder—is still a common headache trigger, except that these days, you're more likely to get a dose of it in a hot dog.

Whether it's a sensitivity to food ingredients like nitrates, a change in the weather, or simply lack of sleep, some kind of trigger is usually responsible for the throbbing, intense pain of a migraine. Whatever the trigger, however, it isn't actually the cause but rather a factor that aggravates an inborn tendency for this type of headache. Pulling the trigger sets off a chain of chemical and electrical events in the brain that inflames the blood vessels and increases sensitivity to pain.

"We are clearly dealing with a biological problem, not a psychological one," says Fred Sheftell, M.D., founder of the New England Center for Headache in Stamford, Connecticut. Unlike tension headaches that simply annoy you, a migraine completely interrupts normal activity and often requires you to shut off all input from the outside world by closing yourself off in a dark, quiet room with a soft bed.

You can't cure your predisposition to migraines, but you can try to get fewer headaches, says Dr. Sheftell. First, get to know your triggers and avoid them. For example, if you seem to get headaches after eating foods like hot dogs or aged cheese or drinking wine, chances are good that you've found a trigger, since all of these are high in nitrates. Aside from avoiding migraine instigators, these herbal remedies may help prevent migraines in some people, or at least reduce the frequency of attacks.

Feverfew

To prevent migraines, take 125 milligrams in capsule form every day. If your migraines are the type that is relieved by applying heat to your head, taking feverfew regularly may help prevent them, says Keith Robertson, a member of Britain's National Institute of Medical Herbalists and director of education for the Scottish School of Herbal Medicine in Glasgow. Research also shows that it reduces the nausea, vomiting, and sensitivity to light that normally accompany migraines. It also has an anti-inflammatory action similar to that of aspirin and works as a vasodilator (meaning that it opens blood vessels), which is why it seems to work best for people whose headaches are caused by constricted blood vessels. Look for capsules containing a standardized extract of at least 0.2 percent of the active substance parthenolide, Robertson adds.

Dr. Sheftell adds that you'll need to take this herb every day to get the most benefit.

Flaxseed

Take 1 to 2 tablespoons of fresh, cold-pressed oil daily. There's a good chance that you'll get fewer migraines and less intense ones if you take a daily dose of flaxseed oil, says Brent Mathieu, N.D., a

Fast Facts

Cause: Medical evidence suggests that people who get migraines have slightly different brain chemistries than people who don't get them. Imbalances in the chemical and electrical activity in the brain cause fluctuations in the diameter of the blood vessels around the head and neck. Throbbing, intense pain on one side of the head, accompanied by nausea, vomiting, and sensitivity to light or noise, typically distinguish migraines from ordinary headaches. They are commonly triggered by sensitivities to foods such as chocolate, MSG, alcohol, or caffeine; hormone fluctuations during the menstrual cycle; changes in the weather or seasons; sleeping too much or not enough; bright lights; odors; and stress.

Incidence: Roughly 6 percent of men and 18 percent of women experience migraines. Surveys of migraine patients have shown that this susceptibility is largely hereditary. Between 70 and 90 percent of migraine sufferers have other family members who also have them. Doctors estimate that more than half of the people who have migraines have never been diagnosed.

When to see the doctor: Contact your physician if you have three or more headaches a week; if you must take a pain reliever almost every day; if you need more than the recommended dose of over-the-counter pain medicine to relieve your headaches; if you have a stiff neck or a fever in addition to a headache; if you feel dizzy or unsteady or have slurred speech, weakness, numbness, confusion, or drowsiness with a headache; if exertion, coughing, bending, or sexual activity triggers your headaches; if you have a persistent headache that continues to worsen; or if your headaches began after age 50.

naturopathic physician in Boise, Idaho. A rich source of essential fatty acids, flaxseed oil changes your body chemistry so that you produce fewer harmful prostaglandins. These hormonelike chemicals in the blood can increase your sensitivity to pain and cause constriction of the blood vessels.

You can find flaxseed oil in the refrigerated section of health food stores. This fragile oil turns rancid quickly when exposed to heat or light, so make sure it's packaged in a dark, opaque glass bottle. Good-quality oil should have a pleasant, nutty flavor. Stir it into a beverage or drizzle it over a salad. Don't cook with it, though, since it loses its healing properties when heated.

It's safe to take this dose of flaxseed oil indefinitely. For most people, it is beneficial to take for all of their lives.

Wood Betony

Take 2 to 6 milliliters of tincture three times a day to ease nervous tension. If you develop migraines from a buildup of nervous tension, this herb will help ease it away, says Robertson. Wood betony has a sedative action and a tonic effect that strengthens and feeds the nervous system. A traditional migraine remedy, this perennial herb grows in wooded areas in Europe and Britain. You should be able to find it in tincture form at well-stocked health food stores.

Take wood betony for 3 to 4 weeks. If your symptoms persist, consult a qualified herbalist.

Skullcap and Rosemary

Drink one to three cups a day of tea made from both herbs, depending on your symptoms. When taken together, rosemary and skullcap create a seemingly paradoxical effect that both stimulates and relaxes you, says Gayle Eversole, Ph.D., a certified nurse practitioner and a professional member of the American Herbalists Guild in Everett, Washington. Rosemary works as a circulatory stimulant to bring more blood and oxygen to the brain, she explains, while skullcap is relaxing and helps nourish and support the nervous system. Historically, both have been used to treat pain.

To make the tea, use 1 teaspoon dried (or 1 tablespoon fresh) of each herb per cup of boiling water. Pour the water over the herbs, cover, and steep for 15 to 20 minutes. It's safe to use this remedy until symptoms subside.

Motion Sickness

*P*eople have been using ginger to soothe their queasy stomachs for centuries, but it took an herbalist from Utah to put this traditional motion sickness remedy to the test.

In his book *The Scientific Validation of Herbal Medicine*, Daniel Mowrey, Ph.D., describes how, after discovering that taking a ginger capsule stopped him from vomiting during a bout with 24-hour flu, he recruited a bunch of people to prove its effectiveness. Half of the hapless volunteers were given a dose of dimenhydrinate (the antihistamine in Dramamine) and half were given a gram of powdered ginger. Then—and this was the fun part—they were strapped into a tilting, rotating chair guaranteed to set their stomachs heaving. The result? The ginger kept nausea at bay almost twice as long as the dimenhydrinate did.

You don't have to be strapped into a spinning chair to get motion sickness. A trip down the highway can do it. So can an airplane flight, a sojourn on the high seas, or a spin on one of the scary rides at the amusement park. The reason that some of us get that tied-in-knots, gut-churning feeling has to do with our senses of balance and spatial orientation.

The trouble starts when the central nervous system receives mixed messages from our inner ears, eyes, skin pressure receptors, and muscle and joint sensory receptors. When you're sitting in the back seat of a car reading a book, for example, your eyes don't detect the motion because what you're focusing on is stationary. Your inner ears and skin receptors know that you're moving, though, and your brain is confused by signals that don't jibe. You end up being nauseated.

If you want to avoid the inevitable outcome, you have to act fast once nausea starts to sneak up on you. The American Academy of Otolaryngology–Head and Neck Surgery suggests the following strategies. First, avoid strong odors and spicy or greasy foods immediately before or during travel (definitely not the time to opt for goat curry with pickled jalapeños). Always ride where your eyes will see what your body and inner ears are feeling: in the front seat of the car, up on the deck of a ship, by the window in an airplane or train, facing the direction you're traveling. And don't even think about reading.

Ginger may be the most powerful herbal motion sickness remedy around, but it's not the only one. To help you enjoy the scenery without side effects, try these herbal stomach calmers.

Peppermint

Put 3 to 5 drops of essential oil on your tongue when your stomach starts to rebel. Peppermint has been praised as an anti-nausea herb for at least 2 centuries. You can find peppermint essential oil at local health food stores. The cure couldn't be simpler, either. As soon as you start to feel queasy, just open your mouth, tip the vial, and let a few drops of oil hit your tongue. You can use this remedy up to four times a day, suggests Andrew Lucking, N.D., a naturopathic doctor in Minneapolis. Just think how sweet your breath will be when you're back on terra firma.

Black Horehound

Make a tea and drink it three times a day or as needed. Pour 1 cup of boiling water over ½ teaspoon of dried herb and steep for 10 minutes, then strain, says Australian naturopath Andrew Pengelly, N.D., who runs the Valley Herb Clinic in Hunter Valley, New South Wales. For a long journey, make up a thermos of the tea and take it along. When you feel nausea approaching, sip the tea as you need it. Note that this tea is very bitter, so a small amount of ginger will improve the flavor and the effect, he says.

Distress Express Fizz

Once motion sickness has you in its grip, there's not much you can do to head off the inevitable vomiting. With a little forethought, though, you might just nip that nasty malaise in the bud. Joan Haynes, N.D., a naturopathic physician in Boise, Idaho, swears by this homemade ginger ale, which calms the stomach, stops the churning, and tastes good to boot.

- **1 2" piece fresh ginger**
- **2 cups water**
- **1 cup honey or Sucanat**
- **Carbonated mineral water**

Grate the ginger and add it to the water in a saucepan. Boil for 10 minutes. Add the honey or Sucanat and boil for 10 to 15 minutes. Remove from the heat and let stand for at least 30 minutes. Strain and add more honey or Sucanat to taste, if desired.

Keep this ginger syrup in the refrigerator. To use, add the syrup to taste to a glass of carbonated mineral water and sip as needed. The refrigerated syrup should keep for about a month.

Note: Sucanat is an unrefined sugar product available in health food stores.

Ginger

Make a tea from fresh ginger and drink it before departure. If you're about to set off on a car journey and you know that you'll be feeling green before you reach the city limits, budget about 15 minutes of predeparture time to make this stomach-soothing tea. Grate 1 teaspoon of fresh ginger and add it to 1 cup of warm water. Don't use freshly boiled water, as too much flavor will leach out of the ginger and make the tea taste unpleasantly strong, says Dr. Lucking. Add 1 tablespoon of fresh lemon juice and 1 teaspoon of honey and steep for 10 minutes. For maximum benefit, drink down all of the pieces of ginger floating in the tea, he adds.

Fast Facts

Cause: The chief cause of motion sickness is—you guessed it—motion. It all comes down to your sense of balance. When the messages that your central nervous system receives from your eyes, inner ears, and body are out of sync, you feel dizzy and queasy.

Incidence: Everyone has probably suffered from this malaise at one time or another. The most common medical problem associated with travel, motion sickness is slightly more common in women, particularly Asian women.

When to see the doctor: If you're so dizzy that you can't walk or even sit up, find a doctor. The same applies if you have repeated vomiting and can't keep anything down. Also seek medical advice if your hearing is affected, you have ringing or fullness in your ears, or you experience ear pain, discharge, or bleeding.

Valerian

To calm travel jitters, take a 500-milligram capsule 1 hour before departure. If you're phobic about flying or the very thought of the open sea makes you quake, your pretrip nerves can upset your stomach even before you leave home. It won't take much turbulence or jostling around for those butterflies to turn into full-blown motion sickness. Beware, though: The odor of valerian is, er, unusual, to say the least. You may not want to get a whiff of the capsule before you swallow it, or your efforts may be counterproductive.

Brewer's Yeast

Eat some popcorn topped with 1 tablespoon of powdered yeast ½ hour before you travel. No one really knows why, but it's believed that vitamin B_6 helps to alleviate nausea by somehow helping liver enzymes modulate the brain chemistry. Dr. Lucking suggests taking brewer's yeast, a rich source of the vitamin, for motion sickness. Sprinkling the yeast on popcorn is a nice way of taking it, says Dr. Lucking, and popcorn is a bland food that absorbs some of the stomach acids that may irritate people with motion sickness.

NAIL FUNGUS

Nail fungus is tough to cure, not because it's a hardy foe but because it has carved out an ideal environmental niche for itself.

Hiding out beneath a nail, these microscopic critters are well-protected from the two main avenues of human assault. Salves and ointments have a hard time getting underneath the nail to the source of the problem, while antifungal drugs may take up to 6 months to deliver a knockout punch. "Oral medications are distributed through the body by the circulatory system," says Kathleen Janel, N.D., a naturopathic physician with the Brattleboro Naturopathic Clinic in Vermont, "and there's a very limited blood supply to a nail."

Nail fungi not only hide beneath the nail, they feed on it, so the nail gradually deteriorates. Once a fungal infection sets in, the nail often thickens and turns yellowish brown, and fungal gunk collects under it. It stinks if left untreated, and the nail becomes disfigured and splits from the nail bed.

As unappealing as this sounds, nail fungus is easy to ignore because it's not painful and it lives in such an obscure corner of the body. Women frequently cover up the problem with nail polish and

*L*avender's healing powers have been applied to plenty of skin problems in addition to nail fungus. In fact, lavender played a central role in the modern renaissance of aromatherapy.

The man credited with coining that term was a French chemist by the name of René-Maurice Gattefossé. The story is that in 1910, he was working in his laboratory when an explosion severely burned his hands and arms. Exactly what happened next depends on whose version you believe, but in some accounts he plunged his arms into a vat containing essential oil of lavender. So miraculous was the lavender's healing power that Gattefossé devoted the rest of his life to researching the medicinal properties of essential oils. His 1937 book, *Aromatherapie*, is considered the foundation work in the field.

pretend it's not there—a bad idea. Fungal infections don't go away; they spread from nail to nail and possibly into your skin.

Given how hard these infections are to eliminate, many doctors feel that the only solution is to remove the nail and let the body start over by growing a new one. There are a few herbal alternatives that you can try first, however, especially if the infection is still in its early stages.

Lavender

Rub essential oil on the infected nail at night. Lavender is an herb with antifungal properties, says Michael Traub, N.D., a naturopathic physician in Kailua Kona, Hawaii.

"Nail fungus is stubborn and takes months to cure," he says, "but

Fast Facts

Cause: Various types of fungi live in the world, just waiting to infect the nails of hapless people prone to such invasions.

Incidence: Approximately 10 percent of the American population is affected by nail fungus each year, but studies suggest that the overall number of people infected is probably several times that high.

When to see the doctor: Although nail fungus is not life-threatening or even painful, an infection can take months and even years to treat successfully at home. See a doctor if you experience itching, redness, or swelling around the site of the infection. Because fungal outbreaks represent some compromise of the immune system, elderly people and children should be evaluated by a professional at the first signs of infection.

---

with consistent applications of lavender, the nail will become healthier as it grows out. It's important to apply it immediately after bathing because the skin is softer and the oil will be better absorbed."

Pau d'Arco

Soak the infected nail in a decoction for 20 minutes twice a day or more. Pau d'arco is the bark of a South American tree known to have strong antifungal properties, says Dr. Janel. To make a strong soak, bring enough water to cover the infected area to a boil. Add 1 to 2 tablespoons of dried herb per cup of water and boil for 10 to 20 minutes. Let it cool, then soak the infected nail in the resulting decoction.

Tea Tree

Apply 1 to 2 drops of oil once or twice a day. Tea tree oil is another potent antifungal medicine, says Dr. Janel. Simply apply the oil directly to the top of the nail.

Garlic

Take capsules equal to 7,500 micrograms of allicin in three divided doses daily. Allicin is the active ingredient in garlic, and it has potent antifungal properties. Be forewarned, however, that the amount of allicin in any given brand of garlic capsules varies widely. Dr. Janel recommends that you make sure you get what you need by reading the label and gauging the appropriate daily dosage by the amount of allicin listed there.

NAUSEA

*E*veryone knows what nausea is. Even the word sounds, well, nauseating. Your stomach churns faster than a farmhand making butter. At its worst, nausea can be accompanied by sweating and vomiting.

Like the warning lights on the instrument panel in your car, nausea is your body's way of signaling that something's not right. It's a way of saying "service required." The problem is, though, that it's a generalized warning. Sometimes the reason for the distress call will be obvious, and sometimes it won't.

At times, to settle your stomach, it's best just to throw up, says Tim Hagney, N.D., a naturopathic physician in Anchorage, Alaska. Frequently, that's all it takes. Unfortunately, that doesn't always work, leaving you with the dry heaves as your body tries to get rid of something that's just not there. And still the nausea persists.

If that's the case, you probably need some good news. Here it is: Herbs have a long, proud tradition of soothing embattled stomachs.

In fact, stomach upsets are as old as stomachs themselves, and many an early healer turned to the plants around him to calm the raging storms of nausea. Here are some time-honored cures to get your gut back in low gear.

Ginger

Slowly sip a cup of tea as needed. Ginger should be your first stop on the way to reducing nausea, says Donald R. Counts, M.D., an Austin, Texas, physician who combines conventional medicine and proven alternative treatments in his practice. Studies have shown that ginger can be even more effective than anti-nausea drugs at calming the waves in your stomach.

You can buy ginger tea bags at health food stores and some grocery stores. Just put a tea bag in a mug, pour boiling water over it, and steep for at least 5 minutes. Let it cool a bit before drinking.

Alternatively, you can make the tea from fresh root if you have some handy or can get to a supermarket, says James S. Sensenig, N.D., distinguished visiting professor at the University of Bridgeport College of Naturopathic Medicine in Connecticut and founding president of the American Association of Naturopathic Physicians. To do that, finely chop or grate 1 teaspoon of fresh ginger. Put it into a mug and fill the mug with boiling water, then cover with a saucer and steep for 10 minutes. Strain and let the tea cool somewhat.

In a pinch, you can even use the powdered ginger in your spice rack. "That's a last resort, though," says Dr. Sensenig. "A lot of the volatile oils are missing from the powdered spice." Use ¼ to ½ teaspoon of ginger per cup of water, steep for 10 minutes, and let cool.

Perhaps best of all is real ginger ale, if you can get your hands on some. Not only will the ginger do the trick, the carbonation can help as well. Don't bother with Schweppes or Canada Dry, though. "The commercially available stuff doesn't even have ginger," explains Dr. Sensenig. Instead, look at health food or spe-

Fast FACTS

Cause: Nausea is a symptom of an underlying problem, not a disorder in itself, and there are many things that can make you nauseated. They range from too much alcohol to the flu, improper digestion, and the effects of medical treatments such as chemotherapy.

Incidence: Do you have a stomach? Well, then, at some point or other, you'll feel the debilitating effects of nausea. Everyone knows what a roiling, tumbling, unsettled stomach feels like.

When to see the doctor: If you are nauseated for several days, have it checked out. It could be a result of something serious. Likewise, if nausea follows a nasty knock on the head, get medical attention immediately. You could have a concussion.

cialty stores for the real McCoy. It should contain real ginger root or its extract, says Dr. Sensenig. Sip it slowly for as long as you're feeling queasy.

Fennel

Take 30 to 40 drops of tincture in a glass of water. Fennel is a carminative, says Dr. Hagney. Literally, the word means "stomach soothing." If it's food that's making you feel queasy, take the tincture before each meal. Otherwise, just take it as needed.

You can often find fennel in something called a Swedish bitters mix, adds Dr. Hagney. Just check the label for ingredients. Bitters are a digestive aid and should be taken before meals, following the dosage above.

You can also get the benefits of fennel by chewing the seeds. Take a small handful and chew them slowly. As your stomach steadies, you can munch on a few more. It's probably not a good idea to swallow the seeds if you're nauseated, however, says Dr. Hagney.

Catnip

Drink tea as needed. Catnip isn't just something that makes your cat crazy, says Dr. Counts. It's also very soothing to ravaged stomachs. Catnip teas are available at any decently stocked grocery store and at most health food stores.

A member of the mint family, catnip also has mild sedative properties, so you may find yourself sleepy as well as relieved. Steep the tea for at least 5 minutes before straining, and let it cool somewhat so that the temperature isn't too shocking to your stomach.

Peppermint

Drink tea as needed. Peppermint is one of the oldest known remedies for nausea, says Dr. Sensenig, and that's because it usually works. "Mint has a very relaxing effect on the gut muscles," he says. That means an end to the roiling you're feeling. Pick up some real peppermint tea at a health food store or grocery store. Just check the label to be sure that it's not just regular tea with peppermint flavoring.

If you have a bunch of fresh peppermint, that will work very nicely as well. Add 1 cup of boiling water to ¼ to ½ cup of fresh, clean leaves. Steep for 10 minutes and strain out the leaves. Sip slowly after it's cooled somewhat.

Anise

Drink one cup of decoction as needed. You may know anise as licorice, and actually, anise is added to many candies and other foods to give them a "licorice" flavor. That's how the decoction tastes, and it's also a good stomach soother, says Dr. Sensenig.

To make the decoction, add 1 cup of boiling water to about 1 teaspoon of aniseed. Steep for 10 minutes, then strain out the seeds. Let the tea cool and sip.

If you just can't wait that long, you can slowly chew and swallow about 1 teaspoon of seeds to get the same benefits.

NICOTINE ADDICTION

*M*ore people than ever before are crushing out their butts for the last time. Just because we're finally getting the message that smoking is bad and quitting is good, though, that doesn't mean that breaking the habit has gotten any easier. It's still an exercise in restraint that involves both your body and your mind.

The physical cravings are what drive you to light up on a regular basis in the first place. Inhaling those plumes of smoke stimulates pleasure centers in your brain, giving you feelings of satisfaction that become hard to live without.

Smoking makes a slave of you psychologically, too. Just knowing that you have a little ritual—lighting up—to turn to can make stressful situations seem easier to get through. And having a cigarette in hand becomes a kind of security blanket or even a crutch during those times when you just don't know what to do with your hands.

Quitting successfully means solving both sides of the problem— the physical and the mental. To address physical cravings, some people turn to synthetic nicotine in the form of patches or gum; others chew on pencils or take up blowing bubbles.

To counter the psychological desire to smoke, experts suggest changing any behavior that you associate with smoking. Some good advice includes throwing away your lighters and ashtrays, moving your furniture around, and even taking a different route to and from work. These tactics can change the scenery and help you avoid the urge to smoke.

Herbs can be a natural part of a do-it-yourself stop-smoking program. Not only can they calm the physical cravings and soothe your psyche, they can actually boost your body's overall health as well, says William Page-Echols, D.O., osteopathic doctor at Full Spectrum Family Medicine in East Lansing, Michigan. Here are the herbs that can help turn you into a nonsmoker, once and for all.

St. John's Wort

Take 300 milligrams of standardized extract in capsule form three times a day. Many people who smoke may also be slightly depressed, says Dr. Page-Echols. Smoking, he says, may be a sign of self-medication. "Nicotine clearly affects mood, and people who smoke are using it to manipulate their moods. It makes sense that herbs could be used in the same way to help a person quit."

That general theory is what's behind the prescription drug buproprion (Zyban), which is used to help people quit. Buproprion's mood-lifting effects are similar to those of another antidepressant medication called fluoxetine, otherwise known as Prozac. The herb St. John's wort has been shown to have similar mood-mending actions.

While there isn't any scientific research to prove it, Dr. Page-Echols believes that the effects of St. John's wort are similar enough to buproprion's to help smokers quit herbally. "I've had great success using it with my patients," he says. "It's less expensive, and there are fewer effects to worry about."

If you'd like to use St. John's wort to help you quit, you'll have to take the same dose that's been deemed effective for treating mild depression. Look for capsules of standardized extract and take 300 milligrams three times a day, for a total of 900 milligrams. The actual number of capsules you'll have to take will depend on the formula you buy.

You should start taking the herb 2 full weeks before your chosen quit date, says Dr. Page-Echols. This will give the St. John's wort time to build up in your body, making quitting easier than it would be without it. Once you're smoke-free, continue to take the herb for 3 to 4 months. After that, you can stop by gradually reducing your dose.

Siberian Ginseng, Licorice, Oats, and Lobelia

Take one dropper of this custom-blended tincture whenever cravings come on. "Herbs that are commonly used for countering addiction are basically adrenal-supporting in nature," explains Nancy

Cause: Nicotine is incredibly addictive. Cigarette smoke enters the body and reaches the brain faster than drugs injected with a needle. A smoking habit is doubly hard to kick because it involves both physical and mental dependence.

Incidence: There are 47 million smokers in the United States alone. Of that number, more than 30 million report that they would like to be able to quit.

When to see the doctor: Smoking-related diseases kill more than 400,000 Americans each year. Cigarette smoking is directly related to lung cancer, emphysema, and bronchitis. It also contributes to heart disease and stroke and is linked to other health problems such as infertility and ulcers. If you smoke, be sure to tell your doctor, and have checkups regularly. Your best health bet: Quit as soon as you can.

Welliver, N.D., director of the Institute of Medical Herbalism in Calistoga, California.

Each adrenal gland (you have two) is a small, triangle-shaped organ that's attached to the top of a kidney. These complex little nuggets are responsible for releasing hormones that go on to stimulate other organs, affecting heart rate, metabolism, circulation, and digestion. Herbalists believe that boosting adrenal gland function is important for recovery from chronic stressors such as nicotine addiction.

Get one 2-ounce bottle each of Siberian ginseng, licorice, and oats tinctures and a 1-ounce bottle of lobelia tincture. If you have high blood pressure, substitute 1 ounce of lemon balm and 1 ounce of hawthorn for the licorice, since licorice may exacerbate high blood pressure.

Empty the contents of the four bottles into a large measuring cup or a bowl with a pour spout. Set the empty bottles aside. Gently stir the liquid to blend the tinctures well, then use a small funnel to carefully refill the bottles with your new custom-mixed, craving-calming tincture.

When a cigarette craving threatens to ruin your resolve, squeeze one dropper of the mixture into half a glass of water and sip. If water's not available, you can take the tincture by putting it directly under your tongue, says Dr. Welliver, but be prepared for a potent taste.

You can take this blend up to 10 times a day. If you feel the need to take it more often, mix half a dropper with an even smaller amount of water and take it up to 20 times a day. After the first couple of weeks, start decreasing the amount of lobelia and increasing the amount of Siberian ginseng. Generally, you can take this mixture for anywhere from 2 weeks to 2 months.

NOSEBLEEDS

*M*ost parts of the human body are surprisingly durable. Whack yourself with the car door, and you'll likely walk away with a bruise that fades in a few days. Tangle with a holly bush, and you'll probably escape with a minor scratch or two. But the edge of a fingernail, a mote of dust or pollen, or even just a change in the air is sometimes all it takes to give you a nosebleed.

As delicate as rose petals, the membranes in your nose don't take abuse stoically. Moreover, it's not the classic head-on collisions with unyielding objects that usually set them off. Mostly, it's the dryness caused by indoor heat in the winter, colds, and allergies that upset the tender inner lining of your nose.

Generally more of a nuisance than a cause for real concern, nosebleeds are embarrassing, alarming, and just plain messy. Although most will stop on their own after a few minutes, it's good to know some ways to stop the bleeding. Luckily, there are several easily prepared remedies that can help stem the tide. The herbs that stop nosebleeds tend to be those that have an astringent effect on the blood vessels and cause them to contract, herbalists say.

Before you reach for the herbs, though, try the simplest remedy of all. Pinch the fleshy parts of your nose together and press firmly toward the facial bones, says Alan J. Sogg, M.D., an otolaryngologist in Cleveland. To help nature along, keep your head higher than your heart, tilt it forward, and hold the pinch for about 5 minutes.

To guard against future nosebleeds, use a humidifier to moisten the air or soak a cotton swab in sesame oil and massage it into the nasal cavity, suggests Sally LaMont, N.D., a naturopathic doctor and licensed acupuncturist in Marin County, California. Consider your diet, too. Nosebleeds can be a sign of weak blood vessels, which may be caused by a shortage of vitamin C. Take 1,000 milligrams of C a day in tablet form, says Dr. LaMont. She also recommends 500 milligrams of bioflavonoids daily. Eat ¼ cup of cherries, blueberries, or blackberries every day, too, says Dr. LaMont. These fruits are rich in flavonoids, compounds that help to strengthen the capillary walls.

When the faucet's on and you're running out of tissues, though, what you need is an immediate solution. Try these herbal remedies to stop the bleeding in its tracks.

Yarrow

Use an astringent nasal wash. An ancient medicinal herb, yarrow has been used for centuries as a dressing for wounds. The plant's common names alone—soldier's woundwort, nose bleed, bloodwort, and staunchweed—tell a graphic story. According to legend, Achilles used yarrow to stanch the bleeding wounds of his soldiers, hence yarrow's botanical name, *Achillea millefolium*.

To make a nasal wash, pour 1 cup of boiling water over 2 tablespoons of dried herb, steep for 10 minutes, strain, and let it cool. Roy Upton, vice president of the American Herbalists Guild and executive director of American Herbal Pharmacopeia, an herbal education foundation based in Santa Cruz, California, recommends tilting your head back and squirting the wash into your nose with an eyedropper. "If you can stand it, it stops the bleeding really fast," he says.

Otherwise, soak a washcloth in the wash, tip your head back, and squeeze the solution into your nose a little at a time. If you are prone to nosebleeds, you can make this infusion and store it in the refrigerator for up to a week, says Upton.

Fast FACTS

Cause: Dry air, vitamin C deficiency, colds, or allergies are often to blame for nosebleeds. Certain types of drug abuse (such as snorting cocaine) and overindulging in alcoholic beverages also make nosebleeds more likely. Daily aspirin use, which thins the blood and decreases its clotting abilities, can also lead to recurrent nosebleeds.

Incidence: According to one study, nosebleeds are twice as common in men as in women up to the age of 49, but after age 50, the discrepancy disappears. Overall, they are more common in people over 40.

When to see the doctor: If you can't stop the bleeding after 15 minutes, or it keeps starting again, call your doctor. You should also seek medical attention if blood is gushing out of your nose or running down the back of your throat. If your nosebleed is the result of an accident such as a fall, see a doctor to rule out the possibility of internal bleeding.

Shepherd's Purse

Take 60 drops of tincture three times a day. So called because its seed pods look like old-fashioned leather purses, shepherd's purse is a powerful astringent that has long been used in traditional medicine to stop bleeding. Irene Catania, N.D., a naturopathic doctor in Ho-Ho-Kus, New Jersey, advises taking the dose above in a shot glass of water on the day of the nosebleed and then taking 30 drops three times the following day. Watch out, though; it's bitter. Mixing it with orange juice instead of water will make it taste better.

Bayberry and Cayenne

Take one dose of 20 drops of bayberry and 10 drops of cayenne. Combine the tinctures on a saucer, pick up the liquid with an eyedropper, and drop it on your tongue. The effect is dramatic, says Steve Horne, president of the American Herbalists Guild and owner of an herb shop in Roosevelt, Utah.

"Your tastebuds are linked to your nerves, so if you put something on your tongue that's astringent, it sends a message through the nervous system that causes the tissues to tense and the bleeding to stop," he says. Usually, one dose will do the trick, says Horne. Cayenne is super-hot, so brace yourself.

English Oak

Sniff 1 teaspoon of bark infusion or decoction. You can find spring-harvested, dried bark of the young oak tree in powder form at health food stores. To make an infusion, boil 1 cup of water and pour it over 2 tablespoons of dried bark. Steep for 10 minutes, then strain out the bark. A decoction is similar, except that you bring the water to a boil with the herb in the pot, then let it simmer on low heat for 10 minutes. Before using the liquid, make sure it is cool enough that you don't burn your nose, then lie down with your head back and gently sniff the liquid up your nostril. You can prepare this remedy ahead of time and store it in the refrigerator for up to a week.

The astringent properties of the oak bark should stop the bleeding within 10 minutes, says Christopher Robbins, a member of Britain's National Institute of Medical Herbalists who practices herbal medicine in Ross-on-Wye, Herefordshire, England, and has written several books, including *The Natural Pharmacy*. Don't blow your nose afterward, or it may start bleeding again, he adds.

OILY HAIR

*O*ily hair is really a problem of oily skin, albeit in a very specific place. When oil glands in the scalp become overactive and produce too much lubricating oil, it can build up on the hair shafts. The results are often obvious—greasy-looking, flat, heavy hair.

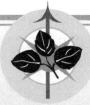

ADVENTURES IN HERBALISM

HEMP FOR HEALTH?

*T*he flowering tops of the lowly hemp plant, *Cannabis sativa*, have earned this annual a bad reputation under a list of aliases, including ganja, grass, dope, and marijuana. But other parts of this five-leaved, weedlike plant have many noble uses that have nothing to do with recreational mind alteration.

In the past (and today, in places where its cultivation is legal), hemp was an alternative source of pulp for paper making and fiber for the manufacture of cloth. Hempseed contains high-quality protein and healthy fats, making it a nutritious food source.

Food-grade hemp oil is currently becoming more available. You can get it at health food stores and via mail order. For now, the sterilized seeds used to produce the oil must be imported (legally) from Canada. Perhaps in the future, hemp will once again become known as a helpful herb rather than a harmful one.

Oily hair may be more prevalent in teens (due to hormone fluctuations), but it isn't restricted to the young. Washing oily hair daily is a good step to take, but you should lather up only once, says Diana Bihova, M.D., a dermatologist in New York City. Sudsing twice, as some shampoo labels direct you to do, might seem to remove more oil, but it can also dry your hair and make it coarse, dull, and full of static. Don't lather twice every day, she advises.

Once your mane is squeaky clean, try these herbal approaches to combat oiliness from inside and out.

Hempseed or Flaxseed

Take 1 tablespoon of hempseed oil or ground flaxseed daily. Eating a certain type of oil to combat oily hair may seem like a con-

Fast FACTS

Cause: Oily hair is caused by overactive sebaceous glands located in the scalp. Hormone changes, poor hygiene, and stress can all be to blame.

Incidence: Oily hair is more common in teenagers due to the hormone fluctuations they are subject to, but it can occur later in life as well.

When to see the doctor: If daily washing and herbal treatments are not enough to keep oily hair in check, see a dermatologist for an evaluation.

---

tradition, but it works, says Monique Martin, D.O., a doctor of osteopathic internal medicine at American WholeHealth in Littleton, Colorado. The seeds of both hemp and flax contain beneficial oils in the form of essential fatty acids.

Hempseed oil is considered the best source of the type of essential fatty acids known as omega-3's, which are known to promote skin health as well as protect against heart disease and many cancers. Ground flaxseed also supplies a good amount, along with a healthy dose of fiber.

You can purchase hempseed oil at health food stores (look in the refrigerated section) or through mail order. (Just for the record, while hempseed does come from the cannabis plant, known for producing marijuana, the seeds do not generate a mind-altering effect.) You can swallow the oil straight or use it on salad or bread.

Flaxseed is also available at health food stores. If you opt for flax, use a clean coffee grinder to grind 1 tablespoon of seeds, then sprinkle them over cereal or yogurt. You can also mix ground flaxseed with ½ cup of water, stir thoroughly, and drink it down.

Rosemary

Make some strong tea and use it as a rinse after every shampoo. The potent essential oils in rosemary can actually help control overproduction of oil on the scalp. "Besides pulling out excess oil, rosemary is great for hair health in general," says Steven Rissman, N.D., a naturopathic physician at American WholeHealth in Cherry Creek, Colorado. And the herb smells wonderful while it does the job.

Use 2 tablespoons of dried rosemary to 1 cup of boiling water. Steep for 20 minutes, then strain and cool. If you like, you can add a few drops of rosemary essential oil to the brew. Then use a funnel to transfer your hair tea to an empty, clean shampoo bottle. Keep the bottle in the shower and splash your hair with the tea as a final rinse. There's no need to rinse again.

OILY SKIN

*I*f your skin has a shine instead of healthy glow, blame it on your glands. Specifically, your sebaceous glands, which can crank out an overabundance of an oily substance called sebum. While having just the right amount of this waxy goo helps keep your skin and hair lubricated, you may be all too familiar with the consequences of its excess—acne-prone skin and enlarged pores.

The oil glands slip into dormancy shortly after birth. Then, stimulated by the hormones of puberty, they awaken just in time to complicate those image-conscious, tumultuous teen years. If all goes well, just about the time you start settling into real life, your hormones settle down, too. And, although they grow larger as you age, the sebaceous glands also produce less and less sebum.

That's the scenario for most people. For some, though, it seems that their skin never grows up. If you have oily skin, proper cleaning is an obvious solution. By that we mean gentle cleansing with gentle ingredients like those listed here. Instinct may tell you to strip away every molecule of excess oil, but this can actually make your skin worse by sending your body a signal to make more sebum, not less, says Jennifer Brett, N.D., a naturopathic physician in Stratford, Connecticut.

Instead of investing a small fortune in specialized cosmetics to care for your skin, follow a cleansing, toning, and moisturizing regimen using the herbal remedies listed here.

Flaxseed

Take 1 tablespoon of oil every day. Your skin is a reflection of your diet. Increasing the amount of healthy oils you consume, such as flaxseed, which is rich in omega-3 essential fatty acids, has been shown to help many skin conditions, including oily skin, says Dr. Brett. Taking flaxseed oil every day helps normalize sebum production.

Shop for fresh, cold-pressed, refrigerated flaxseed oil packaged in a dark, opaque bottle. The oil turns rancid quickly when exposed to light or heat, so you can't cook with it. Instead, stir it into a glass of juice in the morning or drizzle it on salad or vegetables. It should have a pleasant, nutty flavor, says Alan M. Dattner, M.D., a holistic dermatologist in New Rochelle, New York.

Oats or Rice and Witch Hazel

Use a cleansing paste. Herbalists make facial scrubs by combining finely ground dry ingredients with a liquid—everything from plain water to maple syrup. The pasty formula gently cleans and polishes the skin. Scrubs also tend to nourish the skin by stimulating circulation.

"A scrub is used like a soap-and-water wash, but it tends to leave the skin smoother and less stripped of its protective oils," says Dina Falconi, a medical herbalist, author of *Earthly Bodies and Heavenly*

Marvelous Mask

Cypress and lemon essential oils and the fruit and leaves of strawberry help normalize overactive oil glands, says Kathi Keville, director of the American Herb Association, in her book Herbs for Health and Healing. *Try her fragrant mask once a week. Leave it on for 5 to 10 minutes, then rinse it off before your skin begins to feel tight and itchy.*

- **1 tablespoon witch hazel**
- **1 teaspoon bentonite or other facial clay**
- **1 strawberry, mashed (optional)**
- **2 drops cypress essential oil**
- **2 drops lemon essential oil**

Combine the witch hazel, clay, strawberry (if using), cypress oil, and lemon oil in a small bowl.

Hair, and founder of Falcon Formulations in upstate New York. "If you generally use soap on your face, you may want to replace it altogether with a scrub. They contain no harsh detergents or artificial scents."

This simple recipe for a grain scrub, developed by Falconi, absorbs excess oil and helps shed dead skin cells that can clog pores. To make three to four applications, grind and sift 2 tablespoons of oats, brown rice, or other grain. For each application, moisten 1 to 2 teaspoons of dry ingredients with enough witch hazel to form a paste. Smooth it on your skin, then massage thoroughly and gently with your fingertips for about a minute. "Rubbing too hard or too long will irritate delicate facial skin," says Falconi. Rinse with warm water.

For oily skin, she recommends starting your skin-care regimen with the grain cleansing, then following with an astringent while your skin is still moist and finishing with a moisturizer appropriate for oily skin. You can use an astringent toner and skip the moisturizing step if you don't think you need it.

Sage and Thyme

Make a cleanser with herbs and buttermilk to use up to three times a week. Sage and thyme have an antiseptic effect and are good for skin that is acne-prone or has large pores, says Falconi. Buttermilk breaks down dead skin cells and lifts dirt off the surface of the skin. Its astringent action tightens pores and tones the tissue. Check the label to be sure that the buttermilk contains active cultures, which have "good" acids, she says. And always look for freshly dried herbs that are strongly fragrant and have vibrant color.

To make two applications of cleanser, combine ¼ teaspoon each of dried sage and thyme and 1 tablespoon of buttermilk. Cover and let stand for 1 hour at room temperature or overnight in the refrigerator. Using your fingertips, apply it to your face in a gentle, circular motion. Leave the mixture on for 3 to 5 minutes, then remove with a warm, damp washcloth.

Witch Hazel

Blot oily areas with distilled witch hazel twice a day after cleansing. A no-frills toner that Grandma probably used, witch hazel is still a very good astringent, says Dr. Brett. Using it daily kills bacteria on the skin and helps remove excess oil and dead skin cells that can clog pores. Do this for no more than 2 to 3 weeks because it's very drying. After that, she recommends a once-a-day application followed by a light moisturizer. You can use this regimen indefinitely, says Dr. Brett.

Leaves and young twigs of the witch hazel tree are distilled to make the inexpensive bottled astringent that you see on store shelves. The herbal solution contains large quantities of tannins, which have a drying, astringent effect that causes the proteins of the skin surface to tighten.

Chamomile, Elder, Comfrey, and Nettle

After cleansing, mist with a soothing, anti-inflammatory astringent. Falconi often teaches this recipe to students who attend her herbal classes.

Fast FACTS

Cause: Heredity and hormones influence how oily skin is. Tiny glands located along hair shafts all over the body produce a thick, oily substance called sebum, which lubricates the skin. The glands are most numerous and productive on the scalp and face, with the largest located on the forehead, nose, and upper back. Male hormones called androgens stimulate sebum production. Hormone imbalances—common during adolescence, the menstrual cycle, and pregnancy—can trigger overactivity of the glands.

Incidence: Nearly everyone has a bout with oily skin as their bodies weather the hormone fluctuations of puberty.

When to see the doctor: Oily skin can be a sign of certain glandular disorders, so see your doctor if your oily skin is accompanied by unusual constipation, weight gain, or fatigue.

Combine equal parts of dried chamomile and elder flowers, comfrey root, and nettle leaf to equal a hefty handful or 1 ounce (by weight) and place the blend in a covered teapot or mason jar with a tight lid. Pour in 16 ounces of boiling water and steep for 4 hours. Chamomile oils will evaporate with steam, says Falconi, so it's important to keep the container covered while steeping. Strain and pour 8 ounces of the mixture into a 16-ounce jar with 8 ounces of 80-proof vodka. Stir in 2 teaspoons of glycerin, then cap the jar and shake well. Store the mixture in a spray bottle for easy misting.

Rose

Moisturize oily skin twice a day with a glycerin-and-rosewater lotion. Just because your skin is oily doesn't mean that it's moist. "Your skin can have plenty of oil but not a lot of moisture," says Dr. Brett.

To moisturize skin without adding oil, she recommends using an old-time favorite—glycerin and rosewater. "It's probably the most elegant light moisturizer that you'll ever find," she says. Glycerin is softening because it is soluble in water, while the volatile oils in the rose-water are soothing. You can buy it ready-made in drugstores or make your own by mixing equal parts of glycerin and rosewater. Apply it with your fingers to clean, wet skin. Plain glycerin is also available in drugstores, and you can find rosewater in ethnic grocery stores.

OSTEOPOROSIS

We tend to think that bones need to be strong, and they do. But that's not the whole story.

"A healthy bone is like green wood: strong, but also flexible," says C. Leigh Broadhurst, Ph.D., a nutrition consultant and herbal re-searcher based in Clovery, Maryland. "If you take a fall, a brittle bone will probably break. It has to be able to give a little."

Osteoporosis is a disease in which bones become fragile and more likely to break. People who have it need a doctor's care, dietary supplements, and often medication, but a wide variety of vitamins and minerals can contribute to healthy bones over the course of a lifetime.

A diet that emphasizes whole foods, especially fresh vegetables and unrefined grains, is key, Dr. Broadhurst says. Root vegetables such as turnips, carrots, parsnips, radishes, and beets are especially important as sources of boron, she adds, while leafy green vegetables such as fresh spinach, kale, cabbage, basil, and Romaine lettuce are the best sources of vitamin K. Dairy products are by far the best sources of calcium, the basic building block of bones. For those who find it difficult to eat any of these foods on a regular basis, Dr. Broadhurst recommends a supplement of at least 1,000 milligrams of calcium and 500 milligrams of magnesium a day.

Herbs are another route toward giving your bones the nutrients they need over the long haul. Here are the best bone builders that herbalists have to offer.

Horsetail

Take two droppers of extract in 1 cup of water or 700 to 800 milligrams in capsule form twice a day. Horsetail is a reasonable source of silicon, one of the minerals that helps give bones flexibility as well as strength, Dr. Broadhurst says. To ensure that you get a pure, strong dose, she recommends using the liquid extract. Take it on an empty stomach, if possible, in the morning and in the evening.

Horsetail is also available in capsules, says Allan Warshowsky, M.D., a gynecologist on staff at the Long Island Jewish Medical Center in New Hyde Park, New York. He recommends using capsules of standardized extract.

Nettle

Drink one dropper of extract in 1 cup of water once or twice a day, or take a 500-milligram capsule twice a day. Nettle is an excellent source of magnesium and calcium, Dr. Warshowsky says, which are two of the most recommended minerals for building bones.

Another way of taking nettle is to buy standardized extract in capsule form. People who have already developed signs of osteoporosis can double either dosage, he adds.

Oats

Drink one to four cups of infusion a day. Oats infusion is an excellent source of calcium and magnesium, according to master herbalist Susun Weed of Woodstock, New York, author of *Menopausal Years: The Wise Woman Way*. (Pills and tinctures are not good sources.) One particularly effective way to extract those min-

Fast FACTS

Cause: Bones can weaken with age, leading to fractures and serious spinal problems. Risk factors include heredity and lack of calcium in the diet, as well as smoking, alcohol abuse, and lack of exercise, all of which can compromise bone strength and durability.

Incidence: Osteoporosis affects some 25 million Americans, mostly women. Due to hormonal changes after menopause, women are four times more likely than men to develop the condition. They have a 50/50 chance of experiencing an osteoporosis-related fracture in their lifetimes.

When to see the doctor: The first symptom of osteoporosis is usually a broken bone. If you are a woman at menopause and you break a bone or know that you have one or more risk factors, it's a good idea to have a bone-density evaluation. Have a second checkup a couple of years after the first to track any signs of significant deterioration. Regardless of risk factors, all women age 65 and over should be tested for osteoporosis.

---

erals from the herb is to make a strong infusion, rather than a tea. Here are Weed's instructions.

Put 1 ounce (by weight) of dried oats in a quart mason jar. (If you don't have a scale, fill the jar approximately one-third full of herb.) Pour boiling water into the jar right to the top (approximately 4 cups), put a tight lid on it, and let stand for at least 4 hours. Strain out the plant material and drink from 1 cup to 1 quart a day as you like it, either hot or cold, Weed says. The taste is mild and mellow, but you can mix it with anything, even tea or coffee, if you wish. Refrigerate what you don't drink right away, but use it within 48 hours.

Dandelion

Take extract according to package directions twice a day. Dandelion leaf has an abundance of minerals, including calcium, according to Dr. Warshowsky. He recommends looking for a standardized extract.

Asian Ginseng and Ginger

Take one 500-milligram capsule of each herb three times a day. Like other root plants, ginseng and ginger can absorb plenty of minerals from the soil, says Dr. Broadhurst, especially boron. Ginseng has the added benefit of being an energy booster. Having energy can boost your enthusiasm for exercise, which is another important element of bone health.

Alfalfa

Take four 500-milligram capsules of extract daily. The freshest way to ingest leafy green plants—your prime sources of bone-helping vitamin K—is to frequent the salad bar, but an alfalfa supplement can help salad-phobic people get the green nutrients they need. Take two capsules in the morning and two at night, Dr. Broadhurst suggests.

Another easy way to get more leafy greens in your diet, she adds, is to use the "green drink" mixtures sold in health food stores, which combine everything from barley grass to various types of seaweed.

Soy

Take a daily supplement according to package directions. Soy supplements, made from ground soybean sprouts, are rich in substances called isoflavones, which are chemicals that imitate the function of estrogen in the body, Dr. Broadhurst says. That's important, since the decline of estrogen in a woman's body after she goes through menopause is a major reason that osteoporosis is far more prevalent in women than it is in men.

Preparations of isoflavone supplements vary according to the product, Dr. Broadhurst says, so follow the dosage instructions on the package. Mixed isoflavone supplements, which use any number of plants, from black cohosh to kudzu, are also available and are just as effective as the soy versions.

OVERWEIGHT

$\mathcal{W}$alk into any health food store, and you're sure to see a shelf lined with products touting their power to help you lose weight naturally. The truth is, there is no magic formula—herbal or otherwise—to shed those unwanted pounds. If there were, 97 million of us wouldn't be walking around with layers of excess fat stored on our frames.

Even the herbal supplements and teas lining store shelves aren't very helpful. In fact, it's better to avoid them, says Silena Heron, N.D., adjunct professor at Southwest College of Naturopathic Medicine and Health Sciences in Tempe, Arizona, and vice president of the Botanical Medicine Academy. They typically rely on stimulants, diuretics, or laxatives to drain away pounds, and none of these tactics should be included as part of a healthful weight-loss plan. In fact, such potent herbs can often do more harm than good.

"There are dozens of theories on weight loss," says Dr. Heron. "Some people try to lose by limiting grams of fat, others by adjusting their ratio of carbohydrates and protein." But weight loss boils down to one simple principle: You must burn more calories than you consume. Exercise is vitally important. Start with gentle stretches, isometrics, and light weights. Then, with a doctor's approval, move on to some type of aerobic exercise, advises Dr. Heron.

Combine your exercise routine with the herbs we've listed here to safely help promote weight loss in a variety of ways, such as curbing your appetite, defusing cravings, or revving up your metabolism.

Psyllium

Take 1 to 2 tablespoons of ground husks before meals (up to 6 tablespoons a day). Although it's typically used as a laxative, psyllium can also curb a too-hearty appetite, says Dr. Heron. Taken be-

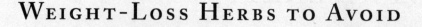

WEIGHT-LOSS HERBS TO AVOID

Some natural weight-loss products contain herbs that are potentially dangerous. Others simply don't do what they claim to do. Because the Food and Drug Administration (FDA) classifies weight-loss products as dietary supplements, not drugs, manufacturers don't need FDA approval to market them. This means that the effectiveness of many of these products is not proven. As tempting as it may be to try a quick fix, you're better off avoiding the following herbs, says Connie Catellani, M.D., medical director of the Miro Center for Integrative Medicine in Evanston, Illinois.

Ephedra. Commonly referred to by its Chinese name, ma huang, ephedra can raise blood pressure, increase heart rate, and overstimulate the central nervous system, which controls the brain. "It's kind of like taking speed. Your whole body is working faster and burning more calories," says Paula Ceh, Pharm.D., assistant professor of pharmacy at Butler University College of Pharmacy and Health Sciences in Indianapolis. Use of this herb has been linked to heart palpitations, stroke, chest pain, heart attack, and, in at least two instances, death. There's no question about this one: Avoid it.

fore meals with lots of water (two to three 8-ounce glasses), the fiber-rich plant swells like a sponge in your digestive tract. That full feeling in your stomach sends a signal to your brain, telling you not to eat as much. The water is critical to this regimen, cautions Dr. Heron, because if you're dehydrated, psyllium can cause digestive tract blockages.

What's more, several studies on weight loss have shown that diets high in fiber (in these studies, it was about 35 grams a day) can re-

Garcinia cambogia. Products containing hydroxycitric acid (HCA), which is obtained from the fruit of the *Garcinia cambogia* plant, won't harm you, but research shows that they may not help you, either. HCA is supposed to help control appetite and reduce absorption of fat by the body. A study with 135 overweight men and women, however, showed that HCA had no significant effect on weight loss or fat loss. Given the controversy regarding the effectiveness of HCA, it is probably better to wait until we know more about it, says Dr. Catellani.

Herbal laxative teas. There's nothing like a cup of hot tea to soothe the soul—but some herbal teas can make you sick. Dieter's teas that contain senna, aloe, buckthorn, cascara, and other plant-derived laxatives produce the illusion of weight loss through dehydration. They can cause diarrhea and stomach cramps and decrease your body's ability to absorb nutrients. If you use such laxative teas too frequently, your bowels may no longer function without them, warns Dr. Catellani. These products can also deplete levels of potassium in your blood, which can lead to paralysis and irregular heartbeat.

duce the number of calories absorbed by the body each day by 30 to 180 calories. That can add up to 19 pounds a year. One study of 52 people found that those who dieted and also took 7 grams of fiber supplements a day lost nearly double the weight—12.1 pounds versus 6.6 pounds—of those who only dieted.

To lose weight, Dr. Heron recommends consuming 40 to 50 grams of fiber a day in your diet. Ideally, you should get that fiber from vegetables, fruits, and whole grains. Apples are excellent sources, with

3.5 grams each; ½ cup of carrots or one potato each has 2.5 grams of fiber, and a slice of whole-wheat toast has 1.5 grams, says Dr. Heron. Getting fiber from food is always preferable, but if you fall short, fiber supplements can help, she adds.

Asian Ginseng

Take a daily dose of 200 milligrams. Known as a feel-good herb to boost vitality, ginseng's ability to regulate blood sugar suggests that it may be useful in helping people lose weight, says Robert Rountree, M.D., a holistic physician at the Helios Health Center in Boulder, Colorado.

"Experts in the field of bariatrics (obesity) feel that continual high levels of the hormone insulin lead to obesity," he explains. When you eat a starchy meal or drink a sugary beverage (which are carbohydrates), your blood sugar rises, and your pancreas reacts by releasing insulin to bring it back down. Insulin receptors in the body allow glucose to enter cells, lowering blood sugar levels, explains Dr. Rountree. As we age, these receptors move less glucose into the cells, and the resultant high levels prompt the pancreas to produce more insulin. Insulin then instructs the fat cells to convert the excess glucose and fatty acids into fats called triglycerides, which are stored until needed. As long as glucose levels—and thus insulin levels—are elevated, the fats remain in storage. Too much of this fat results in obesity.

"If you can control insulin levels, maybe you can stem the fat-storing process from the beginning," says Dr. Rountree. He estimates that half of his overweight patients have abnormally high levels of insulin in their blood.

Research shows that Asian ginseng, also known as panax, Korean, or Chinese ginseng, can help correct blood sugar levels. In a study in Finland, 36 people with type 2 (non-insulin-dependent) diabetes who took a daily dose of 200 milligrams of ginseng for 8 weeks lowered their fasting blood sugar levels and lost weight. Even more important, they reported that they felt better and were able to exercise more.

Bitters-to-Burn Beverage

In Traditional Chinese Medicine, overweight is an indication that your digestion is weak. This means that your digestive fires aren't burning hot, so it's easier for your body to transform food into extra water and fat than to convert it into muscle, blood, and energy, says fourth-generation herbalist Christopher Hobbs, a professional member of the American Herbalists Guild, a botanist and licensed acupuncturist in Santa Cruz, California, and author of many books on herbs, including Handmade Medicines: Simple Recipes for Herbal Health. *Take 1 teaspoon of this bitter tonic recipe, made from a combination of tinctures, in a glass of water before meals to stoke your digestive fires and help shed those pounds.*

- 4½ teaspoons artichoke leaf
- 3 teaspoons ginger rhizome
- 1½ teaspoons angelica root
- 1½ teaspoons cardamom pod
- ¾ teaspoon gentian root
- ¾ teaspoon licorice root

In a small bowl, combine the artichoke, ginger, angelica, cardamom, gentian, and licorice. Store in an amber glass dropper bottle or a dark glass jar.

Bladderwrack

Grind and sprinkle 1 teaspoon over food or add it to soups and stews. In rare cases, an underactive thyroid gland is to blame for overweight. If you have little hormone from this regulating gland, your body runs in slow motion—kind of sluggish and cold.

"Eating this type of seaweed may help you lose weight only if your thyroid is iodine-deficient," says Dr. Heron. A little iodine-rich bladderwrack (a type of kelp) can rev up a lazy metabolism by stimulating the production of thyroid hormones, she explains. You may find the fishy taste unpleasant, but if you cook the seaweed with grains, soups, or stews, you'll hardly notice it.

Fast Facts

Cause: When you take in more calories than your body needs, the thin walls of cell membranes expand—sometimes to 20 times their normal size—to accommodate the growing globules of pure fat in their centers. Family history, eating patterns, metabolism, cultural factors, and activity levels all influence body weight.

Incidence: Approximately one in three people in the United States is overweight or obese. At any one time, 30 to 40 percent of women and 20 to 25 percent of men are trying to lose weight. Men tend to accumulate excess weight in their midsections, while women tend to become heavy around the lower parts of their bodies.

When to see the doctor: If you're worried about your weight, see your doctor to determine whether you have any risk factors for any of the numerous chronic health conditions associated with overweight, such as high blood pressure or elevated levels of cholesterol or sugar in the blood.

Gymnema sylvestre

When you have the urge to indulge in something sweet, squirt a few drops of tincture on your tongue. Used for centuries in Ayurvedic medicine to treat diabetes, this herb, also known as gurmar, can help fend off a craving for sweets. "It has the unusual property of blocking sugary tastes," says Nancy Welliver, N.D., director of the Institute of Medical Herbalism in Calistoga, California. Squirting the tincture directly onto your tongue will block the taste of sugar for about 15 minutes. Look for it in health food stores, says Dr. Welliver.

Stevia

Sweeten coffee and baked goods naturally with a smidgen of this South American herb. Artificial sweeteners like saccharin and aspartame offer calorie-free alternatives to sugar, but both have been linked with health problems, says Connie Catellani, M.D., medical director of the Miro Center for Integrative Medicine in Evanston, Illinois.

Stevia is a noncaloric herbal sweetener sold as a dietary supplement in health food stores. Since it's 200 to 300 times sweeter than sugar, you need only a pinch to satisfy your sweet tooth, says Arthur O. Tucker III, Ph.D., research professor at Delaware State University in Dover. And, unlike aspartame, you can also cook and bake with it. Some recipes call for substituting 2 tablespoons of stevia powder for 1 cup of sugar. The extract form is much sweeter, so if you use that, you'll need only about ¼ teaspoon for every cup of sugar, says Dr. Tucker.

PET PROBLEMS

*E*ver wonder why your dog or cat starts grazing like a cow in the backyard every once in a while? Animals seem to have an innate sense about which plants can help them stay healthy. In fact, some of our own knowledge about herbal remedies has come from watching animals in the wild treat themselves with plants—a science called zoopharmacognosy.

Using herbs is a natural way to better your pet's health by supplying vitamins, minerals, and antioxidants that help fend off disease. Before you begin using herbs for your pet, though, there are a few things that you should know.

Herbalists and holistic veterinarians stress the importance of feeding your dog or cat a home-prepared diet that combines lean meat, whole grains like brown rice, and raw vegetables.

"If we don't have that foundation, we're simply wasting the herbs," says Gregory Tilford, a member of the American Herbalists Guild and developer of Animals Apawthecary, manufacturers of glycerin-based herbal extracts for dogs and cats, in Conner, Montana. "The medicinal activities of herbs work in concert with the quality of food that goes into your pet."

Half the battle of using herbs is getting them into your pet, says Tilford. For the most part, though, botanical remedies are easy to incorporate into a holistic health plan. For a supportive, tonic effect, sprinkle fresh or dried herbs on food. If you're looking for a more therapeutic effect, make an herbal tea to pour on dry food or mix with your pet's drinking water. If your dog likes ice cubes, you can freeze some herbal tea. "Don't be afraid to be creative," says Tilford.

For fast absorption, tinctures are the best options. Dogs and cats prefer the taste of glycerin-based tinctures to that of alcoholic tinctures. "If you give cats an alcohol tincture, they'll foam at the mouth. They're quite dramatic," warns Tilford. He advises against using capsules, unless you break them open before you feed them to your pet. Because dogs and cats are carnivores, their digestive tracts are too short to adequately absorb capsules.

Use only one or two herbs at a time, and watch how your pet reacts to them. Some animals may have allergies or other health conditions that prevent them from consuming certain herbs, while the same herbs won't bother other animals at all. Cats, in particular, are highly sensitive. Michael W. Lemmon, D.V.M., a holistic veterinarian in Renton, Washington, and past president of the American Holistic Veterinary Medical Association, emphasizes that if anything makes your pet foam at the mouth, stop using it.

Armed with this knowledge, here's how to treat 10 common health concerns with herbs.

ANXIETY

Many pets experience anxiety, stress, and downright terror whenever they are exposed to anything out of their normal routine.

Whether it's the rumble of a distant thunderstorm, firecrackers on the Fourth of July, or simply a car ride, just how worked up your pet becomes depends on his disposition, not his size or breed.

Herbs can provide a safe, effective way for your pet to mellow out, says Tilford. It may take some trial and error to determine which herbs work best for your pet, though, since not all animals react the same way to calming herbs.

Valerian

Put 12 drops of a tincture of valerian root on food, or squirt 12 drops of valerian extract per 20 pounds of body weight directly into the animal's mouth. The sedative action of valerian reduces excitability, tension, anxiety, and even full-blown hysteria, says Tilford. Most animals don't seem to mind that it tastes like dirty socks. Valerian is also available in tablets and capsules. With capsules or tablets, dosage recommendations are based on a 150-pound human, so you'll need to adjust it according to your pet's weight. You would use one-fifteenth of the human dosage for a 10-pound cat, for instance.

Chamomile

Relax your pet with a calming cup of chamomile tea. This is an ideal herb to give before a long car trip. Not only does chamomile soothe your pet to sleep, it calms the stomach, says Mary Wulff-Tilford, a professional member of the American Herbalists Guild, a holistic animal care consultant in Conner, Montana, and author of *Herbal Remedies for Dogs and Cats*. Pour 1 cup of boiling water over one tea bag or 1 teaspoon of dried chamomile flowers, steep for 10 to 15 minutes, then let it cool. You can put the whole cup of tea in your pet's water bowl or soak a treat in the tea and feed it to him.

ARTHRITIS

Pets, like people, tend to be a little stiff and creaky as they age. Usually, it's because of arthritis, a painful condition that occurs when the cartilage that cushions the joints begins to wear down. Younger dogs occasionally get arthritis, either from an injury or infection or because they have a condition called hip dysplasia, in which the joint simply isn't put together the way it should be.

In many cases, you can control arthritis pain and stiffness with some simple home remedies. First, make sure that your pet is getting moderate exercise. Twenty minutes of walking each day can keep him limber. Also, help your pet maintain a healthy weight. Extra pounds only add to the wear and tear on joints that are already failing. To slow cartilage breakdown and help repair the joint, give your pet a daily dose of glucosamine sulfate, a nutritional supplement derived from cartilage, says Jeanne Olson, D.V.M., a holistic veterinarian in North Pole, Alaska. Check with your vet for the proper dosage.

The herbs listed here can help reduce pain, swelling, and inflammation.

Alfalfa, Burdock, Yucca, and Licorice

Give cats and dogs this pain-relieving blend two or three times a day. Wulff-Tilford developed this herbal formula to treat arthritis and other rheumatoid conditions that are accompanied by pain. Herbalists believe that alfalfa and burdock act together to provide mild liver support that helps the body eliminate excess waste materials and water from the joints, while yucca and licorice have anti-inflammatory actions. For a chronic condition like arthritis, the four herbs work best when combined, says Wulff-Tilford. A single dose should be 12 drops per 20 pounds of body weight.

You can buy the blend in some health food stores or mix your own compound with 2 parts alfalfa, 2 parts burdock, 1 part yucca, and 1 part licorice. It's important to use smaller proportions of yucca and licorice to reduce the risk of adverse side effects. Excessive use of yucca can interfere with the absorption of fat-soluble vitamins in the intestines, while long-term use of licorice can cause high blood pressure and water retention. Do not use licorice if your pet has high blood pressure, liver or kidney damage, or diabetes.

Turmeric and Boswellia

Start with a daily dose of 150 milligrams of each herb in tablet or capsule form. These two herbs naturally fight joint inflammation and pain, says Dr. Olson. In studies, boswellia has been shown to improve blood supply to the joints and prevent the breakdown of tissues affected by all types of arthritis. Curcumin, the powerful anti-inflammatory substance in turmeric, isn't a drug, but it can act like one.

When compared to the popular nonsteroidal anti-inflammatory drug phenylbutazone in clinical studies, curcumin was found to be as effective or more effective in treating arthritis.

Alfalfa

Mix ¼ to ½ cup of alfalfa tea in your pet's drinking water, or sprinkle dried leaf on food daily. Alfalfa works as a gentle nutritive tonic and anti-inflammatory for the musculoskeletal system, says Tilford. When used over the long term, it's been shown to reduce joint pain and stiffness. Use ⅛ to ¼ teaspoon of dried leaf for cats or 1 teaspoon for every 30 pounds of body weight for dogs.

BAD BREATH

Imagine how your breath would smell if you ate bowl after bowl of kibble and never brushed your teeth. Bad breath is generally caused by a combination of bad diet and poor dental hygiene, says Junia Borden Childs, D.V.M., a holistic veterinarian in Ojai, California. By the time they are 5 years old, 60 to 80 percent of pets will have gingivitis or some other dental problem if they have never had dental care. The evidence? Foul breath.

The first step in dealing with bad breath is to take care of your pet's teeth and gums. Some veterinarians recommend feeding more dry food than canned and providing dogs with hard chew toys and raw carrot snacks to help clean the teeth and gums with their abrasive action. Dental care doesn't stop there, though. You should also brush your pet's teeth once a week, says Dr. Childs.

If your pet is not used to brushing, start by dampening a washcloth with a little beef broth and rubbing his teeth and gums. Later, you can graduate to a toothbrush made especially for pets. Use a toothpaste formulated for the four-legged since conventional toothpaste ingredients can upset your dog or cat's stomach, advises Dr. Childs.

That done, try these herbal remedies to keep odor-causing bacteria at bay and freshen breath.

Thyme

To fight gingivitis, swab tincture directly onto your pet's teeth and gums, or add strong tea to his drinking water. Swollen, red gums provide a breeding ground for foul-smelling bacteria. "Thyme is an excellent disinfectant for the mouth and gums. It contains the same active constituent as Listerine," notes Tilford. For established cases of gingivitis, apply the tincture directly to your pet's teeth and gums.

"For bad breath and early signs of gingivitis, a small amount of tea made from thyme can be added to the animal's drinking water," Tilford says. To make it, steep 2 teaspoons of dried thyme in 1 cup of boiling water and let it cool. Mix 2 ounces of tea per quart of water. If your pet will not drink it this way, you can squirt ¼ teaspoon directly into his mouth.

Parsley

Feed your pet a few sprigs of nature's breath freshener. Like a Certs mint, parsley will temporarily freshen your pet's breath, but it won't fix the underlying causes of foul breath, says Tilford. It can, however, help boost your pet's overall health. Considered highly nutritious, the fresh leaves are natural vitamin and mineral supplements in their own right. Do not give parsley to a pet with kidney disease.

FLEAS

Fleas are tough to fight. In her lifetime, one flea can lay 2,000 eggs. Since fleas have been doing this for millions of years, you have to approach the battle against them with this basic but grim truth in mind: No matter what you do, they will come back.

The following herbal remedies can help eliminate the flea problem without exposing your pet or your family to harmful chemicals.

Aromatic Flea Repellent

Pennyroyal is an easy-to-grow, natural flea repellent, but if taken internally, it can be toxic to pets, especially cats. This recipe, developed by Pat Zook, D.V.M., a holistic veterinarian in private practice in Stone Mountain, Georgia, is a safe way to take advantage of the herb's natural repellent properties.

About once a week, use the mixture to mop your floors, baseboards, and any other areas where fleas may multiply. (Dr. Zook advises testing the repellent on an inconspicuous area first to make sure that it will not stain.) Let it dry without rinsing; the smell of the herbs will repel fleas. Be sure to keep pets away from the treated areas until they are completely dry.

- 1 **quart boiling water**
- 2 **tablespoons dried pennyroyal**
- 1 **tablespoon peppermint or spearmint leaves**

Place the water in a large saucepan and bring it to a boil. Remove from the heat, add the pennyroyal and mint, and cover the pan so that the aromatic properties of the herbs don't escape. Steep for 15 minutes and cool before using.

Feverfew

Bathe your dog in tea. Part of the difficulty in getting rid of fleas is the fact that they're constantly hopping around; they can leap up to 150 times their body length. For us, that would be like jumping the length of three football fields. Feverfew tea will temporarily paralyze them, explains Tilford.

Prepare the tea by steeping 6 to 8 teaspoons of dried feverfew per quart of boiling water. Make enough tea to completely soak your dog. (You'll need at least a gallon for a 40-pound dog.) After soaking, rinse the tea (and the fleas) off. It's better to use this method in the bathtub, where the fleas will flow right down the drain, than in the backyard. "Keep in mind that eventually, the fleas will wake up, and when they do, they'll be hungry and hop right back on your pet," says Tilford.

Neem

Apply oil or lotion to the animal's skin. An Indian herb called neem repels fleas and soothes sore skin, says Dr. Lemmon. One popular brand of lotion, available from some holistic veterinarians, is PhytoGel, which contains neem along with other essential oils. Some animals are sensitive to neem, so Dr. Lemmon recommends using the lotion, which isn't as strong as the oil. "Test a small area on your pet first to make sure he doesn't have a reaction," he says, "and only use it for 2 or 3 days in a row."

Neem has a bitter taste that fleas dislike. Dogs and cats dislike it, too, which means that they're less inclined to bite and chew at their skin, says Dr. Lemmon.

HAIRBALLS

Cats can spend hours a day grooming, but what's good for their coats can eventually gum up their insides. With every lick of their rough, brushlike tongues, they swallow a little fur. Although some hair is eliminated in the stool, some stays in the stomach, forming a gooey wad. Eventually your cat chucks it up, leaving an unpleasant, hairy mess—usually on your best carpet.

Regular brushing can prevent your feline from swallowing large amounts of fur, says Dr. Childs. The following herbal remedies can aid digestion so that any hair that the cat does swallow moves quickly through the digestive tract instead of staying in the stomach.

Oats

To speed hair through the system, feed your cat a laxative made with oats, honey, and olive oil. One way to eliminate hair from the intestines is to give a natural laxative. Combine 4 parts of plain, uncooked cereal-type oatmeal with 1 part each of honey and olive oil and make a paste. Offer 1 to 2 tablespoons as a treat when hairballs are a problem, suggests Kathleen Carson, D.V.M., a holistic veterinarian in Hermosa Beach, California. For cats who suffer from hairballs regularly, you can give the mixture two or three times a week.

Pumpkin

Add ½ teaspoon of canned plain pumpkin to your cat's food once a day while the problem continues. Fiber-rich pumpkin is another way get a hairball moving, says Robin Cannizzaro, D.V.M., a holistic veterinarian in St. Petersburg, Florida. Mix it into wet or dry food. Most cats enjoy the taste.

Slippery Elm

Give one dropper of diluted tincture three times a day. Hairballs can irritate the stomach and intestines, causing constipation or an upset stomach. "Slippery elm bark can reduce the discomfort," says Dr. Carson. To make the proper strength, dilute 20 drops of slippery elm tincture in 1 ounce of spring water. Give the mixture 20 minutes before morning and evening meals and again at bedtime. You can use this remedy daily if the problem is severe; if it's mild, give it one or two times a week as long as the problem persists.

HOT SPOTS

Hot spots are red, raw, painful sores that form when bacteria spread rapidly among the hair follicles in the area that your dog is scratching, usually behind the ears and around the tail. They cause intense itching that can literally drive your dog into a frenzy.

The bald circular patches can grow alarmingly fast, from the size of a dime to that of a dinner plate in 12 to 24 hours. Although they look scary, they involve only the top layer of skin, but they don't usually heal on their own. They just get worse.

Your vet may recommend a short-acting cortisone spray or gel to relieve the intense itch of hot spots. But to develop an effective treatment plan, herbal or otherwise, you need to have your vet test your dog's skin and blood to determine the cause so that it can be eliminated. Anything from bacterial or fungal infections to nutritional or hormone imbalances, allergies, or parasites can trigger the incessant scratching that leads to hot spots, "but typically, hot spots develop when skin problems caused by allergies or fleas get out of control," says Dr. Childs. "If caught early enough, they respond well to herbal treatments," she says. Try these herbal remedies to naturally relieve the itch and promote healing.

Calendula, Grindelia, Plantain, and Comfrey

Spritz the spot with tea made with these herbs every 3 to 4 hours. Your canine will breathe a sigh of relief as this cooling spray instantly relieves itching, says Dr. Cannizzaro. And while he is relishing the respite, the antiseptic and healing properties of the herbs will go to work to speed the repair of red, inflamed skin.

First, mix equal parts of dried calendula flowers, grindelia leaves and flowers, plantain leaves, and comfrey leaves. You can add 1 teaspoon of goldenseal, if desired. To make the tea, pour 1 pint of boiling water over 1 tablespoon of the herb blend and steep for 10 to 15 minutes. Put it in a spray bottle and chill before applying it to the inflamed skin. Do not use comfrey on deep wounds, however, Dr. Lemmon cautions, because it might impede healing.

Aloe

Smooth fresh gel liberally on the hot spot. The clear gel inside the leaf of the aloe plant speeds up the rate of healing and reduces the risk of infection. Between treatments with the calendula tea, Dr. Childs suggests applying cooling aloe gel as needed.

You can grow your own household first-aid plant or purchase the gel already bottled at a drugstore. Look for products that contain at least 90 percent pure aloe vera gel. Do not use it on deep wounds, says Dr. Lemmon.

Witch Hazel

Cool the heat with witch hazel two or three times a day. As the name suggests, hot spots can be literally warm to the touch. Witch hazel evaporates almost instantly, making hot spots feel more comfortable, says Lowell Ackerman, D.V.M., a veterinary dermatologist in Mesa, Arizona, and author of *Guide to Skin and Haircoat Problems in Dogs*. It contains a large amount of tannins, which will help the sores dry and heal.

ITCHING

Itching can drive even the most placid pet into a veritable frenzy of thumping paws and jingling collars. Without relief, your pet may continue to scratch and bite until his skin becomes raw and inflamed.

"There are so many causes," says Dr. Childs. The culprit could be allergies to fleas or food, dry skin, or simply dirty fur. "Itching is more likely to be a problem when your pet's overall health isn't what it should be," she says. The herbal remedies listed here will help ease the itch, but consult your vet to determine the underlying cause.

Chickweed or Plantain

Apply an herbal lotion or a soothing compress dipped in tea made from either of these herbs. Chiefly used to treat irritated skin, chickweed or plantain may soothe severe itchiness when other remedies have failed, says Dr. Lemmon. You can buy a lotion of either herb in health food stores. Apply it three or four times a day, covering the affected area completely, until the itching is relieved.

You can also use bulk leaves to brew a tea. Boil a pint of water, remove it from the heat, and pour it over 1 tablespoon of either dried herb. Cover and steep for 10 to 20 minutes, let the tea cool to room temperature, and strain. Dip a cloth in the solution and apply it to areas of itchy, irritated skin for 5 to 10 minutes a few times a day.

Flaxseed

Mix fresh, cold-pressed oil into your pet's food daily. Flaxseed oil is rich in essential fatty acids, which can help reduce itching and inflammation caused by flea and food allergies, says Dr. Lemmon. You can buy fresh flaxseed oil at health food stores. To guard against rancidity, look for brands that are stored in the refrigerated section, packaged in dark glass or plastic to block out the light and stamped with a date, advises Dr. Lemmon. Give 1 teaspoon a day to cats and small dogs and 1 to 2 tablespoons a day to large dogs, he says. Pets usually like the nutty flavor of the oil.

Burdock

Add 2 to 3 ounces of fresh, grated root to your pet's food every day. "A classic skin remedy and blood purifier, burdock is as much a food as it is a medicine," says Tilford. Its diuretic, antibiotic, and bitter properties help eliminate toxins so that the body is better able to deal with whatever is causing the itching. "It has good antioxidant properties and is believed to scavenge free radicals before they can cause damage to the cells," he explains. If you have a 40-pound dog, start with the dosage recommended above. You can adjust the amount to suit the size of your pet. For a cat or small dog, for example, use 1 to 2 ounces.

Lemon

Pour a rinse over your pet's fur. A lemon rinse will temporarily relieve itching, says Dr. Olson. Steep a thinly sliced lemon in 1 quart of boiling water, let it cool, strain, and pour it over the area of itching skin. Do not rinse; blot or towel dry your pet.

OVERWEIGHT

Overweight is as much an epidemic among U.S. pets as it is among their owners. About one in three pets is overweight. And as with us,

The Dosing Dilemma

*P*ets come in all shapes and sizes, which makes it difficult to answer the very basic question, "What's the right dose?" Unfortunately, there are no easy answers when it comes to dosage. Throughout this chapter, we've provided the basic guidelines, and Gregory Tilford, a member of the American Herbalists Guild and developer of Animals Apawthecary, manufacturers of glycerin-based herbal extracts for dogs and cats, in Conner, Montana, recommends the following strategies.

Do your math. Dosage recommendations on herbal tinctures, capsules, and tablets are typically based on a 150-pound human animal. Figure out your pet's weight and adjust the dose accordingly. A 10-pound cat, for example, is one-fifteenth the size of a typical person.

Start small. You're working with a small body. Use small doses, and use them often. Dogs and cats have much faster metabolic rates than we do.

Follow the 10 percent rule. To find the effective dose if the starting dose doesn't seem to be working, increase dosage levels in increments of 10 percent. Don't increase by more than 75 percent of the original starting dose, however.

Take the weekend off. Generally, it's best to take at least a 2-day break from herbal therapies each week. That's 5 days on, then 2 days off. This allows you to monitor your pet's response and determine whether there are any tolerance or toxicity problems that may develop as a result of long-term use.

Know when to quit. If results don't begin to materialize after you have given your pet the maximum dosage of an herb for 10 days, it may be time to try another herb.

Keep a pet-care diary. As you experiment with different herbal treatments, remember to write them down. It will eliminate the element of mystery the next time around.

their formula for weight loss can be summed up simply. "Eat less. Exercise more," says Wulff-Tilford.

How can you tell if your pet is overweight? The best rule of thumb is to feel around his ribs. If you look down on a standing cat, his body should look like a straight line from shoulder to tail. A dog viewed from the same angle should curve at his midsection to form a waist. You should be able to feel the animal's shoulders as well. If you cannot find his ribs but can grab handfuls of fat, it's time to put your pet on a weight-loss program.

That task is nearly impossible if you're using commercial food, say holistic vets. Low-fat, high-fiber "lite" pet foods may set the stage for health problems such as a dull coat; dry, flaky skin; and a more serious condition called pancreatitis, which can lead to diabetes, says Dr. Olson. "I don't see many pets losing weight with commercial weight-loss diets, but I haven't seen one yet who failed to lose weight by using a well-balanced homemade diet," she says.

Here's one recipe that Dr. Olson uses for her own pets. The proportions are for a 50-pound dog, but they can be adjusted to suit any pet.

Put half of your pet's normal dry food in a bowl. Add about $\frac{1}{3}$ cup of raw lean ground or lightly sautéed turkey and approximately 1 tablespoon of low-fat cottage cheese. Add $\frac{1}{2}$ to 1 cup of a favorite frozen vegetable, such as green beans, broccoli, spinach, mixed vegetables, carrots, or cauliflower. If your pet is taking supplements, herbs, or medication, you can add them to this "stew," which disguises any unpleasant flavors. Stir in enough hot water to thaw the vegetables and produce the desired consistency.

The following herbs can work in conjunction with a healthy diet to help your pet lose weight. If diet and exercise don't work, contact your vet to see if there is some underlying chronic problem such as hypothyroidism, says Dr. Olson.

Hawthorn

Give 10 milligrams of extract in capsule form for every 10 pounds of body weight three times a day. Hawthorn is an herb that can reduce body fat. It improves liver function, which helps reduce the amounts of fat and cholesterol in the blood, says Ihor Basko, D.V.M., a holistic veterinarian in Honolulu and Kilauea, Hawaii. Do not use hawthorn for pets who have heart disease, however.

Catnip

Give cats ¼ to ½ teaspoon of dried catnip. Some cats are content to be doorstops, and it can be a real challenge to entice them to exercise, says Dr. Basko. "If they're really lethargic, you may have to get them stimulated with catnip first." Catnip, both fresh and dried, lowers their inhibitions, he explains, so "they'll be more willing to play games and exercise when they've had some catnip."

URINARY TRACT INFECTIONS

Urinary tract infections are just as uncomfortable for pets as they are for people, and they get them nearly as often. Suspect an infection if your pet cries or strains while urinating, needs to go out more often, or is having accidents in the house.

Caused by bacteria in the bladder or urethra—the tube through which urine flows—these infections can make urination very painful. And if the infections aren't caught early, they can spread upward to the kidneys, causing serious problems.

To prevent infections, ask your vet to suggest ways to provide your pet with a diet high in animal protein to keep the urine acidic, suggests Dr. Olson. Bacteria will not thrive in an acid environment.

Both holistic and mainstream veterinarians treat urinary tract infections with antibiotics, so be sure to see a vet if you see any of the symptoms occur. Holistic vets also recommend a variety of herbs to soothe the urinary tract, discourage the growth of bacteria, and help infections heal faster.

Couch Grass

Give 12 drops of glycerin-based herbal extract per 20 pounds of body weight twice a day or 1 teaspoon of herb tea three times a day. Because it works on so many different levels, couch grass is the best single herb to use for urinary tract problems, says Tilford. This common garden weed soothes the urinary tract, fights bacteria and inflammation, and works as a diuretic.

If your health food store or pet supply store doesn't carry glycerin-based herbal extracts, you can substitute a tea made from the dried herb. Prepare it by placing 1 heaping teaspoon of couch grass in 8 ounces of boiling water. Remove from the heat and steep until cool.

If your pet is prone to infections, include the fresh green leaves of the plant as part of his regular diet to discourage bacteria growth and promote overall health of the urinary tract.

Cranberry

Feed your pet one 400-milligram capsule of extract for every 20 pounds of body weight daily. Cranberry stops bacteria from adhering to the walls of the bladder and acidifies the urine, says Dr. Olson. It works best to prevent an infection, so if you suspect that your pet already has one, see your vet. When there is already a huge number of bacteria rapidly multiplying in the urinary tract, your pet may need antibiotics to bring the infection under control.

"Avoid giving your pet commercial cranberry juice. It contains sugar, which negates the effect of the cranberries," says Dr. Olson.

Marshmallow, Corn Silk, and Dandelion

Give cats and small dogs 1 teaspoon of strong tea mixed with salt-free chicken or beef broth twice a day. Marshmallow and corn silk contain a substance called mucilage, which coats and soothes irritation in the urinary tract. Dandelion leaves have a strong diuretic action that helps flush away bacteria, says Wulff-Tilford.

To make a strong tea with dried herbs, use 1 teaspoon of each per cup of water. Pour 1 cup of just-boiled water over the herbs, steep for at least 15 minutes, and let cool. Start with 1 teaspoon twice a day for cats and small dogs. Larger dogs will need more. Increase the dose by 1 teaspoon of tea for each 10 pounds of body weight.

WORMS

Many puppies and kittens are born with worms or develop them within the first few weeks of life, while adult pets get worms from the soil, fleas, or by eating rodents and other animals.

It certainly isn't pleasant to discover that your pet has a colony of writhing vermin dwelling in his intestines. Worms can cause serious symptoms, such as diarrhea, weight loss, weakness, anemia, and nutritional deficiencies. Any kind of worm, if it multiplies long enough, can make your pet ill, so it's important to get rid of them.

Some holistic care providers discourage the use of conventional medicines that work by killing the worms. "Anything that can kill a parasite is not good for the host," says Tilford. The following herbal remedies are safer for your pet. "They work by creating a less hospitable environment for the parasite and helping the body expel them more readily," he says.

Sometimes, however, the problem requires a prescription, says Dr. Olson, so you should check with your vet before trying to solve the problem on your own.

To get rid of the worms in 2 to 3 weeks, Tilford suggests using both pumpkin seeds and garlic along with a daily dose of digestive enzymes, such as Dr. Goodpet or Prozyme.

If your pet's health declines during the treatment, or if worms are still present after 3 weeks, see a holistic veterinarian, advises Dr. Cannizzaro. Their presence may indicate a weakness in the overall health of the animal.

Pumpkin

Sprinkle a liberal amount of ground raw, dried seeds on your pet's food. Pumpkin seeds are a safe, nontoxic way to help your pet's body expel tapeworms, which look like short grains of white rice in the stool, says Dr. Olson. Early settlers in North America mixed the seeds with milk and honey to make a remedy for worms. The practice later became so widespread that doctors began prescribing it. You can buy raw, dried, unsalted seeds at a health food store and grind them in a food processor or coffee grinder. Use 1 to 2 teaspoons of ground seeds for smaller dogs and cats and 2 or more tablespoons for larger dogs.

Garlic

Add fresh, chopped garlic to your pet's food. Known for its ability to fight microscopic invaders such as bacteria and fungi, garlic also has the power to push out bigger organisms like worms. Give dogs over 20 pounds one clove a day. "For cats, it's a much smaller amount," says Wulff-Tilford. Give them ½ clove just once or twice a week.

PHLEBITIS

*B*eing ordered by your doctor to stay off your feet after a heart attack or major surgery can get old pretty quickly. It can also make you a sitting—or lying—target for phlebitis. Although that sounds alarming, it's just a general term for inflammation of a vein, usually in the leg, that happens when immobility causes stagnation of the blood.

Pregnant women and people with varicose veins are also susceptible. Even people on long airplane flights or car rides can develop phlebitis.

The first thing to know about phlebitis is that there are two kinds, one minor and one serious. Superficial phlebitis affects a vein near the surface of the skin. It's a benign, though often very painful, condition that shows up as a red streak along a vein that's surrounded by a swollen, tender area.

Deep-vein thrombophlebitis, which affects the larger veins deep beneath the skin's surface, often has no symptoms at all, but it can be life-threatening. In this disorder, a blood clot forms within the vein. The danger is that it may break away, enter the bloodstream, and make its way to the lungs, where it could block one of the major vessels and lead to a pulmonary embolism.

If you've been diagnosed with superficial phlebitis, you're not in danger, but you may be in a lot of pain. Take heart; there are ways to calm that hot, throbbing vein in your leg and ease the discomfort. Herbal remedies for phlebitis work best in tandem with such simple measures as resting with your leg elevated, applying heat, doing gentle exercise such as stretching and walking to get the circulation moving, and wearing elastic support stockings to reduce swelling, says Connie Catellani, M.D., medical director of the Miro Center for Integrative Medicine in Evanston, Illinois. You'll also want to try the following herbs.

Horse Chestnut and Calendula

Smooth an herbal cream directly onto the inflamed area two or three times a day. "Horse chestnut is a very good and very well established anti-inflammatory for the veins," says British herbalist Christopher Robbins, a member of Britain's National Institute of Medical Herbalists who practices herbal medicine in Ross-on-Wye, Herefordshire, England, and has written several books, including *The Natural Pharmacy*. Studies have shown that horse chestnut extract significantly reduces the sensation of heaviness and swelling in the legs of people with this painful condition. Calendula is known for its anti-inflammatory properties.

To make the cream, mix together 4 parts calendula cream and 1 part horse chestnut tincture, and store the cream in a jar with a tight-fitting lid. You can find calendula cream in most health food stores. Just check the label to be sure it's herbal cream, not the homeopathic version.

If there is swelling in the leg from fluid accumulation, pull on a not-too-tight elastic bandage or support stocking to help rev up your circulation and get the blood flowing again. Be sure that it extends from the site of the phlebitis to the foot, otherwise you may stop the blood from flowing back up the leg from below the bandage or stocking. You can use the cream for as long as you like.

Arnica

Smooth cream or lotion onto the swollen vein up to four times daily until the pain subsides. Germany's Commission E, which evaluates herbs for safety and effectiveness, gives arnica its seal of approval for treating phlebitis. Arnica's bright yellow flowers contain anti-inflammatory and pain-relieving compounds. This herb also keeps the blood moving by stimulating the circulation, says Roy Upton, vice president of the American Herbalists Guild (AHG) and executive director of American Herbal Pharmacopeia, an herbal education foundation based in Santa Cruz, California.

Arnica lotion, generally sold as a remedy for soothing bumps and bruises, is easy to find in health food stores.

Calendula, Yarrow, and Echinacea

Take 3 to 5 milliliters of this tincture blend in 2 ounces of water three times daily. This formula combines anti-inflammatory calendula with infection-fighting echinacea and the herb yarrow, which tones the blood vessels.

Mix 2 milliliters of each tincture and add the recommended dose to some water. Drink the slightly bitter-tasting brew with a small glass of juice, says Australian naturopath Andrew Pengelly, N.D., who runs

Cause: Veins can become inflamed for several reasons. Direct injury to a blood vessel can do it, as can the use of intravenous needles and catheters. Sluggish blood flow due to immobility is a common cause of phlebitis in bedridden patients, especially those who have undergone major surgery. Even a long-haul flight on an airplane can be enough to cause inflammation. Pregnancy and varicose veins both appear to increase the risk of phlebitis, and heredity can also play a part.

Incidence: Superficial phlebitis is a common condition that seems to occur more frequently among women and older people.

When to see the doctor: If you have swelling and tenderness around a reddened area, usually on your leg, and you suspect phlebitis, see your doctor to rule out a more serious ailment. Any unexplained swelling in an arm or leg also merits a visit to the doctor's office.

the Valley Herb Clinic in Hunter Valley, New South Wales. As long as you have periodic checkups with a qualified practitioner, he says that it is safe to take this as long as needed for pain and inflammation.

White Oak

Make a hot infusion of bark and apply it with a wet cloth once a day three times a week until the pain subsides. To ease the pain of an inflamed vein, mix 3 tablespoons of white oak bark powder with 1 cup of water in a saucepan, bring it to a boil, and simmer for 10 minutes, says Upton. Let the liquid cool just a little, until it's comfortable to the touch. Soak a cloth in the tea, then press it gently onto the tender area. Leave it in place for 20 minutes with your legs elevated.

Bromelain

Take 500 milligrams in capsule form three times a day between meals. Bromelain has a twofold effect, says Mark Stengler,

N.D., a naturopathic doctor in Oceanside, California, and author of *The Natural Physician: Your Health Guide for Common Ailments*. An enzyme derived from the pineapple plant, bromelain acts as a powerful anti-inflammatory agent, and it breaks up plaque formation in the blood vessels, he says. You can take it for as long as needed.

POISON PLANT RASHES

*L*eaves of three, let them be," goes the old saying, and it's a good maxim to follow when you're out in the woods.

Like most popular sayings, though, it's only partially correct. The problem is, poison oak and poison ivy look different depending on where they're growing, and the number of leaves ranges from groups of three to groups of five, seven, or even nine. With poison plants, then, the best preventive advice is "Know your enemy."

Poison oak is found mostly in the West and Southwest, and it can grow as a shrub or a small tree. In either case, you can spot it because of its oaklike leaves and yellow berries. Poison ivy, a denizen of the eastern part of the country, also plays the chameleon, appearing as either a shrub or a vine. Whatever its guise, it sports yellow green flowers and white berries. Poison sumac, which grows in swamps in the South and peat bogs in the North, is the only consistent one of the bunch. It's a tall shrub with groups of 7 to 13 leaves and cream-colored berries.

What makes people break out in an itchy, blistery rash when they come in contact with these plants is a substance called urushiol that's found in the sap. It's an almost colorless oil that seeps out from any part of the plant that's crushed or cut. You don't even have to touch the plant to get a rash: This stuff spreads like wildfire, and you could just as easily get a dose from petting your dog after he's been running through the woods.

Not everyone is allergic to urushiol, but if you are, you'll know it. "You may see streaks where the plant scratched you and blistery lesions running all along it," says dermatologist Nia Terezakis, M.D., clinical professor of dermatology at Tulane University School of Medicine and Louisiana State University School of Medicine, both in New Orleans.

"It may break out over a series of days," she says, "and often, people think they're spreading it by scratching." That's not the case, according to the doctor. What's happening is that it can take your body several days to say, "Oh, yes, that pesky plant touched me there and there and there."

In a few days, the blisters crust over and begin to scale, and within a couple of weeks, the rash will usually heal on its own. That's small consolation, though, for anyone suffering the miserable itch of poison plant rash.

One very simple remedy that can stop a rash before it's begun is cool or cold running water. As soon as you think that you may have come in contact with a poison plant, wash every exposed area thoroughly with water. You can actually deactivate the urushiol and stop it from spreading if you catch it within 5 minutes of the encounter, says Dr. Terezakis.

If you couldn't get to that mountain stream in time, your battle with the itch has just begun. Over-the-counter hydrocortisone creams won't make it call a truce, either. They're just not strong enough. You do have some allies in the plant world, though, which can weaken the enemy and make life bearable while nature runs its course. Here's the herbal anti-itch brigade.

Jewelweed

Rub juice from the crushed stems and leaves over the affected part. Simply rub the sap on the areas that came in contact with the poison plant as soon as possible, writes Varro E. Tyler, Ph.D., Sc.D., distinguished professor emeritus of pharmacognosy at Purdue University in West Lafayette, Indiana, in his book *Tyler's Herbs of Choice*.

Also known as impatiens and touch-me-not, this bushy plant with spotted, salmon- or yellow-colored flowers sometimes grows near poison ivy and oak. Herbalists swear by this common succulent, and in clinical trials of its effects on poison ivy, it worked just as well as prescription cortisone creams.

Oats

Take an oatmeal bath before bed to soothe the itch. "If someone has a really annoying itch, which is what you'll have if you're sensitive to poison ivy, I suggest an oatmeal bath," says Beverly Yates, N.D., a naturopathic physician with the Natural Health Care Group in Portland, Oregon, and Seattle. Simply take a cup of oats, put them in a handkerchief, tie it over the faucet, and let the warm water run through it. Stay in the tub for 20 to 30 minutes. If you take a bath before you go to bed, says Dr. Yates, "you'll get some sleep and not wake up in the middle of the night with that crazy itch."

Peppermint

Make a paste with cosmetic clay and peppermint oil to stop the itch. Fourth-generation herbalist Christopher Hobbs, a professional member of the American Herbalists Guild, a botanist and licensed acupuncturist in Santa Cruz, California, and author of many books on herbs, including *Handmade Medicines: Simple Recipes for Herbal Health*, says in his book that this lotion will swiftly bring an end to your poison plant–induced misery.

Dissolve ½ teaspoon of salt in ½ cup of water and add enough cosmetic clay to make a creamy paste. Stir in 25 drops of peppermint oil

Fast FACTS

and apply the paste to the affected area. In an emergency, says Hobbs, you can add 30 drops of peppermint oil to a full bottle of calamine lotion, shake well, and apply as needed.

Passionflower, Oats, Skullcap, and St. John's Wort

Take two droppers (40 drops) of blended tincture four times a day to nourish the nervous system. Dr. Yates prescribes this tincture combination for her patients whenever the nervous system is overstimulated, and that can be an understatement when you've brushed up against a poison plant. Passionflower, skullcap, and oats are all nervines, or herbs that support the nervous system and help to balance things out. St. John's wort has a mildly sedative effect.

Make a blended tincture with 2 tablespoons of passionflower, 2 tablespoons of skullcap, 1 tablespoon of oats, and ½ tablespoon of St. John's wort. Measure your dose into a small juice glass and dilute it with water or orange juice to make it more palatable. Use this remedy until your rash heals.

PREMENSTRUAL SYNDROME

*T*o understand exactly how herbs can be used to curb the symptoms of premenstrual syndrome (PMS), it helps to turn back the clock. Not to ancient times, when herbs were considered conventional medicine. No, you need only go back to 5th-grade hygiene class, when the boys were discreetly ushered out of the room and the girls were shown that long-awaited movie about the mysteries of womanhood. For those of you who didn't take notes the first time, here's a quick refresher.

As your body goes through the menstrual cycle, hormone shifts occur. Estrogen gradually tapers off, while progesterone production rises. By the 19th day of your cycle, the two are balanced at roughly equal levels. Then, estrogen and progesterone production taper off together during the last 10 days of the cycle. This is the stage when most women begin to feel premenstrual symptoms, of which there are literally hundreds.

Typically, women with PMS have elevated estrogen levels relative to reduced progesterone levels in the 1 to 2 weeks before their periods, says Joel Evans, M.D., a holistic physician and founder and director of the Center for Women's Health in Darien, Connecticut. This imbalance can trigger mood swings, bloating, breast pain, headaches, fatigue, and appetite changes, to name just a few.

As hormone levels shift in your thirties and forties, you may find that PMS consumes more of your life, coming on as early as 2 weeks before the start of your period. Doctors aren't sure why this happens, but poor diet may play a role. Studies show that women who experience many of the emotional symptoms of PMS eat more sugar, salt, and fat than women who don't, notes Dr. Evans.

Natural practitioners start by recommending a diet low in fat and sugar and high in complex carbohydrates like whole grains, rice and beans, fruits, and vegetables—a diet very similar to the one promoted by the American Heart Association. Dr. Evans suggests taking a daily multivitamin along with 50 milligrams of vitamin B_6, which is a natural diuretic and hormone balancer. To reduce anxiety and cramps and help promote serotonin production, he recommends 400 milligrams of magnesium daily. (If you have heart or kidney problems, check with your doctor before taking supplemental magnesium.)

That done, you can turn to these herbal remedies to help restore hormone balance. Try them for three full cycles. If they don't work by then, you may want to consult a doctor or professional herbal practitioner.

Chasteberry

Take one or two 225-milligram capsules standardized for 0.5 percent agnuside every day. Used for more than 2,500 years to treat menstrual disorders, chasteberry relieves PMS symptoms by stabilizing and regulating hormones, says Robert Rountree, M.D., a holistic physician at the Helios Health Center in Boulder, Colorado. Doctors and herbalists consider it *the* herbal remedy for PMS.

In one German study of 175 women with PMS, a chasteberry extract relieved six typical complaints of PMS—breast tenderness, bloating, headache, constipation, depression, and inner tension—more effectively than vitamin B_6. One-third of the women who took chasteberry for three menstrual cycles experienced complete relief of their symptoms.

"The balancing effect of the herb is gradual and typically occurs over a 3- to 6-month period," says Beverly Yates, N.D., a naturopathic physician with the Natural Health Care Group in Portland, Oregon, and Seattle. Once your symptoms have improved, you should stop taking the herb. Like a mechanic giving a car a tune-up, chasteberry should reset your switches so that your body maintains the new hormonal rhythm on its own.

Black Cohosh

Drink two to four droppers of tincture in some water or tea three times daily, or take two 20-milligram capsules of standardized extract daily. Like chasteberry, black cohosh has a balancing effect on female hormone production.

"Instead of stimulating progesterone, black cohosh acts as a mild estrogen promoter," says Dr. Yates. If your estrogen levels are too low, plant estrogens pick up the slack and make you feel a little better. Also, when your estrogen levels are too high, the same weak estrogens take up spots that would normally be occupied by your body's own, much stronger estrogen. Since that estrogen has nowhere else to go, your body excretes its own overproduction as waste.

Widely used in Europe and recommended by Germany's Commission E, which evaluates herbs for safety and effectiveness, for treating PMS, this North American plant was first used for menstrual problems by Native Americans, who called it squawroot. In more recent times, one study of 110 women showed that black cohosh reduced feelings of depression, anxiety, tension, and mood swings associated with PMS. For most women, once hormone balance is restored, the herb can be discontinued.

Devil's Claw

Ease sugar cravings with ½ teaspoon of liquid extract three times a day. Your body is more sensitive to insulin during the last 2 weeks of your menstrual cycle. As a result, there is less sugar in the blood, explains Dr. Evans. For some women, this decrease in blood sugar triggers intense cravings for sweets.

Devil's claw can help you resist temptation by normalizing blood sugar levels, says Dr. Evans. Start taking it around the time of ovulation and continue until your period starts. Eat more complex carbohydrates and avoid foods with simple sugars.

Evening Primrose

For bloating and breast tenderness, take 3 to 6 grams of oil, in capsules or gel caps, daily with meals. Some studies show that evening primrose oil significantly eases breast pain and tenderness as well as mood swings and irritability, notes Paula Ceh, Pharm.D., assistant professor of pharmacy at Butler University College of Pharmacy and Health Sciences in Indianapolis. You should take this supplement throughout the month, not just when symptoms appear.

Dandelion

To rid your body of excess hormones that can cause anxiety, insomnia, and irritability, take $\frac{1}{2}$ teaspoon of root tincture in a glass of water three times a day. Not only do our bodies produce too much estrogen at times, but we can also absorb it from the food we eat, particularly chicken and beef from animals that are fed estrogens, says Dr. Yates. For this reason, it's important for the digestive system to function more effectively to discourage a buildup of hormones.

Dr. Evans suggests using dandelion root to keep your hormone levels in check during the last 2 weeks of your cycle. A detoxifying herb, dandelion stimulates bile production and helps the liver metabolize estrogen so that it can be eliminated from your body efficiently. It's also important to have regular bowel movements so that excess estrogen can be excreted. Plenty of fiber and water will keep things moving.

Nettle

To decrease swelling and bloating, take a 100-milligram capsule three times a day or $\frac{1}{4}$ teaspoon of tincture one to three times a day. Recommended by the Greek physician Dioscorides in the first cen-

Fast Facts

Cause: An imbalance of the hormones estrogen and progesterone can be responsible for any of the literally hundreds of symptoms that have been attributed to PMS. Typically, women with PMS have elevated levels of estrogen combined with diminished levels of progesterone. Stress and poor diet seem to play a significant role in the hormone shift. Some studies also suggest that PMS may be linked to low thyroid function.

Incidence: Premenstrual symptoms affect up to 40 percent of menstruating women, most often occurring between the ages of 26 and 35. The most serious cases of PMS, in which symptoms can become debilitating, affect 1 to 5 percent of all women.

When to see the doctor: If the physical or psychological symptoms of PMS consistently impair your daily life or relationships, consult your physician.

---

tury A.D. to bring on menstruation, nettle is a useful diuretic for easing PMS symptoms.

Rich in potassium and flavonoids, nettle increases urine production and the elimination of waste products from your body. For a change of pace, eat the fresh leaves as a tonic vegetable. The leaves have a flavor similar to spinach and are quite tasty sautéed in a little olive oil and garlic, says Dr. Evans.

Geranium

Put a drop of hormone-balancing essential oil on your pillow at night and add 5 to 8 drops to your bath twice a week. Geranium oil is thought to balance hormones by acting on the adrenal glands, which are involved in everything from regulating sodium levels to influencing sexual development. The oil may also be a diuretic.

If the scent of geranium doesn't agree with you, Jeanne Rose, San Francisco herbalist and author of *The World of Aromatherapy*, recommends trying the same approach with equal parts of lavender and chamomile essential oils.

Bergamot

To ease tension, put a drop of essential oil in a bowl of just-boiled water and inhale. Daily use of a pure scent can relieve feelings of tension, anxiety, fatigue, and anger, says Rose. Research shows that linalool, one of the components in citrusy-smelling bergamot essential oil, has a relaxing effect on the body. To take you through the day, put a drop on a cotton ball and keep it in a plastic bag so the essential oil doesn't evaporate. Whenever those anxious feelings start, open the bag and take a sniff.

Licorice

On the 14th day of your cycle, begin taking 1 teaspoon of 1:1 liquid extract or one 250-milligram capsule three times a day for 10 days. This sweet-tasting herb has been used for centuries to treat menstrual problems. It is believed to lower estrogen levels while raising progesterone levels. It also helps reduce water retention, says Dr. Evans—but if you take too much, it can actually cause it. For this reason, he doesn't normally include it in his first line of treatment. If you've tried chasteberry and black cohosh, though, and they don't seem to work, licorice may be worth a try.

PROSTATE PROBLEMS

Nothing is certain but death and taxes. And, if you're a man, prostate problems.

It's not really a question of if your prostate gland will start acting up; it's more a matter of when, says Steven L. Bratman, M.D., medical director for Prima Health publishing in Fort Collins, Colorado, and author of *The Alternative Medicine Ratings Guide.*

ADVENTURES IN HERBALISM

HIS PROSTATE PROVED THE POINT

*I*n the early 1990s, James A. Duke, Ph.D., laid his butt on the line.

Dr. Duke, an herbalist and ethnobotanist in Fulton, Maryland, who is one of the world's leading authorities on herbs, publicly bet his own prostate gland that herbal remedies for an enlarged prostate would work as well as the newly approved prescription drug finasteride (Proscar). To make sure that his wager was heard, he made it in front of dozens of officials, including some from the Food and Drug Administration (FDA), the government agency that approved the drug. And for good measure, members of the National Institutes of Health were also present.

The reason that Dr. Duke made such a dramatic wager was to prove a couple of points: first, that some herbs could do just as good a job as pharmaceuticals, and second, that they could do it for less money. One of Dr. Duke's long-standing goals is to have the FDA test synthetic drugs against herbal alternatives to see how they compare. That way, if an herb turns out to be as effective or nearly as effective as a drug, people would have a cheaper alternative. So far, that hasn't happened.

But Dr. Duke still has his prostate.

By age 45, 10 to 15 percent of men have enlarged prostates, a condition known medically as benign prostatic hyperplasia (BPH). For men over age 60, it's 50 percent, and if a man makes it past age 80, the number rises to 90 percent or more, adds Dr. Bratman.

Unexplained growth is not the prostate's normal job description. It's a small gland that sits next to your rectum and produces some of the fluid in semen. The prostate surrounds the urethra, the tube that carries urine from your bladder along its journey out of your body and into the toilet.

When the prostate enlarges, it puts the pinch on the urethra. That leads to the symptoms of BPH, which include difficulty getting the urine flow going, a dribbling stream when it does start, and a feeling that your bladder is still partly full even after you're done. It also causes men to get up often during the night to stand in frustration over the toilet. Occasionally, there's some abdominal pain.

Conventional medicine treats BPH in either of two ways. The first is surgery, in which a portion of the gland is removed to open the urethra. The second treatment is prescription medications such as finasteride (Proscar). Surgery works, but it's invasive, and recovery takes a while, says Donald R. Counts, M.D., an Austin, Texas, physician who combines conventional medicine and proven alternative treatments in his practice.

The prescription medications allow you to avoid surgery but are less effective in some cases, he adds. Plus, there can be some troubling side effects with either surgery or medication, such as a decreased interest in sex, ejaculatory problems, and erection difficulties. With the herbs commonly used to treat prostate enlargement, no such side effects have been reported, according to Dr. Counts. However, he adds, there may be mild gastrointestinal side effects such as nausea in some men.

Since the B in BPH stands for benign, there's no health risk in trying herbal remedies once a proper diagnosis has been established by your medical doctor, says Dr. Counts. Given their high success rate, using them could save you the cost of expensive prescription medications and the risk of surgery. Here are the top choices in herbs for prostate enlargement.

Saw Palmetto

Take 160 milligrams in capsule form twice daily. If you haven't heard of saw palmetto, welcome back from your interplanetary voyages. There's been a lot of hubbub over this extract from the berry of the saw palmetto tree—and for good reason, says Dr. Bratman, since it usually works.

No one knows for sure how it works, although one theory is that it prevents your prostate from converting testosterone, the male hormone, into a related hormone that stimulates cell production. Whatever the mechanism, though, evidence tells us that saw palmetto can actually shrink a growing prostate. Look for a standardized extract that contains 85 to 95 percent fatty acids and sterols.

Be advised, however: Saw palmetto, like other herbs and even prescription drugs, is not a permanent cure. You have to take it on a continual basis. The good news is that in studies, saw palmetto has been associated with milder side effects than finasteride. In his practice, Dr. Counts has found that the herb is as effective as the prescription drug but without the side effects.

Nettle

Take 200 to 400 milligrams of dried root extract in capsule form three times a day continually. Also known as stinging nettle, this root also works to shrink your prostate. "Nettle has all the same possibilities as saw palmetto," explains Dr. Bratman.

Be sure to look for root extract. Capsules of dried leaves are also available, but they contain far different compounds and are used for treating conditions like allergies.

Pygeum

Take capsules supplying 50 to 100 milligrams twice a day continually. Pygeum is an extract from the bark of an African tree. "It is extremely well researched, and it's effective," says Dr. Bratman.

If you have tried a couple of herbal remedies and haven't had much luck, don't give up quite yet, says Dr. Counts. Sometimes, herbs can work better in combination than they do alone. Saw palmetto and pygeum are good examples.

Look for a brand that combines the two herbs (Solaray and Jarrow are two), he recommends. The capsule should have about 320 milligrams of saw palmetto and 100 or so milligrams of pygeum.

Fast Facts

Cause: Among others, two things tend to keep growing after a man reaches adulthood—his waistline and his prostate. What causes benign prostatic hyperplasia (BPH) is unknown, but the male hormone testosterone plays a role. The result is an enlarged prostate.

Incidence: BPH is largely inevitable if a man lives long enough. By age 80, 90 percent of men have symptoms. But it doesn't affect only those of advanced years. Even at age 45, a small number of men experience some of the symptoms.

When to see the doctor: If you have difficulty getting your urine flow started and then have only a dribbling stream, plus the sensation that your bladder is still partly full even after you're done, see a doctor right away. These symptoms, along with a need to get up often during the night to urinate and occasional abdominal pain, can be signs of BPH. But prostate cancer can cause similar symptoms, and so can prostatitis (an infection), so you need to have a doctor's diagnosis.

Pumpkin

Eat 5 grams (about 1 tablespoon) of seeds a day. Pumpkin seeds were once used as a traditional remedy for BPH in countries like Bulgaria, Turkey, and the Ukraine. Now, they're used globally, says Tim Hagney, N.D., a naturopathic physician in Anchorage, Alaska.

Pumpkin seeds have multiple actions. They provide essential fatty acids, which have an anti-inflammatory effect and can help relieve the symptoms of a swelling prostate, says Dr. Hagney. They also seem to confound the mechanism that turns testosterone into a prostate-enlarging hormone. On top of that, they are rich in zinc, a mineral that promotes a healthy prostate.

One problem, though, is that the fatty acids are fragile and easily destroyed by heat and even light. Grind fresh raw seeds and sprinkle them over cereal and other foods. If you prefer the taste of roasted seeds, look for some that are already roasted or roast them yourself in the oven, the way you did at Halloween when you were a kid. Spread the seeds on a shallow pan and slide the pan into a 350°F oven for 5 minutes, or until the seeds are very lightly browned. "When they're roasted, they're pretty good," says Dr. Hagney. "They taste a lot like sunflower seeds, and you will still get the benefits of the zinc in them, since heat doesn't affect it."

Grass Pollen

Take 25 to 40 milligrams in tablet form three times a day. Once upon a time, grass pollen was available only through mail-order companies. Now, with increasing demand for the herb, it's available in some health food stores and drugstores, says Dr. Bratman.

Usually, the tablets contain rye pollen, but sometimes the herb can be based on other grasses, such as timothy or corn. Bear that in mind and don't use these pollens if you have allergies to grasses. Otherwise, this herb may work well for you if none of the others seems to free up your flow. "That's the good thing about all of these herbs that are used to treat BPH," says Dr. Bratman. "If you don't get results with one, you can try another. They're all quite safe and take about the same amount of time— 1 to 3 months—before you see an improvement in BPH symptoms."

PSORIASIS

*W*hen you cut yourself, your body responds by ordering the skin-cell factory to speed up production to help heal the wound. If you have psoriasis, though, that accelerated wound-healing mode is in full swing all the time, literally causing too much of a good thing.

How so? Consider this: In the normal course of things, it takes about 28 days for a skin cell to go through its life cycle. If you have psoriasis, though, it can take as little as 3 to 4 days for a cell to be created in the deepest layer of the skin, rise to the surface, and flake off. Your poor skin just can't slough those flakes off fast enough. As a result, dead skin cells pile up, causing red lesions covered with a dry, silvery white scale.

Not all psoriasis is created equal, though. "Most people just have a few itchy, scaly patches on their knees and elbows and don't even realize they have psoriasis," says dermatologist Nia Terezakis, M.D., clinical professor of dermatology at Tulane University School of Medicine and Louisiana State University School of Medicine, both in New Orleans. "In a few people, it can be so severe and painful that they can hardly walk, especially if they also have psoriatic arthritis." Psoriatic arthritis is caused by severe psoriasis and affects the joints of the fingers and toes.

Psoriasis also tends to wax and wane. It's a chronic disease, so you may have it for months or even years, but it can inexplicably go into remission and then flare up again with a vengeance.

Because there's no known cause, finding an effective treatment can become a series of frustrating, time-consuming, expensive shots in the dark. Conventional medicine favors steroid creams, ointments with vitamin A and D derivatives, controlled exposure to UV light, and other medications, some of which carry serious side effects. The search for a safe, effective treatment continues.

What works for one person with psoriasis may not work for another, so you'll need to try different approaches to see what works best for you. How you carry out the remedy is at least as important as what you do, says Dr. Terezakis.

"Keeping the skin hydrated is the single most important thing," she says. "That helps to soften the scaly patches and also relieves itching." Take long baths, swim every day, and slather on the moisturizer. Applications of any treatment that you may use will also be absorbed more effectively on moisturized skin.

There are some herbs that can help, too. Herbalists tend to see psoriasis as the external manifestation of an internal problem, such as poor digestion or liver function, and to address that as well as treating the skin topically.

Dandy De-Itching Dandelion Coffee

Dandelion has a stellar reputation for stimulating the liver and cleansing the blood, which are both useful actions when you're dealing with skin disease. Douglas Schar, a medical herbalist in London, editor of the British Journal of Phytotherapy, *and author of* Backyard Medicine Chest, *uses this recipe to indulge his coffee habit while being kind to his skin. Here's what you need.*

- **1 salad bowl of dandelion roots and leaves**
- **1 cup ground coffee**

Preheat the oven to 250°F. Wash the dandelion and put it on a baking sheet. Bake for 30 minutes, or until the dandelion is brown and crisp. In a food processor or blender, grind the dandelion to a powder.

In a resealable plastic bag, mix 1 cup of dandelion powder with the coffee, then use the mixture to make your morning brew.

Christopher Robbins, a member of Britain's National Institute of Medical Herbalists who practices herbal medicine in Ross-on-Wye, Herefordshire, England, and has written several books, including *The Natural Pharmacy*, sums up the aim of treatment this way. "Rather than seeing the target as completely curing the psoriasis, which is difficult, the target for me is to slow it down, start reversing the process, and stop the spread, which does have a pretty good success rate." Here are some herbal treatments to try.

Calendula and Comfrey

Apply a thin coat of cream to scaly patches twice a day. "Externally, I'd recommend very simple, cooling creams," says Robbins. He advises using a cream rather than an ointment because the latter has a tendency to heat up the skin. Calendula and comfrey, he says, are a good combination because they calm down the skin, keep it from drying out, and help soothe the inflammation and repair the damaged tissues.

Calendula and comfrey are often paired in lotions and creams, so you should be able to find this product easily in most health food stores. Do not use comfrey on your psoriasis if your skin is cracked open or raw.

Aloe

Smooth aloe gel onto the patches three times a day. "There are some old standbys that really work well," says David Richard Decatur, M.D., who runs the Decatur Medical Center, a holistic health facility in Indianapolis, "and aloe vera is one of them. It's really a great moisturizer."

In a study in Sweden, people with chronic psoriasis used an aloe cream three times a day for 4 weeks. After a year, all but five of the people in the study experienced significant reduction of lesions and decreased redness.

Avoid products that contain perfumes, colorants, and other additives, though, warns Robbins. You should be able to find the stabilized, pure gel. "And that's a goody," he says, "because there's no junk in there that might irritate." His rule of thumb is to never put anything on your skin that has any ingredients you don't need.

The other option, of course, is to grow an aloe plant in your kitchen. Cut off about 3 inches of leaf each day, split it open, scrape out the gel, and apply it to the skin.

Burdock, Oregon Grape, Yellow Dock, and Siberian Ginseng

Take 1 teaspoon of blended tincture twice a day in grapefruit juice. Like many naturopathic doctors, Thomas Kruzel, N.D., former president of the American Association of Naturopathic Physicians, who practices in Portland, Oregon, draws a link between psoriasis and a deficiency in the body's ability to rid itself of toxic substances.

Fast Facts

Cause: The cause of psoriasis is still a mystery, but doctors think heredity may be involved. Flare-ups can be triggered by certain bacterial infections, such as strep throat, as well as skin injuries, vaccinations, stress, and some medications.

Incidence: Psoriasis affects 6.4 million Americans. The disease is slightly more common in women than in men, and symptoms usually begin to appear in the late twenties, although it's been seen at birth and as late as age 90. Ten to 20 percent of people with psoriasis also develop psoriatic arthritis.

When to see the doctor: Call your doctor for an appointment if your symptoms do not respond to self-treatment. If you develop psoriatic patches all over your body, or if you experience fever, joint pain, or fatigue, see a doctor immediately.

This tincture combination brings together three traditional detoxifiers, or blood cleansers, all of which have a mild laxative quality.

Dr. Kruzel says that this blend may help rid your body of toxins that contribute to psoriasis outbreaks. To make it, mix equal parts of each tincture, then take the dosage above for 3 to 4 weeks. To prevent further outbreaks, stop taking it for 1 week, then resume and take the same dosage two or three times a week.

Milk Thistle

Take a 150-milligram capsule three times a day. Herbalists recommend milk thistle for the treatment of psoriasis because of its reputation for protecting and repairing liver cells. Its active ingredient, a flavonoid called silymarin, is an antioxidant that acts very specifically on liver tissue, they say. The liver plays a crucial role in eliminating toxins from the body. If this ability is compromised, the blood cannot be cleansed adequately, and the psoriasis will get much worse.

Barbara Silbert, N.D., D.C., a naturopathic doctor and chiropractor who is president of the Massachusetts Society of Naturopathic Physicians and has a family practice in Boston and Newbury, Massachusetts, recommends taking the herb for 3 to 6 months.

Licorice

Take 1 teaspoon of extract three or four times a day during flare-ups. In use for centuries as a sweetener (it's 50 times sweeter than sugar), licorice has powerful anti-inflammatory properties, and research has shown that it compares favorably to conventional anti-inflammatory drugs such as butadione and hydrocortisone.

It's not the candy variety you want, though, says Tammy Alex, N.D., a naturopathic doctor based in Guilford, Connecticut. You need to find pure licorice extract. Thick and syrupy like molasses, it comes in 1- or 2-ounce bottles and is available at health food stores.

RECTAL ITCH

Pruritus ani is the 10-cent term for rectal itch, but even it doesn't capture the maddening feeling that comes with this condition. Rectal itch is often worse at night, just when you most need some sleep, and the more you scratch, it seems, the worse it gets.

If you were of flexible frame and able to peer at the area in which your itch resides, you would likely see something that resembles diaper rash, says Brenda Snowman, M.D., a physician in Cleveland, Tennessee. You would also see irritations caused by your fingernails.

As hard as it may be to resist, that's a cue to try to take it easy on the scratching, since it's only making things worse.

Before you consider herbal remedies, there are a few things that you must do. Because rectal itch forms in a warm, moist environment, you need to make the landscape a little more inhospitable. That means keeping the area dry. After showering and toweling dry, gently spread your cheeks and use a blow dryer set on low to help dry the area, recommends Miles Greenberg, N.D., a naturopathic physician in Kapaa, Hawaii, and president of the Hawaii Society of Naturopathic Physicians. You should also avoid synthetic-fiber underwear and stick with absorbent cotton.

You also need to examine the way you clean the area. Too little cleaning leaves fecal matter hanging around, which contributes to increasing the itch. But some people are too zealous in their scrubbing and end up leaving the area raw and irritated.

To handle both concerns, follow the advice of Dr. Greenberg. "Just wash with water after a bowel movement," he says. Ideally, that means no toilet paper. Climb in the bathtub and use your hand and lots of free-flowing water. Dry carefully. If you're not near a tub, the second best method is to use dampened toilet paper. This cleans well and slides easily over damaged skin. Pat yourself dry afterward.

Unfortunately, long-term solutions to rectal itch are hard to come by. It has a tendency to stump doctors. It's often hard to discover what's causing it, and it's equally hard to treat it in many people. But don't despair quite yet. There are some herbal remedies that may scratch some of your itch naturally.

Witch Hazel

Apply as needed. Witch hazel extract has a long history of use for skin conditions, says Dr. Snowman. It is an astringent and a mild antibiotic and gives the area a nice cooling feeling. Most extracts have an alcohol base, though, so they can sting sensitive skin. If you experience stinging, stop using it.

You can do double duty with witch hazel if you dampen a wad of toilet paper and gently use it to clean yourself.

Fast Facts

Cause: Rectal itch can have many causes or none. Some things that may be to blame are scabies (a contagious skin disease caused by itch mites), fungal infections, yeast infections, warts, psoriasis, ringworm, pinworms, and even excessive sweating. Cleaning your bottom too little can cause itching, as can cleaning too much and irritating the skin. But for as many things as there are that can cause rectal itch, about half of cases have no known origin. This makes it difficult to treat.

Incidence: Although it's hard to put an exact number on the people who live with rectal itch, it is known that many more men than women get the condition.

When to see the doctor: If you can't control your itch with home remedies within a month or so, seek out a health-care practitioner who specializes in ano-genital conditions, such as a gastroenterologist. He may be able to pinpoint a cause that you've missed.

Aloe

Coat the affected area with gel once or twice a day until symptoms subside. Aloe vera is a traditional remedy that has become very mainstream, says Dr. Snowman. The compounds in aloe help promote healing and also act as mild antiseptics.

Many people find that it soothes their itching bottoms. Pick up some pure gel, not a cream with aloe in it, at a health food store or drugstore and test it on a small area. Some people are sensitive to aloe. If there's no additional irritation, you can continue to apply it up to twice a day.

Pau d'Arco

Drink a cup of tea twice a day. Sometimes, rectal itch can be caused by an overgrowth of yeast in your intestinal tract, says Dr.

Greenberg. This spills over into your rectal area and takes root in the moist skin.

If that's the case, hit it with pau d'arco, an herb that contains the yeast-fighting compounds lapachol and beta-lapachone. To make the tea, pour 1 cup of boiling water over 1 teaspoon of herb. Steep for 5 minutes, then sip. Don't sweeten the tea, though, as that can reduce its effectiveness. Yeasts eat sugars.

"If yeast is the cause of your itch, you should see an improvement within a few days. If you don't, yeast is probably not the cause, and you should discontinue use," says Dr. Greenberg.

Clove

Drink one cup of decoction four to six times daily until symptoms disappear. The common kitchen spice clove has anti-yeast compounds, too, says Dr. Greenberg. To make a decoction, use 1 teaspoon of crushed herb for each cup of water you plan to use. Bring the mixture to a boil, let it bubble for 10 to 15 minutes, and strain out the herb before drinking. To save time, you can make one large batch of this in the morning and sip it throughout the day.

SCARS

*F*or a movie star like Harrison Ford, a scar such as the one that Ford sports on his chin can be an imperfection that gives a handsome face even more character.

For most of us, though, a scar isn't something that we want to draw attention to, and often, it serves as an unwelcome reminder of a traumatic accident or surgery. Knowing that a scar is a natural, healthy result of the skin's wound-repair process doesn't help much.

If you have a recent scar, though, take heart in this fact: Scars usually become thicker and more noticeable about 2 months into the healing process. After that, they start to fade gradually. Within 6 months to a year, the scar tissue should thin out and become even with your skin surface.

Some people, though, have a genetic tendency to develop large, irregularly shaped scars called keloids, which are caused by abnormal growth of scar tissue. If the keloid-creating gene is in your makeup, you don't have to have a major wound to develop one. Even a minor scratch or vaccination can result in a keloid.

Conventional medicine has a number of options for reducing scar tissue, including surgery, laser resurfacing, skin grafts, and chemical peels. If those approaches strike you as too aggressive, the natural world has a few gentler remedies that can help. A traditional favorite of naturopaths and holistic doctors is vitamin E. Breaking open a capsule and spreading the gel on a healing scar several times a day may help it to heal faster and leave less of a scar, says David Richard Decatur, M.D., who runs the Decatur Medical Center, a holistic medical facility in Indianapolis.

Herbally, there are some steps you can take, too, to help soften and shrink stubborn scar tissue. Before trying these remedies, be sure to thoroughly clean the wound.

Calendula

Apply a tincture or succus to the wound twice a day until it heals. You can get a head start on vanquishing your scar before it even appears. Thomas Kruzel, N.D., former president of the American Association of Naturopathic Physicians, who practices in Portland, Oregon, suggests using a tincture or succus (a thicker, more concentrated extract) of calendula on the cut to help it heal and cut down

Fast Facts

Cause: Scars are caused by the natural repair process that skin goes through when it's wounded by accident, surgery, or disease. The large, thick scar known as a keloid occurs when there is an abnormal growth of scar tissue.

Incidence: Everyone who suffers cuts is likely to develop scars. Young people end up with larger, more prominent scars than older people because their skin-healing process tends to be overly vigorous. People with darkly pigmented skin are more likely to develop keloids than people with lighter skin.

When to see the doctor: If you have a scar that does not respond to self-treatment and you wish to explore other options to reduce or remove the scar tissue, consult a dermatologist or plastic surgeon.

---

on scar formation. Use enough to cover the wound so it can be absorbed into the skin.

Calendula, or pot marigold, is known as an excellent anti-inflammatory, and it encourages new, healthy cells to grow at the wound site. Germany's Commission E, which evaluates herbs for safety and effectiveness, endorses the herb for wound healing.

Gotu Kola

Make a paste and apply it to the scar twice daily until the scar heals. Dr. Decatur recommends this remedy to reduce scars. Add enough water to 1 tablespoon of gotu kola powder to make a paste and apply it directly to the scar.

A member of the parsley family, gotu kola has drawn much attention for its reputed ability to rejuvenate nerve and brain cells, and it was traditionally used to improve memory and fend off senility. Experiments have also indicated that it soothes inflammation, strengthens wounded tissue, and helps rebuild damaged skin.

Calendula and Cottonwood

Add these infused oils to a salve and apply it to the scar twice a day. Beverly Yates, N.D., knows of what she speaks when she recommends this healing salve. Dr. Yates, a naturopathic physician with the Natural Health Care Group in Portland, Oregon, and Seattle, tried it out on her husband, who had a nasty keloid on the back of his hand. "This salve really seems to soften keloids and help them shrink," she says. She's not sure exactly what the mechanism is, however. "Calendula is anti-inflammatory, but I don't know why the cottonwood works." She does know that when she looks at the back of her husband's hand these days, she has to stare hard to make out any scar at all.

To 100 milliliters (6 tablespoons) of basic skin salve, add 50 milliliters (3 tablespoons) of calendula oil, 40 milliliters (2½ tablespoons) of cottonwood oil, and 10 milliliters (½ tablespoon) of melted beeswax. The cottonwood comes as either a sticky resin or an oil. You should be able to find beeswax at a health food store. Buy a hunk and melt it down.

Apply the salve in the morning and evening. If the scar is on your hand, Dr. Yates suggests wearing a cotton glove to keep the salve in direct contact with the skin. "For an old, thick, lumpy-bumpy kind of scar," she says, "you may need to use it for 2 to 3 months. For a much newer scar, a week or two might be enough. Let your eyes be your guide. You'll know when it's time to stop."

Bromelain

Take a 500-milligram capsule twice a day between meals until the scar heals completely. Tammy Alex, N.D., a naturopathic doctor based in Guilford, Connecticut, recommends taking bromelain internally for scars because of its anti-inflammatory properties. An enzyme derived from the pineapple plant, bromelain helps break down the debris at the wound site, she says, and acts like a cellular cleanup crew.

SHINGLES

*C*hickenpox was bad enough when you were a kid, but when the same virus rears its ugly head again in your adult years, it's just not fair.

Nevertheless, that's what happens when you get shingles. The chickenpox virus that you thought you'd said goodbye to so long ago decided to stick around, and then, after lying dormant for years, it springs back to life to pay you a return visit. Only this time, you don't get itchy brown dots all over your body. Instead, you may feel a burning or tingling sensation in the nerve endings under your skin. Clusters of tiny blisters soon show up on the skin directly above the nerve, often around your torso.

Shingles is definitely no picnic. Those blisters can be horribly itchy as well as painful, but happily, they dry up and scab over quickly. Often within a month, the whole episode is just an unpleasant memory. For some, though, shingles linger longer in the form of sharp, burning, or aching pain in the nerve endings. Called postherpetic neuralgia, this post-shingles pain can make skin so sensitive that even the touch of clothing becomes almost unbearable. In some cases, this can last months or even years.

Herbally, shingles remedies focus on soothing the rash and helping the body fight off the viral attack. "When you have a viral infection like shingles, it's important to boost your immune system," says Dominique Davis, M.D., a physician and member of Britain's National Institute of Medical Herbalists (NIMH) who practices herbal medicine in Berwickshire, Scotland. Some herbs can also help with the pain of postherpetic neuralgia.

Chamomile

Make a compress and apply it to the blisters. Sabine Rickert, an herbalist in Berlin, Germany, advises against using any kind of oil or

St. John's All-Over Nerve Oil

Prepare this oil for the next time shingles strikes. You can begin applying it at the first sign of pain along a nerve, even before the skin has blistered, says Anne McIntyre, a member of Britain's National Institute of Medical Herbalists and co-owner of the Midsummer Cottage Clinic in Oxfordshire, England. The St. John's wort acts as an anti-inflammatory. Lemon balm, traditionally used as an antiviral, may add other properties to this tonic.

Once the blisters have formed, apply the oil very gingerly with a soft cloth or massage it with your fingers around the immediate area. Reapply this mixture in the morning and evening and as needed throughout the day. Use it until your pain is gone.

- **1 handful fresh St. John's wort flowers**
- **100 milliliters sunflower oil (or any other vegetable oil)**
- **20 drops lemon balm essential oil**

Put the St. John's wort in a clear glass jar. Add the sunflower and lemon balm oils, screw the lid on, and leave it on a sunny windowsill for about 2 weeks. You'll know it's ready when the oil starts to turn red. Strain out the flowers and store the infused oil in an amber bottle.

ointment on a wet, blistery rash. "If the blisters burst, it tends to get very sticky," she says, "and then they can't heal properly." Apply a chamomile compress to clean away the stickiness before you proceed with any oil treatments.

To make the compress, brew a double-strength tea by using 2 tablespoons of dried chamomile to 1 cup of boiling water. Let stand for about 20 minutes, then strain, taking care to remove all of the plant material, and soak a cotton cloth in the liquid. Place the cloth on the affected area, lay a clean towel on top of that, and leave it in place for 15 minutes. Remove the compress and carefully

Fast FACTS

Cause: Shingles is caused by the same virus (varicella zoster) that causes chickenpox. The virus can remain dormant within a nerve after the chickenpox has gone away, only to become reactivated many years later. Why this happens is not clear, although it's thought that a weakened immune system—due to age, illness, stress, or the use of certain drugs—plays a role in awakening the virus.

Incidence: Shingles is a fairly common disease that affects one in five adults. Only people who have had chickenpox are susceptible, and it's most common after age 50.

When to see the doctor: Call your doctor if you develop the typical symptoms of shingles, including a burning, tingling sensation in nerve endings, often around your torso, and small blisters in the same area. If shingles occurs near your eyes, see your doctor immediately.

---

wipe the affected area with a clean cotton cloth. You can use this remedy as often as necessary.

Chickweed

Smooth on a thin layer of soothing cream twice a day. Seventeenth-century herbalist Nicholas Culpeper recommended boiling chickweed in hog's grease to calm itching skin. Now you can just go to your local health food store and buy a tube of chickweed cream to ease the itchies, no hog's grease necessary.

Echinacea

Take two 250-milligram capsules three times a day while you have shingles. Echinacea increases the production of white blood cells in the body, which helps you fight infections better, says Dr. Davis. It's particularly effective against viral infections such as shingles.

As a preventive measure against outbreaks during the winter months, you may want to take one 250-milligram capsule twice a day, especially if you are prone to catching colds or the flu easily.

Garlic

Eat three cloves a day. Take up arms against the viral attack by eating raw garlic, suggests medical herbalist Jacqueline Kilbryde, a member of the NIMH in Ballydehob, West Cork, Ireland. Although garlic capsules are readily available in health food stores, Kilbryde prefers the real thing.

If the idea of munching on raw garlic makes you wince, try crushing a medium clove and mixing it with a teaspoon of honey. That way, says Kilbryde, you can swallow it without even having to chew it. Still, it helps to have a glass of water handy to wash away some of the pungent taste. Other ways to get your three cloves a day: Use crushed garlic in your dinner salad or slice a clove thinly and make a sandwich with brown bread.

SINUSITIS

*H*erbal and conventional medicine use similar strategies in treating sinusitis, a congesting and often painful inflammation of the sinuses, the series of cavities behind your eye, nose, and cheek areas. Both herbal and pharmaceutical remedies go straight to the site to loosen the congestion, and both try to eliminate the source of the inflammation, which is often a viral, allergy-related, or bacterial infection. But unlike antibiotics, herbal remedies work with your body's immune system to neutralize the infection, says Lorilee Schoenbeck, N.D., a naturopathic physician at the Champlain Center for Natural Medicine in Shelburne, Vermont.

The following herbal remedies work best when you start them early. "If you catch sinusitis at its height, natural medicine can still shorten the duration and make you feel more comfortable," Dr. Schoenbeck says, "but herbal medicine is most effective at the onset of symptoms."

Eucalyptus

Do a steam inhalation with essential oil at least once a day. "A substance like eucalyptus essential oil will actually get right up into the mucous membranes and loosen the congestion," says Emily Kane, N.D., a naturopathic physician and licensed acupuncturist in Juneau, Alaska. Not only is rising steam an excellent way to get it up there, but the evaporated water itself helps with the job. The treatment can be continued once or twice daily until all symptoms are resolved, says Dr. Kane.

Vials of essential oil of eucalyptus are readily available in health food stores. "It's really strong," Dr. Kane says, "so you just need a few drops." Put those drops at the bottom of a large bowl and carefully fill it with steaming hot water. Immediately put a towel over your head and slowly lean over the bowl to breathe in the steam. Be careful not to get too close to avoid burning your face. "Inhale as deeply as possible through your nose until the water cools down," Dr. Kane advises.

Thyme, Rosemary, and Peppermint

Do a steam inhalation with these herbs at least once a day. Sure, you can use thyme, rosemary, and peppermint essential oils in much the same way as the eucalyptus inhalation above (use just a drop or two of each oil), but fresh leaves picked from the little plants you have growing on your windowsill will release their own oils, notes Dr. Schoenbeck. If you don't have the fresh herbs handy, buy dried leaves or raid your spice rack, she suggests. "The vapor action of the steam

Cause: Viruses cause most acute cases, but sinusitis is often a one-two punch. A cold or flu virus creates hospitable conditions for bacteria to thrive in the sinuses, creating even more inflammation. A lot of other things can set off the nasal reaction, including fungus infections, hay fever, damp weather, intolerance to certain medicines, and even emotional conditions such as grief.

Incidence: More than 35 million Americans suffer from at least one case of acute sinusitis each year.

When to see the doctor: If your nasal secretions are yellow or grayish green and thick, the infection has lasted for 5 to 7 days and doesn't show signs of improvement, or you have continuing fever, see your doctor.

---

inhalation will warm, moisten, and loosen the mucus that's stuck in your sinuses, which will drain a lot after that," Dr. Schoenbeck says.

Put a heaping tablespoon of each of the three herbs into a large bowl and pour hot, steaming water over them, she says. "An important point is not to mix the herbs and water before heating," she advises. "If you heat the herbs, you'll release the volatile oils into the kitchen instead of your sinuses." Cover your head with a towel, lower your nose slowly toward the steaming bowl, and inhale for about 5 minutes. You can repeat the process once or twice a day until your symptoms subside.

Echinacea

Each day, drink six cups of tea, or take a total of 1,200 milligrams in capsule form or four 1-teaspoon doses of tincture. As with any infection, echinacea is a great aid to your immune system's efforts to overcome sinusitis. While any form of echinacea is helpful, taking it as tea allows you to taste and feel the actual herb, a factor that many herbal practitioners, including Dr. Schoenbeck, consider to be conducive to better healing.

Here's how to do it. First, buy some cut-and-sifted echinacea root at a health food store. For sinusitis, Dr. Schoenbeck recommends adding 6 heaping teaspoons of herb to 6 cups of cold water in a saucepan. Cover the pan, bring the water to a boil, lower the heat to simmer, and let the herb decoct for 10 to 15 minutes before straining. You've made a day's supply. Continue taking echinacea until you feel better.

Oregon Grape

Take 1 teaspoon of tincture three times a day. The root of the wild Oregon grape has powerful infection-fighting action, says Dr. Schoenbeck. Take it at the very first sign of sinus symptoms and continue for the duration of the infection.

Garlic

Eat three cloves, or take capsules that supply 10 milligrams of allicin, each day until the infection is gone. Garlic, nature's antibiotic, adds another dimension to overcoming sinusitis by increasing natural killer cell activity against virally infected cells. Since sinusitis often starts out as a viral infection, that's an important tool, Dr. Schoenbeck says.

SNORING

*I*f necessity is the mother of invention, then a cure for snoring must be one of the most needed remedies around. There are at least 140 anti-snoring devices registered with the U.S. Patent and Trademark Office. While none of them works any better than simply staying awake, inventors keep on trying. That certainly says a lot about the difficulty you encounter when you try to silence a snorer.

Simply put, snoring happens when there's an obstruction blocking the free flow of air through the back of the throat and the nose. That respiratory roadblock can be put in place by many things, including flabby throat muscles, a double chin, or even a misshapen soft palate.

Allergies are another big cause of snoring, says Connie Catellani, M.D., medical director of the Miro Center for Integrative Medicine in Evanston, Illinois. That's because food allergies as well as hay fever can cause chronically swollen nasal passages and draining sinuses. These problems—no matter what the cause—are sure sources of snores.

If your snoring is allergy-related, you'll need to figure out what you're allergic to and do your best to avoid it, says Dr. Catellani. Then you can turn to herbs to help open stuffy nasal passages and make snoring nothing more than a bad dream.

Nettle

Drink up to three cups of tea throughout the day. Nettle is sometimes called stinging nettle because of its bristly, spiny leaves. Herbalists consider this mineral-rich plant helpful for various ailments, but it's particularly good for easing the respiratory inflammation brought on by allergies, says Steven Rissman, N.D., a naturopathic physician at American WholeHealth in Cherry Creek, Colorado.

Take nettle as a tea. To make it, pour 1 cup of boiling water over 1 tablespoon of dried nettle leaf, cover and steep for 5 minutes, then strain the tea into a mug. If you have allergies, start with one cup a day for the first few days, since nettle may worsen symptoms. After that, you can drink up to three cups a day. Just be sure to make one of them a nightcap to get the best nose-clearing effects while you sleep.

Oak or Oregon Grape

Use a strong infusion of either herb as a gargle and nasal rinse just before bed. Oak bark is an astringent herb that contains water-

Fast FACTS

Cause: The characteristic sounds of snoring come from the vibration and rubbing of tissues in the back of the mouth, nose, and throat. Snoring is usually caused by poor tone in the muscles of the nose and throat, overly large tonsils or bulky neck tissue, or obstructed nasal passageways due to allergy or illness.

Incidence: About 45 million Americans, or 40 percent of adults by age 50, are habitual snorers. Men and people who are overweight have more snoring problems. Snoring is also worse among the elderly.

When to see the doctor: Snoring can be seriously disruptive to family life, disturbing the sleep of others and sparking resentment. If snoring is affecting your personal relationships, that is reason enough to visit your doctor, but snoring can threaten physical health as well. If you are a snorer, you wake unrefreshed, and you often feel sleepy during the day, you may have sleep apnea. Apnea is a potentially serious condition in which loud snoring alternates with periods of completely obstructed breathing. If you suspect that your snoring may be related to this condition, see your doctor for an evaluation.

---

soluble chemical compounds called tannins. Tannins can protect inflamed mucous membranes in the throat and nose and will help dry up secretions that can contribute to snoring. To target these effects, an infusion of oak bark is often recommended as a gargle and nasal rinse, says Dr. Rissman.

If you can't find oak bark, an infusion made with Oregon grape root works pretty much the same way. Besides being astringent, this herb also possesses an antimicrobial effect, says Dr. Rissman, which is helpful if there is any infection brewing inside your inflamed sinuses.

To make a strong infusion, start with 2 tablespoons of either dried herb and cover with 1 cup of boiling water. Steep for up to 15 minutes, then strain it into a small cup or bowl that has a pour spout. Wait until the infusion cools to room temperature before using it.

Gargling is the easy part: Simply take a small mouthful of the liquid, tilt your head back, and gurgle away before spitting the liquid out. Rinsing your nasal passages (nasal lavage) is a little trickier, but it's also the most effective part of the treatment for snoring. Form a cup with the palm of one hand and fill it with about 2 tablespoons of infusion. Keeping your head upright, bring your hand up to one nostril while pressing the other nostril closed. Gently sniff the liquid into your nose, then release it through your mouth. You may sputter at first, but keep trying. Once you get the hang of it, nasal lavage will actually feel good as it frees your nostrils and sinuses of congestion.

Sore Throat

*O*ne thing about herbal sore throat remedies is that you don't always follow the usual "two or three times a day" schedule. You take some of the preparations every hour or two, and others as often as you want.

What should you do if you miss one of these frequent doses? Congratulate yourself, says Liz Collins, N.D., a naturopathic physician at the Natural Childbirth and Family Clinic in Portland, Oregon. "You start to forget doses as you start feeling better," she says. "That works out perfectly."

Sore throat, or pharyngitis, is sometimes caused by bacteria, including the infamous streptococcus, says Connie Catellani, M.D., medical director of the Miro Center for Integrative Medicine in Evanston, Illinois. A strep throat usually demands conventional antibiotics. Nine out of 10 times, however, a sore throat is the result of a viral infection, a milder, herb-treatable condition marked mostly by—you guessed it—soreness in the throat, she adds. Herbs to soothe this problem are often accompanied by other natural treatments, such as readily available zinc lozenges, which soothe your throat as they boost your immune system, and the time-honored saltwater gargle, Dr. Collins says.

Slippery Elm Soother

Here's a hot fireside drink that's throat-soothing and tastes great. "It's from an old-fashioned recipe that's helped a ton of people over the years," says Cascade Anderson Geller, an herbal educator and consulting herbal practitioner in Portland, Oregon. "It's just amazing how it works."

This simple recipe's star is slippery elm. "For any irritated mucous membrane, slippery elm has a mixed action that's very healing," Geller says. "On the one hand, it's mucilaginous and very hydrating, but it has a lot of tannins that also make it a dehydrating astringent." You can drink this remedy as needed for sore throat relief. Here's how to make it.

1 teaspoon slippery elm powder
½ cup pear juice

In a saucepan, combine the slippery elm and the pear juice. Stir over medium heat until the mixture thickens, about 2 minutes. (To make it thicker, add more powder.) Remove from the heat and pour into a mug.

Echinacea, Oregon Grape, and Myrrh

Combine these three tinctures and take 30 to 60 drops in a little water every 2 hours for 2 days, then reduce the frequency of the dosage by half. This is an easy-to-use variation of a formula that herbalists often rely on for treating throat infections. The Oregon grape inhibits the growth of offending microorganisms, while the echinacea boosts immune function to rid your throat of the infection faster, Dr. Collins says. Myrrh, meanwhile, acts as an expectorant to help clear your throat.

Buy 1-ounce bottles of each tincture and combine them in a larger bottle. This combination is bitter, so it helps to dilute it and have some more water handy as a chaser.

Slippery Elm

Suck on lozenges freely. Natural herbal throat lozenges are available all over the place, and they do indeed work for a sore throat, natural practitioners say. Dr. Collins suggests looking for slippery elm lozenges. "Slippery elm is mucilaginous and soothing to the mucous membranes," she says. "As a lozenge, it can be really nice for a dry throat irritation. It helps you salivate."

The dosage? "You could pretty much suck on them forever," Dr. Collins says. If your throat dryness or irritation is persistent, however, or if you find yourself using these lozenges for relief all the time, see your doctor, she adds.

Echinacea, Goldenseal, and Peppermint

Spray this mixture into your throat once an hour. For simultaneous symptom relief and infection fighting, spray an echinacea-goldenseal combination in tincture form directly into your throat, suggests Shiva Barton, N.D., lead naturopathic practitioner at Wellspace, a complementary health center in Cambridge, Massachusetts. Buy 1-ounce tincture bottles of echinacea, goldenseal, and peppermint. Or, instead of peppermint—which is just used to improve the taste—you can substitute licorice or ginger, Dr. Barton says. You'll also need a medicinal spray bottle, available at any drugstore.

Combine the echinacea and goldenseal in equal amounts in the spray bottle, then add about one-quarter of that amount of the peppermint or other flavoring. "Spray this on your throat and then swallow it," Dr. Barton says.

Sage, Thyme, and Poplar

Do three deep 30-second gargles with this tea blend several times a day. For sore throat, Cascade Anderson Geller, an herbal educator and consulting herbal practitioner in Portland, Oregon,

Fast FACTS

Cause: Most sore throats are viral infections, although about 10 percent are bacterial.

Incidence: Viral pharyngitis is one of the most frequent medical complaints. Strep throat, the main bacterial version, is most common among schoolchildren from ages 5 to 10, usually striking between October and April.

When to see the doctor: Coldlike viral infections in the upper respiratory tract, sore throats included, should not last much more than a week. If the sore throat lingers, see a doctor to rule out something more serious. If your symptoms indicate strep throat—with fever, severe pain, difficulty swallowing, inflamed tonsils, weakness, headache, and stomach discomfort—call your physician immediately.

recommends gargling with a strong tea made from these three astringent herbs. "Thyme is antispasmodic, so it's nice if you have that real achy, tight feeling in your throat," Geller says. "The poplar buds are really antiseptic and very popular in sore throat gargles."

To make the tea blend, mix equal parts of dried sage leaves, thyme leaves, and poplar buds. Steep 1 heaping tablespoon of the blend in 1 cup of boiling water for about 10 minutes. Let it cool just enough to be nice and warm but not hot enough to burn your throat. Take a mouthful of tea and gargle deeply. "To do a really good therapeutic gargle, you need to tilt your head way back, open up the back of your throat as wide as you can, and let the water go back as far as possible without swallowing it," says Geller.

Gargle three times. You can swallow the tea each time, but if you find it too bitter, just spit it out before taking the next mouthful. "You'll notice an immediate improvement in how you feel," Geller says. Put the remaining tea in a tightly sealed jar and reheat it for repeated use. Continue gargling with this mixture as long as your sore throat lasts, she advises.

Usnea, Osha, Marshmallow, and Ginger

Do three deep 30-second gargles with these tinctures every 2 to 3 hours. As a sore throat gargle, tinctures work as well as tea, Geller says. Blend ¼ ounce each of tinctured usnea and the tinctured roots of osha, marshmallow, and ginger. Put about 15 drops of this formula in enough water to make a good mouthful and gargle as described above.

STIES AND CHALAZIA

*P*imples are bad enough on your face, but there's something especially irritating about getting one on your eye. That's essentially what sties and chalazia are: two types of pimples that appear either along the edge of or within the sensitive skin of the eyelid.

Chalazia are the less painful of the two. The name comes from the Greek word for barley corn, says Jay Cohen, O.D., professor of optometry at the State University of New York College of Optometry in New York City, because a chalazion feels like a hard little seed inside the lid of your eye. It starts when an oil gland just under the skin becomes blocked.

A sty, on the other hand, is an infection of an eyelid gland near an eyelash root or follicle that results in inflammation similar to a boil or pimple. "If you can barely touch it without feeling a lot of pain, it's probably a sty," says Alice Laule, M.D., who practices holistic medicine and ophthalmology in Harrison, Arkansas. "If you can mash on it and just say 'ouch' a little bit, it's a chalazion. In fact, a chalazion might not even be that tender."

If you have a tendency toward dandruff and for the edges of your eyelids to be red, you may have a skin condition called seborrhea,

Fast Facts

Cause: Chalazia are the result of blocked or inflamed oil glands; sties are the product of infected eyelash follicles.

Incidence: Anyone can get a sty or a chalazion, but wearing eye makeup and rubbing the eyes can make them more likely.

When to see the doctor: A sty that continues to be sore after 3 to 4 days should be examined by a doctor or an ophthalmologist. A chalazion should be examined if there's a steady increase in size or if you're unsure what it is.

which can lead to more frequent sties and chalazia. In general, both problems tend to go away by themselves. Doctors often prescribe antibiotic drops to treat sties, but Dr. Laule doesn't think that they are particularly helpful. "The drops can't get up into the gland, where they need to be if they're going to do any good," she says. Here's how herbs might be able to help.

Eyebright

Apply a warm compress three or four times a day. This represents an advance on the usual treatment for sties and chalazia, which is to apply a warm compress using plain tap water. The big difference, Dr. Laule says, is eyebright's anti-inflammatory properties, which help soothe sties more quickly.

She suggests that you put a small handful of dried herb in 1 pint of water in a pot and brew it for 10 minutes. When the mixture has cooled enough so that it won't burn you, soak a clean cloth in it and hold it against your closed eyelid for 5 to 10 minutes. "Be meticulous about using this compress several times a day," Dr. Laule says. "Consistency counts." If you tend to get sties regularly, she recommends using an eyebright compress on a regular basis, such as once a week or so, as a preventive measure.

Echinacea

Take a 325-miligram capsule three or four times a day. Since sties are infections, building up the body's internal defense system may help them heal more quickly, says Dr. Laule. Chalazia that are swollen and inflamed may be infected and could also benefit. Echinacea is one of the best immune-stimulating plants in the herbal arsenal. Take as long as necessary to get rid of the infection.

Garlic

Eat one clove a day. Like echinacea, garlic can help you get over sties or infected chalazia by building up your immune system. "Raw garlic is a potent antibiotic," says Andrew Weil, M.D., director of the program in integrative medicine at the University of Arizona College of Medicine in Tucson and author of *8 Weeks to Optimum Health*. "It has antiviral effects as well." He suggests that you mash the garlic or chop it finely and mix it with food.

For people who don't like the taste of fresh garlic, Dr. Laule recommends tucking a diced clove into a corner of a piece of bread. "Dice the clove finely and then wrap the bread around it, squish it together, and swallow it like a pill," she says. Be careful that you don't make the wad so big that you choke on it.

STOMACHACHES

*I*n the medical textbooks of yesteryear, a stomachache was called dyspepsia. It was kind of a generalized term for a generalized ache. Nowadays, dyspepsia has largely disappeared from medical textbooks as doctors try to identify specific disorders like ulcers or heartburn or irritable bowel problems. As far as modern medicine is concerned, a stomachache doesn't exist.

Too bad they forgot to tell your stomach that.

Since there's a good chance that your stomachache was caused by something you ate or how you ate it (namely, too quickly), one of the first things that you may want to do is get up and take a walk, says Robert Jay Rowen, M.D., a holistic physician at the Complementary Medicine Center in Anchorage, Alaska, and a pioneer in the effort to have alternative medicine recognized in Alaska. There's a reason that so many people go for a walk after dinner—it aids digestion.

Once you get back from your walk, there's a nice handful of herbs that can help out if your tummy is still troubling you.

Ginger

Drink tea as needed. Ginger is a powerful stomach soother, says Dr. Rowen. Pick up the tea at any health food store or well-stocked supermarket and let it steep for about 10 minutes, then sip it slowly.

You can also make tea from fresh ginger. Finely chop or grate 1 teaspoon of the root, put it in a mug, and fill the mug with boiling water. Cover it with a saucer and steep for 10 minutes. Let the tea cool slightly and sip slowly.

In a pinch, you can even make tea from the powdered ginger in your spice rack. (A lot of the volatile oils are missing, though, so use the other methods if possible.) Add $\frac{1}{4}$ to $\frac{1}{2}$ teaspoon of powdered ginger to 1 cup of boiling water, steep for 10 minutes, let it cool, and sip slowly.

Peppermint

Drink tea as needed. Peppermint is great for comforting the stomach, says James S. Sensenig, N.D., distinguished visiting professor at the University of Bridgeport College of Naturopathic Medicine in Connecticut and founding president of the American

Cause: Stomachaches are often caused by stress, eating too much or too quickly, or even a lack of exercise. They are by-products of a too-busy, too-rushed life.

Incidence: Almost everyone is susceptible to a stomachache once in a while. Only those with the most cast-iron of stomachs escape the pangs of dyspepsia.

When to see the doctor: If you chronically suffer from stomachaches that last for more than 3 days or you don't get relief from home remedies, have yourself checked by a physician. You could have a condition such as an ulcer. And remember, aches are just that—achy. If you have stabbing pains, it's something else. Call your doctor.

Association of Naturopathic Physicians. "Mint has a very relaxing effect on the gut because it stops muscle spasms in the digestive tract," he says.

Pick up some real peppermint tea at a health food store or grocery store. Check the label to be sure it contains real peppermint, not just peppermint flavoring, and make it according to package instructions. For tea from fresh leaves, add 1 cup of boiling water to $\frac{1}{4}$ to $\frac{1}{2}$ cup of leaves, steep for 10 minutes, and strain out the herb. Sip it slowly after it cools slightly.

Aloe

Take 1 to 3 teaspoons of juice daily. Taking a small amount of aloe juice every day can be very soothing to the stomach, says Dr. Rowen. Be sure to buy fresh aloe juice, not the kind made from concentrate, he recommends, since the concentrate contains fewer active ingredients. Refrigerate the juice after opening. There are also aloe gel products available at health food stores. (Check the label to be sure you're getting gel that's meant for internal use.) Follow the dosage instructions on the label. Be careful not to exceed the recommended dose of juice or gel, as aloe can be a powerful laxative at too high a dose.

Cabbage

Drink the juice as needed. Cabbage juice and/or sauerkraut is an old-time remedy for stomachaches, says Dr. Rowen. Old-time though it may be, there's no time like the present to put it to work. Sip some juice or eat some sauerkraut until you start to feel better.

Chamomile

Drink up to three cups of tea daily. Chamomile tea is a great all-around soother, says Dr. Sensenig. Since many stomachaches are caused by a hurried meal tossed on top of a stressed stomach, chamomile can help slow things down.

Pick up the tea at a health food store or well-stocked grocery store and steep for about 5 minutes. Drink it before you eat if you want a nice, relaxing way to start your meals, or have it afterward if you're feeling the pangs of a stomachache.

STRAINS AND SPRAINS

*I*n his fight for justice, Plastic Man—that malleable superhero of cartoon and comic book fame—could stretch and bend his way through any precarious situation. Whether squeezing through a crack in the door or reaching three stories above his head, flexibility was his weapon as he helped rid the world of supervillains.

Mere mortals that we are, our bodies erupt in pain when they encounter unexpected twists and turns. A sudden pull on a muscle or ligament can injure and inflame real flesh and bone. We end up hobbled by pain.

Herbal Sprain Soother

This warming homemade liniment promotes circulation and helps heal strains, sprains, and bruises. "After you put it on, you're going to feel better," says Phoebe Reeve, a professional member of the American Herbalists Guild and an herbalist in Winchester, Virginia. She is a big fan of using everyday herbs to make home remedies.

The vitamin E in this formula helps keep the oil from oxidizing and going rancid. You can apply this mixture to sore areas as often as needed, either warmed or at room temperature.

> 4 ounces safflower or canola oil (or any other fresh vegetable oil)
>
> 2 tablespoons dried peppermint leaves or 4 tablespoons fresh, chopped
>
> 2" piece fresh ginger, coarsely chopped
>
> 8–10 cloves
>
> 1 capsule vitamin E

Put the vegetable oil, peppermint, ginger, cloves, and the liquid from the vitamin E capsule in a wide-mouth glass jar and shake to mix. Place the jar on a sunny windowsill or in a warm, dry place for 7 to 10 days to let the herbs infuse the oil. Shake the jar now and then. Then strain, rebottle, and keep refrigerated.

If you want to speed the process, heat the vegetable oil over low heat, then add the peppermint and ginger and simmer very gently for 20 minutes to 1 hour. Let cool before adding the vitamin E, then strain, rebottle, and refrigerate.

While lactic acid, a muscle waste product that builds up after exercise, commonly takes the rap for achy muscles, your body purges this acid quickly, within an hour. The feeling that starts a day or two after strenuous activity is caused by tiny tears in the muscle that become inflamed as your body attempts to heal. Fitness experts call it delayed-onset muscle soreness, says Andrew J. Cole, M.D., assistant clinical professor in the department of physical medicine and rehabilitation at the University of Washington in Seattle and medical director of the Spine Center at Overlake Hospital in Bellevue, Washington. One way to avoid it is to be sure to include warmups and cooldowns with strenuous workouts.

When you overstretch or tear a ligament—the ropy tissue that connects bone to bone or a joint capsule—it causes a sprain. Pain and swelling in the joint are normally the first symptoms, says Dr. Cole. In some cases, you may not be able to move the affected limb. The skin and muscles around the joint may also become swollen and bruised. A strain involves stretching or tearing of a muscle and tendons and also causes pain and swelling. Only a doctor can tell you for certain whether you have a sprain or a strain.

To minimize inflammation, rest and apply ice during the first 24 hours, says Jacob Schor, N.D., a naturopathic physician in Denver. After that, you can promote healing by alternating hot and cold treatments on the sore area. The contrasting temperatures work like a pump to increase the flow of blood in the injured area. Improving circulation is one way to help your body heal faster.

"What you want to do is go in there and hose the area out with fresh blood," says Dr. Schor. This actually accomplishes two things: It flushes away tiny fragments of debris and damaged cells, and it brings in oxygen and nutrients to promote healing.

It may take only a few days for sore muscles to feel better, but a more serious injury, like a sprain, can take 4 to 6 weeks to heal. To speed the process and help ease the pain of a sprain or a strain, try these herbal remedies.

Arnica

Rub an ointment, oil, or cream-based formula directly on the affected area three times a day. "Arnica is the best first-aid to speed healing of sprains," says Gayle Eversole, Ph.D., a certified nurse practitioner and a professional member of the American Herbalists Guild in Everett, Washington.

The healing powers of this potent anti-trauma herb come from its ability to stimulate peripheral blood flow when applied externally. Germany's Commission E, which evaluates herbs for safety and effectiveness, has approved the topical use of arnica for its pain relieving, anti-inflammatory, and antiseptic properties.

If the pain or related problems, such as unresolved swelling, redness, or heat, continue after the first 3 days, discontinue use and see your health-care provider.

Bromelain

Take 500 milligrams in capsule form 1 hour after meals three or four times a day until the injury heals. One of nature's best antidotes for a speedy recovery is bromelain, an enzyme derived from the pineapple plant. "If I've spent the day skiing, and I know my muscles are going to be sore from overexertion, I take bromelain before I get sore and for about 3 days afterward," says Dr. Schor.

Because its enzyme activity breaks down protein, bromelain helps you digest food when you take it with meals. When you take it on an empty stomach, however, it scarfs up the cellular debris generated by the inflamed tissue like the cleanup crew after an all-night party. The result? You heal faster. In a classic study conducted with 74 boxers, most of the group who took bromelain healed twice as fast from their injuries as those who didn't take it.

Researchers know that bromelain improves circulation, a key factor in speeding the healing process. But the enzyme also seems to offer pain relief. In clinical trials, people who took bromelain also reported that they had less pain.

The labeling on a bottle of bromelain capsules can be confusing, though, says Jacqueline Jacques, N.D., a naturopathic physician in Portland, Oregon, who specializes in pain management. Bromelain strength is standardized in measurements called milk-clotting units (mcu) or gelatin-dissolving units (gdu), which literally means how much of the enzyme is needed to curdle milk or dissolve gelatin. Since 1,200 gdu equal roughly 2,000 mcu per gram, Dr. Jacques recommends looking for a product with a strength between 1,200 and 2,400 mcu or 720 and 1,440 gdu.

Dr. Schor advises patients to avoid bromelain supplements that don't list the strength on the label. It could mean one of two things, he explains. Either the product is so weak that the manufacturer doesn't want you to know it, or the company simply doesn't know what it's doing. In either case, avoid products that are not clearly labeled. It's safe to take bromelain for long periods of time.

Turmeric

Take 1,000 to 1,600 milligrams of extract a day, divided into three or four doses, for as long as needed for inflammation. Like bromelain, turmeric helps to break down the tiny bits of protein that circulate in damaged tissue. "It has a very strong antioxidant effect and may be useful in many chronic health conditions," says Dr. Schor.

The chemical at work in turmeric is curcumin, which is found in small amounts in the dried, yellow orange spice. While you can use 1 or 2 tablespoons a day of the spice in food or stirred into juice to ease inflammation, the most practical way to take advantage of the herb's pain-fighting powers is to take capsules of standardized concentrated turmeric extract.

Combining bromelain and turmeric is one of Dr. Schor's favorite remedies in natural medicine. He usually suggests taking them in a 1:1 ratio, that is, 400 milligrams of bromelain and 400 milligrams of standardized turmeric extract three times a day.

Your body can absorb turmeric better when you take it with bromelain, since the latter is a digestive enzyme, says Dr. Schor. To get these nutrients from foods, consider combining fresh pineapple juice, a little turmeric powder, and fresh grated ginger.

Lavender, Peppermint, and Rosemary

Massage a blend of 4 drops of each essential oil and ½ ounce of safflower oil into the injured area as needed. This make-it-yourself mixture of oils will help relieve inflammation and pain and relax muscles, says Dr. Jacques. To help your skin better absorb the healing properties of the oil, you can warm it first.

Cause: Activities such as heavy lifting, repetitive and prolonged use of a limb, or a sudden pull or twist can cause a strain or sprain. Tiny tears in the muscle or ligament inflame the surrounding tissue, causing pain and swelling.

Incidence: Virtually everyone will suffer a muscle strain or sprain at some point in their lives. Athletic folks are more vulnerable to these injuries because of how often they use or overuse their muscles. For less active people, jarring their muscles with a sudden burst of activity makes strains and sprains more likely. Body parts heading up the most-likely-to-be-injured list are ankles, backs, fingers, knees, and wrists.

When to see the doctor: In most cases, strains and sprains heal on their own, but if you notice increasing pain, swelling, weakness, or instability, consult a physician.

When you buy lavender essential oil, make sure that it is labeled as *Lavendula officinalis* or *L. angustifolia*. Some manufacturers don't use the actual plant but rather reproduce the aroma from a chemical formula. The two may smell the same, but they don't produce the same effects in your body.

One way to test for the real thing, says Dr. Jacques, is to put a drop of oil on a piece of heavy construction paper and let it evaporate for a few minutes. Because essential oils are volatile, they tend to evaporate quickly and don't leave an oily ring. If the oil you're testing does leave a ring, it may have been made with a vegetable oil.

Comfrey

Apply a compress soaked in a strong decoction four times a day until you're better. Comfrey is a powerful healing agent for sprains, strains, and even broken bones when applied externally, says Dr. Eversole. Also known as knitbone, the herb contains a substance called allantoin, which stimulates connective tissue growth.

A decoction is simply a strong tea made from the root of the plant. To prepare it, make a double-strength tea by bringing 1 cup of water and 2 teaspoons of dried root to a boil, then simmering for 20 minutes. Let the tea cool somewhat, then dip a clean white cloth or unbleached muslin in the warm liquid. Wrap the wet cloth around the strain or sprain bandage-style. Don't apply the compress to broken skin or open wounds, however, since comfrey's ability to knit tissue together can close a wound prematurely, says Dr. Eversole.

Although there are some safety concerns about using comfrey internally, Commission E has approved its use externally to treat pulled muscles and sprains. It should not be used more than 4 to 6 weeks per year.

STRESS

*B*ack in medieval times, life was stressful, what with all those feudal lords bossing people around and no Saturdays off. Fortunately, the monks who doubled as doctors back then knew how to treat stress—they had tense patients rest on beds of chamomile, an herb known for its soothing scent.

Modern-day studies confirm what those monks figured out centuries ago—chamomile and other herbs are effective tension relievers. And it's lucky for us, because our day and age is plenty stressful, too.

With no stress at all, life would be hopelessly boring. But too much stress is also bad. It undermines not only your sense of well-being but your health, too, lowering your immunity and raising your risk of heart disease.

While herbs can help when you're overstressed, they're only part of the solution. To ease out from under, you also need to whittle down the list of stressors in your life. If you're stressed because you're always overbooking yourself to run errands, contact people, or attend extra meetings, for instance, you need to set priorities and cut back on the nonessential stuff. At the same time, you have to make sure that you get enough sleep and cut back on stimulants like caffeine, says George Milowe, M.D., a holistic physician in Saratoga Springs, New York. You should also get some stress-relieving exercise, practice stress-management techniques such as meditation, and try one or more of the following herbal remedies whenever you would like to combat stress.

Chamomile

Drink one cup of tea three times daily and use aromatherapy oil. Calming and exceptionally safe, chamomile is a good choice for stressed-out people, says Anne Cowper, a medical herbalist in Morisset, Australia, and a member of the National Herbalists Association of Australia. To brew a calming cup of chamomile tea, stop at a health food store and buy some dried chamomile flowers that are yellow and white, says Cowper. (If they're straw-colored, they're too old.) Add 2 teaspoons of bulk flowers or 1 teaspoon of finely ground flowers to a mug, pour in 8 ounces of boiling water, cover, steep for 15 minutes, and strain.

To give yourself a stress-beating chamomile aromatherapy treatment—almost like the monks used to prescribe—pick up some chamomile essential oil at a health food store. Sprinkle a couple of drops on a tissue and inhale the soothing aroma for 5 minutes, suggests Jane Buckle, R.N., of Hunter, New York, author of *Clinical Aromatherapy in Nursing*.

Valerian, Passionflower, and Skullcap

Take two droppers of mixed tincture in ½ cup of water three times daily. This common herbal combination, found in many health food stores, can help you relax, too, says Dr. Milowe. Passionflower is a popular stress remedy throughout Europe; Romanian shops even

Fast Facts

carry tension-easing passionflower chewing gum. Both skullcap, a member of the mint family, and valerian have been shown to have mild sedative effects as well.

Be sure to dilute this remedy as recommended, since many tinctures contain alcohol that may be hard on your stomach if they are not diluted.

Valerian

Take 150 to 300 milligrams in capsule form twice a day. Valerian is a particularly good choice if stress is keeping you up at night, says Cowper. This is an herb that will help you calm down, doze off, and get a good night's rest so you're more relaxed come morning. The higher dose is especially for insomnia.

Siberian Ginseng

Take 15 drops of tincture daily or 100 to 200 milligrams in capsule form three times a day before meals. Ginseng can also help you stay calm in chronic high-stress situations, says Lise Alshuler, N.D., chair of the botanical medicine department at Bastyr University in Kenmore, Washington.

You can find ginseng in tincture and capsules. Look for a 25:1 tincture. You can also pick up capsules that are standardized to contain 1 percent eleutherosides, suggests Dr. Milowe. It is best to take this remedy for 60 days at a time, then take a rest period of 2 to 3 weeks between courses.

Kava Kava

Take 200 milligrams of root extract in capsule form three times a day or 1 teaspoon of tincture twice daily. A popular stress remedy in Germany, kava contains active ingredients called kavalactones that act like muscle relaxants.

If you buy capsules, look for a product that contains 30 percent kavalactones, says Dr. Alshuler. In a 1:5 tincture form, take no more than 1 teaspoon twice a day, she says. You can take kava as needed during periods of high stress, but you shouldn't take it for long periods of time.

STUFFY NOSE

A stuffy nose isn't an ailment. It's a symptom—usually of an upper respiratory infection such as the common cold or sinusitis, or of an allergy, says Connie Catellani, M.D., medical director of the Miro Center for Integrative Medicine in Evanston, Illinois. But the fact that stuffiness is a symptom doesn't make it any more pleasant to have to breathe through your mouth and pronounce your *n*s like *d*s.

You should try to determine what's causing the stuffiness so you can get at the real culprit, especially if the problem is a recurrent allergy and not an isolated cold, says Dr. Catellani. Then try the following herbal remedies, aimed specifically at your plugged proboscis, no matter what the cause.

Thyme

Do occasional steam inhalations with essential oil. Sniffing thyme-treated steam helps your stuffy nose in lots of ways. First and foremost, it relieves congestion immediately. But thyme is also one of the most antiseptic of herbal essential oils, so it can help overcome whatever infection might be stopping up your nose, says Dr. Catellani.

Add a drop or two of thyme essential oil to a bowl of steaming hot water. Drape a large towel over your head and lower your face no less than 12 inches from the surface of the water to avoid burning yourself. Inhale the fragrant herbal steam for at least 5 minutes. You can repeat the treatment daily.

Sage and Rosemary

Drink ½ cup of this tea blend twice a day. "Astringents like sage and rosemary are very good for cleaning the nose," says Cascade Anderson Geller, an herbal educator and consulting herbal practitioner in Portland, Oregon. Buy sage and rosemary in dried-leaf form at a health food store.

Make an infusion by pouring 1 cup of boiling water over 1 teaspoon of each herb and steep, covered, for 10 minutes or so. That leaf-to-water ratio may not seem strong until you taste the tea; these are bitter and extremely drying herbs.

Fast FACTS

"You're not going to want to drink a lot of it," Geller says, suggesting that you drink a half-cup at a time and limit that dosage to a day or two.

Sage

Douche your nose occasionally with strong tea. Don't use all of your dried sage leaves for the sage-and-rosemary tea, because there's another use for sage that will help unblock your nose faster. It's called a nasal douche, and it consists of nothing more than putting a few drops of strong sage tea up each nostril and letting it run down into your throat.

"It's very soothing and helps dry things up," Geller says. "Do this instead of using an antihistamine. It doesn't work the same way, but the effect is similar."

For a nasal douche, make sage tea that's stronger than one that you'd drink. "Use 1 good heaping tablespoon per cup of water to make a strong infusion," Geller says, then wait for the tea to cool. "It should be a good, pleasant temperature, not too cold and not too hot," she says. Tilt your head back and use an eyedropper to put just a few drops into each nostril, then sniff. Use the nasal sage drops for occasional relief, but not for more than a day or two.

Chamomile

Douche your nose regularly with tea. Chamomile is a great nasal douche, and you can use it this way for the duration of your stuffy nose problems.

Make the chamomile tea very strong. Use at least 2 tablespoons of dried chamomile flowers and steep for 15 to 20 minutes. "If you want to use tea bags, that's fine," Dr. Catellani says, "but use just ½ cup of water and really squeeze the bag to get all the good stuff out of it."

Try putting a couple of drops of the cooled tea up your nose, she says. If you can't tilt your head back far enough to make sure the drops run into your throat instead of dribbling back out of your nostrils, try it lying down. It may be helpful to wrap a towel around you, especially when you try this for the first time, says Dr. Catellani.

SUNBURN

*M*ost of us know the dangers of too much sun. Age spots and wrinkles are at the benign end of the spectrum. Skin cancer, which affects about a million Americans each year, is at the other, scarier, end. Nevertheless, the appeal of sun-kissed skin endures for many.

The sneaky thing about a sunburn is that you probably won't notice it while you're lying on the beach. It takes 2 to 4 hours for skin damaged by the sun's ultraviolet rays to heat up and turn that attractive shade of beet red. What's more, it takes a full 24 hours for the redness, pain, and swelling to reach their peak.

Obviously, it's best to try to avoid a sunburn. Slathering on sunscreen with an SPF of at least 15, wearing dark-colored fabrics with

Mindy Green's Sunburn Spray

The next time the sun gets the better of you, try this soothing spray, courtesy of Mindy Green, a founder and professional member of the American Herbalists Guild, director of educational services at the Herb Research Foundation in Boulder, Colorado, and co-author of Aromatherapy: A Complete Guide to the Healing Art. *She says that the ingredients will promote new cell growth and healing while reducing inflammation.*

Refrigerate the sunburn spray to make it extra soothing and cooling, says Green, and be sure to shake the bottle vigorously before use. Otherwise, the lavender essential oil and vitamin E will separate from the juice. It is okay to spray your face, but avoid contact with your eyes.

50 drops (½ teaspoon) lavender essential oil
4 ounces aloe juice
1 teaspoon vitamin E oil
1 teaspoon vinegar

Combine the lavender, aloe, vitamin E, and vinegar in a spray bottle. If you plan to store the spray for any length of time, make half of the recipe in a 2-ounce bottle and store it in the refrigerator for up to 4 months.

---

tight weaves, and avoiding the sun whenever your shadow is shorter than you are (between about 10:00 A.M. and 3:00 P.M.) are all wise moves.

If the sun has gotten the better of you, the best thing is to keep your cool, says William Dvorine, M.D., former chief of dermatology at St. Agnes Hospital in Baltimore and author of *A Dermatologist's Guide to Home Skin Treatment.* "If the sunburn is limited to a leg or an arm, you can try cold compresses. If it's the entire torso, you're better off soaking in a cold tub." Either way, there are herbs that can also help take the burn away. Take your pick.

Aloe

Dab on some gel. You've seen it on the drugstore shelf right next to the sunscreen, and maybe you've wondered, "Does this stuff really work?" An emphatic "yes" is the answer from Eric A. Weiss, M.D., assistant professor and associate director of emergency medicine at Stanford University Medical Center and founder of Adventure Medical Kits, an Oakland, California–based company that makes first-aid kits that include both conventional and herbal remedies.

"It's great for sunburn," he says, "because the pain of a sunburn is produced through the release of substances called prostaglandins, and aloe counteracts those substances, thereby reducing the pain. It also facilitates healing of the sunburn."

When buying aloe gel, take the advice of Earl Mindell, R.Ph., Ph.D., a pharmacist and nutrition professor at Pacific Western University in Los Angeles and author of *Earl Mindell's Herb Bible*. Read the label, he says. "It should say 98 to 100 percent aloe vera. If it doesn't say that, don't buy it. You want it as pure as possible."

Prickly Pear

Slice a piece of cactus and lay it on the burn. The gel inside the leaf of a prickly pear (also known as Nopal cactus) works a lot like aloe, says Connie Catellani, M.D., medical director of the Miro Center for Integrative Medicine in Evanston, Illinois. Cut the leaves in half and press the pulpy flesh of the cactus against the sunburned areas.

Prickly pears are available in some supermarkets, but they're more often found in Spanish-American grocery stores, where they are called by their Spanish name, *Nopalitos*.

Black Tea and Peppermint

Brew a pot of tea, let it cool, add peppermint oil, and spray it on. The ingredients in this remedy couldn't be easier to find, and they

Fast FACTS

Cause: A sunburn is the visible evidence that your skin cells have been damaged by ultraviolet light. Prolonged exposure to the sun can also cause long-term problems that build up over the years, such as sagging skin, wrinkles, and even skin cancer.

Incidence: Most of us have stayed out in the sun longer than we should at least once. People with fair skin tend to burn easily and are twice as likely as their olive-skinned friends to develop the skin cancer known as melanoma. Having red or blond hair, blue or green eyes, and freckles also puts you in a higher risk category. Geography plays a role as well. States or regions closer to the equator receive more of the sun's damaging rays than more northern areas.

When to see the doctor: If you experience a severe reaction marked by extreme tenderness, pain, swelling, and blistering, often accompanied by fever, chills, nausea, and delirium, within 12 hours of overexposure, see a doctor.

---

make a fabulous sunburn soother, says Dr. Catellani. Just brew a pot of black tea and set it aside to cool. Pour the tea through a strainer into a spray bottle. Then, for every 4 ounces of tea, add 4 drops of peppermint oil. Shake the bottle well and spray the blend on your sunburn as often as needed.

The astringent tannins in the tea will help calm down your inflamed skin, and the peppermint oil adds cooling, healing properties. One drawback of this remedy, however, is that black tea may stain your clothes, says Dr. Catellani.

Because you should avoid spraying this solution near your eyes, Dr. Dvorine suggests using tea bags for a sunburn on the delicate tissue of the eyelids. Soak the tea bags first in ice water, then use them as compresses.

Comfrey

Make a root decoction and apply as a compress. To make the decoction, place 1 ounce of dried comfrey root, available in health food stores, in a saucepan, add 1 pint of water, and bring to a boil. Simmer for 20 minutes, then remove from the heat. Cool the liquid in the refrigerator and strain.

If you've burned just your nose or hands or other small area of your body, soak small cotton pads in the decoction, says Dr. Catellani. Wring them out and lay them over the burned areas. If your whole back or torso is lobster-hued, use a washcloth. Don't use comfrey on badly burned skin with broken blisters, she says.

Potato

Cover your sunburn with a smashed-potato poultice. If you slice a potato in half and slide it over a kitchen counter, the juice will dry and leave a white coating. Put that same substance on your skin, and it's almost like a natural bandage, says Dr. Catellani.

Potatoes have been part of folk-remedy lore for centuries, and although it's not clear exactly why they work, Dr. Catellani believes that complex carbohydrates, vitamins, and trace minerals contribute to their healing properties.

You can either cut a potato in half and smooth it over your sunburn or apply thinly sliced pieces or coarsely grated shreds as a poultice.

SURGERY RECOVERY

Like an impending IRS audit, the prospect of having to undergo surgery evokes a feeling of dread among even the most stout-hearted of souls.

After it's all over, you may feel perfectly fine or completely drained. It all depends on what type of surgery you've had, your general state of health, and whether the operation went as expected. Don't be surprised or disappointed if you feel less than 100 percent, says Robert Rountree, M.D., a holistic physician at the Helios Health Center in Boulder, Colorado.

In the hours and days following surgery, you may experience sluggishness, nausea, an increase in abdominal gas, or pain at the site of the incision. Long before you feel up to it, your doctor will encourage you to get up and move around. Even if you're a little weak-kneed, walking around the bed or other short distances stimulates your circulation and discourages the formation of blood clots, explains Dr. Rountree. Movement also helps you to breathe deeply to avoid contracting a case of pneumonia.

Sometimes, you just need to put your faith in modern technology, but that doesn't mean that you have to abandon natural measures. After you've had surgery, herbs can play a helpful role when it comes to healing. Herbalists treat surgery as a wound-healing situation, says Alan Tillotson, a professional member of the American Herbalists Guild and a medical herbalist at the Chrysalis Natural Medicine Clinic in Wilmington, Delaware. The herbs recommended here will help control the pain and inflammation that often follow surgery as well as promote healing of the incision.

San Qi Ginseng

Take two 500-milligram capsules twice a day for 3 to 4 weeks. This Chinese herb, which you can find in health food stores and some Asian grocery stores, can help speed healing, says Dr. Rountree.

According to Chinese herbal medicine texts, san qi has an unusual ability to simultaneously reduce bleeding and promote circulation. Herbalists also use it to treat internal bleeding of almost any kind.

Animal studies indicate that after it helps stop the bleeding, the herb may work to help your body absorb the clot and rebuild the capillaries at the incision site. The result? You'll have less swelling and pain, says Tillotson, who has seen these effects in his clinical practice.

Tillotson suggests looking for san qi that comes from the Yunnan province in China, which is known for being of the best quality.

Grape Seed

Take one 100-milligram capsule of standardized extract twice a day for 2 to 4 weeks following surgery. The wound created by the surgical incision will heal more quickly if you take grape seed extract, says Dr. Rountree. Naturally occurring flavonoids in grape seed strengthen and repair connective tissue, including that of the cardiovascular system. They also help control inflammation.

Gotu Kola

To speed up the repair process, take four 500-milligram capsules or 60 drops of extract twice a day for 3 weeks following surgery. Gotu kola helps your skin build a bridge to close the wound sooner, says Tillotson. Used since ancient times in Indian medicine as a revitalizing herbal remedy, gotu kola has gained popularity in Western medicine for its ability to heal skin and help repair connective tissue.

"Gotu kola seems to regulate fibroblasts, the cells that enhance wound healing," says Dr. Rountree. "What's more important is that it may also improve the quality of healing so there is less scarring."

Bromelain

To help control inflammation, take two 500-milligram tablets three times a day at least 30 minutes before meals for 2 to 3 weeks. After the anesthetic wears off, your body's first-aid team goes to work flooding the injured area with blood to bring in repair supplies.

"The swelling created by the increased fluid can cause secondary damage that interferes with wound healing," says Dr. Rountree. Bromelain, a protein-digesting enzyme derived from the pineapple plant, reduces swelling and helps your body break down the proteins that cause inflammation. "If you keep the swelling down, you're going to heal faster," he says.

When taken with food, bromelain's protein-digesting action goes to work on the contents of your stomach, not your wound, so be sure to take it on an empty stomach.

Labeling for this enzyme can be confusing, says Dr. Rountree. That's because bromelain strength is standardized in measurements called milk-clotting units (mcu) or gelatin-dissolving units (gdu), which indicate how much of the enzyme it takes to curdle milk or dissolve gelatin. He recommends looking for products standardized to either 2,400 mcu or 1,600 gdu per gram. They're about the same strength.

Boswellia

To ease pain and inflammation naturally, take 400 milligrams one to three times a day for 2 to 4 weeks after surgery. An extract from the frankincense tree can help reduce pain, swelling, and discomfort almost as well as ibuprofen, says Dr. Rountree.

Grown on the dry hills of India, the bark of this fragrant tree provides an aromatic gum resin that is used to make a standardized extract. Research suggests that phytochemicals in the bark, called boswellic acids, interrupt the inflammation process early on and keep our bodies from producing the chemicals that cause pain, says C. Leigh Broadhurst, Ph.D., an herbal researcher and nutrition consultant based in Clovery, Maryland.

Turmeric

To relieve pain and inflammation, take six to eight 500-milligram capsules of extract a day for 2 to 3 weeks. Curcumin, the powerful anti-inflammatory substance in turmeric, isn't a drug, but it can act like one, says Dr. Broadhurst. Research shows that the active substance in this Indian spice reduces postoperative inflammation. The problem is, your body has a hard time absorbing it. Turmeric me-

Fast Facts

Cause: Although surgery is ultimately meant to help heal the body, cutting through skin and muscle causes deep-tissue trauma that can make the cure feel worse than the condition. Knowing what to expect helps. As your body works to regenerate tissue, it is typical to experience some pain, swelling, and inflammation. Recovery times will vary depending on the type of procedure and your age, nutritional status, and general state of health.

Incidence: More than 46 million people undergo some type of surgery each year. In the United States, the most frequently performed procedure is cataract surgery.

When to see the doctor: Whether you're in the hospital for a week or go to your doctor's office for a simple outpatient procedure, your doctor will undoubtedly send you home with a set of detailed instructions. Contact him if you experience fever, shortness of breath, nausea to the point of vomiting, severe constipation or persistent diarrhea, painful urination, increased bleeding, or pain, especially in the calves of your legs, all of which are signs of possible complications during the recovery period.

tabolizes so quickly in the liver and intestine that blood levels of curcumin remain low. To enhance absorption, take 5 milligrams of a standardized piperine extract each time you take the turmeric. An alkaloid derived from black pepper, piperine increased bioavailability of this anti-inflammatory herb by 2,000 percent in one clinical trial.

Aloe

Once the wound has closed completely, apply fresh gel twice a day until all of the inflammation is gone. Coating the closed incision with aloe will speed healing, explains Dr. Rountree. Extensive research since the 1930s has shown that the clear gel has a dramatic ability to heal wounds. This action is due in part to a substance in the plant called aloectin B, which stimulates the immune system.

"For healing power, it's hard to beat the fresh plant," says Dr. Rountree, but if you don't have one, look for a product that is at least 90 percent pure aloe vera.

SWIMMER'S EAR

*Y*ou have to hand it to bacteria: They're resourceful little buggers, and they'll take up residence in just about any cozy spot they can get into. When there are bacteria in water and you go swimming in it, your ear might as well have a big sign on it that says "Open House."

You'll know you have a case of swimmer's ear because the infected ear will hurt, often a lot, says William Warnock, N.D., director of the Champlain Center for Natural Medicine in Shelburne, Vermont. Because it's an infection of what doctors call the outer ear—meaning the part of the ear on this side of the eardrum—someone looking into your ear probably will be able to see that it's red and swollen. Sometimes the ear will give off a watery discharge as well.

Swimmer's ear tends to go away with home treatment within 48 hours or so, says Richard Barrett, N.D., who teaches eye, ear, nose, and throat medicine at the National College of Naturopathic Medicine in Portland, Oregon. But there are steps you can take to hasten its departure.

The first step, Dr. Barrett says, is to rinse the infected ear (or ears, if both are infected) with a 50/50 mixture of warm water and hydrogen peroxide, using a bulb syringe. Wrap a towel around your neck and tilt your head toward the shoulder opposite the infected ear. Squirt some of the solution into your ear, then wait about 5 seconds before lifting your head upright.

Fast FACTS

Cause: Swimmer's ear is a bacterial infection of the ear canal.
Incidence: This problem occurs most often in people who have been swimming in pools, lakes, or the ocean during warm weather, because bacteria flourish in warmer water.
When to see the doctor: If symptoms become worse or don't clear up within 48 hours, let your physician know. If the pain in your ear increases and then suddenly lets up, or if you notice any discharge, that's also a cue to see your doctor.

The hydrogen peroxide wash serves to clean out the infected discharge and other bacterial "gunk," Dr. Barrett says. At that point, you can enhance the healing process with the following herbal remedies. Use them until your symptoms subside and then for 2 more days to make sure that the infection is completely gone.

Garlic

Use garlic oil eardrops twice a day. Garlic kills bacteria, thus making garlic oil an excellent weapon to enlist in your battle against bacterial infections like swimmer's ear. You can buy garlic oil ready-made in health food stores, but it's not hard to make your own at home, says Dr. Warnock.

"Grate two large cloves or three medium gloves of garlic and put them in a shallow dish or cup," he says. "Cover them with olive oil and let the mixture stand overnight. Strain out the pieces of garlic, and you've got garlic oil." He recommends putting 3 drops in the infected ear (or ears). "Let it stay for about 5 minutes so it really coats the ear canal," he says.

Calendula, Garlic, and Mullein

Use eardrops made from oil extracts of these three herbs every 2 to 3 hours. You can buy herbal eardrops in health food stores that may contain slightly different ingredients, but you don't need to be a master herbalist to mix up this simple recipe at home, according to Connie Catellani, M.D., medical director of the Miro Center for Integrative Medicine in Evanston, Illinois.

Calendula and mullein will both work to soothe the irritated tissues of your infected ear, Dr. Catellani says, while the garlic will help fight the growth of bacteria. Look for extractions of each herb in an olive oil base. Mix them in equal parts, lie down on your side, and put 4 to 6 drops of the mixture in the infected ear. Lie in the same position for 5 minutes to give the drops a chance to soak into the infected tissues.

Apple Cider Vinegar

To avoid getting swimmer's ear, use vinegar eardrops regularly after swimming. Apple cider vinegar diluted in water can be the ounce of prevention that will keep the bacteria you encounter while swimming from gaining a foothold in your ear, says Dr. Barrett. That's because the vinegar is acidic, and bacteria won't take up residence in an acidic ear environment. Simply dilute a small amount of vinegar with an equal amount of distilled water and use 1 drop in each ear after swimming. The mixture should stay fresh for about a week.

TICK BITES

*T*icks don't fly or jump. They only crawl. Mammals crawl—or walk or run or gallop—much faster than ticks do. So how do these blood-sucking parasites get hooked up with their hosts? They lie in wait, hanging out on the tip of a grass blade or the edge of a leaf until an unsuspecting victim happens to brush by.

Getting a good meal may be of paramount importance to a tick, but chances are that you won't even be aware of the feast. Most ticks are tiny—often no bigger than a pinhead—and their bite is usually painless. So why worry?

"You can develop three problems from a tick bite," says Eric A. Weiss, M.D., assistant professor and associate director of emergency medicine at Stanford University Medical Center and founder of Adventure Medical Kits, an Oakland, California–based company that makes first-aid kits that include both conventional and herbal remedies. "One is a local wound infection caused by a tick bite allowing bacteria that live on the skin to enter the wound. The second thing is tick paralysis, temporary paralysis caused by a tick bite, which is cured by simply removing the tick. The third is tickborne diseases."

Lyme disease and Rocky Mountain spotted fever are probably the best-known of the tickborne diseases, and they can cause all sorts of problems, from fatigue to joint swelling. Other diseases—such as ehrlichiosis and babesiosis—are on the rise, too. When you consider that the numbers of deer (the tick's favorite host) in the United States have shot up from an estimated 500,000 in 1900 to 30 million today, it's not surprising that reported cases of tickborne diseases have increased dramatically, too.

Before you decide to never again venture into the wilds of nature, take comfort in the fact that not all ticks carry disease, and even those that do may not make you sick. A lot depends on how long the tick remains on your body. The longer the critter is attached, the greater your chance of becoming infected. That's why it's so important to remove a tick as soon as you notice it. Grasp it on the head with tweezers as close as possible to your skin and, in one gradual upward movement, pull it out, says Dr. Weiss. Be careful not to squeeze the body of the tick, as that may cause it to push body fluid into the wound and spread the infection. Don't mess around with petroleum jelly, fingernail polish, rubbing alcohol, or hot matches. They don't work and can be dangerous.

If you receive a diagnosis of Lyme disease or other tickborne illness, you'll almost certainly be put on a course of antibiotics. Meanwhile, herbal poultices and immune-boosting herbs can help.

Plantain, St. John's Wort, Oregon Grape, Comfrey, and Lavender

Make an herbal salve and apply it to the bite as soon as possible. If you live in a tick-infested area, it makes sense to be prepared. Make up a batch of this drawing salve and apply it as soon as you think you've been bitten to help draw out the infected saliva, advises Cathryn Flanagan, N.D., a naturopathic physician in Old Saybrook, Connecticut.

To make the salve, place ¼ cup each of dried plantain, St. John's wort flowers, Oregon grape root, and comfrey in a slow cooker and cover with olive oil. Let the oil warm over very low heat, checking to be sure that it doesn't burn, for 1 to 6 hours. You'll know it's ready when the oil has picked up some of the color from the herbs.

Remove the herbs from the oil by carefully straining the mixture through a piece of cheesecloth, gently squeeze the remaining oil from the herbs, and discard the herbs. For every cup of oil, add 1 ounce of grated beeswax and stir until melted. Put the salve into a wide-mouth jar, add a couple of drops of lavender essential oil or vitamin E oil to keep it from spoiling, and let it cool. You can store the salve in a cool, dark place for up to a year.

Potato

Apply raw potato to the bite as a poultice. If nothing else is handy, Dr. Flanagan suggests making a simple, drawing poultice by grating a potato and adding just enough flour to hold it together. Apply the poultice to the bite and tape it in place.

Cat's Claw

Take two 500-milligram capsules three times a day. "*Uña de gato*, or cat's claw, which comes from the stem and root of an Amazonian vine, is a really great herb for helping the immune system," says Whitney Miller, N.D., a naturopathic doctor who has a family prac-

Fast FACTS

Cause: There are 82 species of ticks found in the United States, and between them, they cause nine major diseases, including Lyme disease. Ticks bite because they are hungry, not because they want to make you sick.

Incidence: The most common tickborne disease is Lyme disease, with about 7,000 cases reported each year. The highest incidence has been in Connecticut (where the disease was discovered in 1975), New Jersey, Maryland, Pennsylvania, and New York. Rocky Mountain spotted fever, human granulocytic ehrlichiosis, and babesiosis are less common, but they appear to be on the rise. Prime tick season in the United States occurs from late April through September.

When to see the doctor: If you are bitten by a tick and are unable to remove it, or you have removed the beast but its head remains attached, call your doctor. You should also consult a doctor if you think that you've been bitten by a deer tick or if you have been bitten while in an area where Lyme disease is known to occur. If you develop flu-like symptoms and the telltale circular rash that radiates from the bite site like a bull's-eye, see a doctor; you could have Lyme disease.

---

tice in New London and Colchester, Connecticut. Look for a standardized extract of the herb that contains 3 percent oxindole alkaloids, and try to find a brand that is grown in South America rather than the United States, she says. Some people believe that cat's claw grown south of the equator, where it is a native plant, may have better medicinal properties.

Tea Tree

Soak an adhesive strip bandage in oil and apply it over the bite. Even if the tick that bit you wasn't carrying a disease, you still run the risk of getting a localized infection around the bite. Dr. Miller, whose Connecticut practice is in the middle of prime tick country, says that when people don't successfully remove the whole tick, there's a high risk of the bite becoming infected. She's found this to be particularly common with bites from large brown wood ticks.

Using tea tree oil on an adhesive bandage can help fend off infection. You may keep the same bandage on all day, but change it if it gets wet. Put a freshly soaked bandage on the bite daily until it has healed.

Dandelion

If you have been diagnosed with Lyme disease and experience swelling, drink a cup of tea three times a day. Dr. Miller often sees Lyme disease patients with severe swelling. "It tends to be in the lower limbs," she says. "Sometimes, it's so bad that their shoes don't fit." For those patients, she prescribes dandelion tea, which acts as a diuretic.

To make the tea, pour 1 cup of boiling water over 1 tablespoon of dried dandelion leaf, steep for 10 minutes, and strain. Keep drinking the tea until the swelling subsides.

TINNITUS

*I*n an era of amplifiers, airplanes, and leaf blowers, ringing in the ears, medically known as tinnitus, is a malady that you hear a lot about.

Different people with tinnitus hear different sorts of sounds, ranging from a low roar to a high squeal or whine, in one or both ears. For some people, the ringing can be continuous, while for others, it comes and goes. The effect ranges from annoying to maddening.

Lots of things can cause tinnitus, but the most common is damage to the nerve endings in the inner ear. The deterioration is usually prompted by age or noise, says Thomas J. Balkany, M.D., chair of the

Fast FACTS

Cause: Prolonged exposure to loud noise and deterioration of nerves in the inner ear due to aging are the most common causes, although tinnitus may also be caused by allergies, high or low blood pressure, and certain medications, such as aspirin. Tumors, problems with blood circulation, diabetes, thyroid problems, and drug reactions can also be responsible.

Incidence: Some 36 million Americans have some form of tinnitus, according to the American Academy of Otolaryngology–Head and Neck Surgery; more than 7 million have severe cases.

When to see the doctor: If you have persistent ringing, if the ringing is worsening, or if hearing loss worsens, see an ear, nose, and throat (ENT) specialist for an auditory evaluation.

hearing and equilibrium committee of the American Academy of Otolaryngology–Head and Neck Surgery. Often, it's a combination. People who are exposed to loud noise for long periods of time—rock musicians and factory workers are the classic examples—are especially susceptible.

"The key is the duration and loudness of the exposure," says Dr. Balkany. "Many of us have left rock concerts with our ears ringing. By the next day, the ringing usually stops. It's when you have that sort of exposure time and time again that the ears lose their ability to recover."

To help manage your tinnitus, there are lifestyle changes that you can make, says Dr. Balkany. Decrease the amount of salt you use and cut down on coffee, tea, cola, and tobacco, which can overstimulate the auditory nerve endings and make the problem worse. Exercise daily to improve your circulation. Try to work in relaxation exercises, and make sure you get enough rest. Herbal remedies may also help.

Ginkgo

Take 180 milligrams of standardized extract a day. Ginkgo can help reduce tinnitus symptoms in two ways, says William Warnock, N.D., director of the Champlain Center for Natural Medicine in

Shelburne, Vermont. First, it improves blood circulation to the tiny capillaries of the ear, thereby helping the tissues there flourish. Second, it actually works to repair damaged nerve cells. "Exactly how that happens isn't certain," he says, "but ginkgo can definitely help prevent an increase in the ringing and can sometimes actually reduce it."

Buy an extract that has 24 percent ginkgoflavoglycosides, Dr. Warnock suggests. He recommends taking a 60-milligram capsule three times a day on an empty stomach, although two 90-milligram capsules a day, morning and night, would also be fine. Ginkgo is a slow-acting herb, so you will need to take it for at least 6 months. You can take it indefinitely, but Dr. Warnock suggests that three times a year, you take a break from it for 1 week.

Bilberry

Take a 40-milligram capsule of standardized extract or 40 drops of tincture in ¼ cup of water four times a day. Like ginkgo, bilberry promotes circulation in the tiny capillaries of the ears, says Dr. Barrett. It also stimulates the growth of new connective tissues. That makes it an ideal tonic for the intricate mechanisms of the inner ear. Tincture of bilberry is as effective as capsules, he adds. Use it until your symptoms subside.

TOOTHACHE

A toothache hurts so much that it's almost the universal symbol of excruciating pain. Just think of the poor, downcast comic strip character with a rag tied around his face and little lines of pain shooting out from his jaw. If you're that character, the last thing you want to hear about is what you could have done to prevent it. You want it to stop hurting, and you want it to stop hurting *right now*. Herbs can give you that relief.

"There are lots of herbs that work as pain relievers," says Flora Parsa Stay, D.D.S., a dentist in Oxnard, California, and author of *The Complete Book of Dental Remedies*. "You still have to deal with whatever's causing it by going to a dentist, but in the meantime, you can deal with the pain herbally."

A great thing about herbal remedies for toothache pain is that most of them work by being applied directly to your aching tooth. Some are essential oils of common herbs that you usually apply with cotton. It's important to remember, though, that all essential oils are potentially toxic and should never be ingested. Other remedies are strong teas that you use as rinses, either cold or warm, whichever seems to work best for you. "As long as the herb soaks into the tooth, it will help," Dr. Stay says.

Remember, though, that the following herbal remedies are for temporary pain relief while you arrange to see a dental professional as soon as possible. None are for long-term use, but if your tooth is aching, it's precisely short-term relief you want. These herbs will deliver it.

Clove

Apply oil as needed for pain relief. Clove is as useful around your mouth as it is in the kitchen. For toothache relief, it has no peer among herbs, says Dr. Stay.

The little clove balls that you keep in your spice cabinet are actually the dried flower buds of a tropical evergreen. Those same buds yield a volatile essential oil with remarkable medicinal properties, including a mild local anesthetic. For your toothache, buy that essential oil in a little vial at a health food store. "Then take a cotton swab, saturate it with 1 drop of the oil, and apply it directly to the tooth," says Dr. Stay.

White Willow

Use tea as a mouthwash several times a day as needed. Aspirin can work for toothache pain, but dentists warn against applying crushed aspirin directly to an aching tooth; it can burn the gums and damage enamel. Neither of those problems can occur with white willow, the "natural aspirin" that's been used as an analgesic for thousands of years.

The bark of the willow contains the same salicin constituents that are synthesized to make aspirin. To exploit this natural wonder for pain relief, Dr. Stay recommends decocting a strong tea by simmering 1 tablespoon of the bark (bought cut and sifted at a health food store) in 1 cup of water for 30 minutes. After you strain it and let it cool to room temperature, use the liquid to rinse your mouth thoroughly, giving it a good chance to soak into the problem tooth before spitting it out.

Peppermint

Rinse sore gums as needed for pain relief. A nice bonus with herbal toothache remedies is that they can be pretty darn good-tasting. You can steep 1 teaspoon of dried peppermint leaves in 1 cup of boiling water for about 20 minutes. Let it cool and use as a mouthwash once a day. Peppermint is an age-old folk remedy that's good for a lot of things, but we tend to associate it with our teeth since it's a common flavoring in toothpastes and breath fresheners.

Marjoram

Drink one or more cups of tea a day as needed. An alternate route to toothache relief is to actually drink certain herbal teas rather than just swishing an extra-strong version around in your mouth. One tea that Dr. Stay recommends is marjoram, a kitchen herb that can relieve toothache pain (as well as the headache that sometimes accompanies it).

Buy the dried herb at a health food store. Steep 1 full tablespoon in 1 cup of hot water to make a strong but drinkable tea. "Drink it while it's comfortably hot," Dr. Stay advises.

Fast FACTS

Cause: Cavities or oral infections such as periodontitis are the most common causes of toothaches. Sometimes, a toothache is a temporary reaction to certain dental work, and it can even be a symptom of some non-dental conditions, such as angina.

Incidence: Virtually everyone experiences some kind of tooth pain at some point in their lives. People who don't visit their dentists regularly, don't brush frequently, and don't floss every day have a much higher incidence of the problems that lead to toothaches.

When to see the doctor: Any toothache is a sign that you need a checkup to determine the source of the problem. Swelling of the face or jaw may indicate infection, so see a dentist immediately.

Hops

Drink one or more cups of tea a day as needed. Hops is a pain reliever with the added benefit of promoting sleep and relaxation, which are welcome side effects for anyone with a toothache. Yes, this is the same hops used in breweries, but—as you've surely guessed—Dr. Stay insists that hot hops tea is a better bet than Budweiser.

Look for the dried fruits at a health food store, and make an infusion by steeping 1 tablespoon of the herb for 10 minutes or more in 1 cup of water. Strain, drink, and relax.

Aloe and Clove

Apply salve to your tooth as needed. Often, your tooth aches because it's cracked. If you know that to be the case, Dr. Stay suggests a little salve made of aloe gel, baking soda, and clove essential oil as your best pain-relieving strategy. Aloe gel is what comes right out of the thick leaves of this juicy succulent, so the best way to obtain it is to get a plant, break open a leaf, and help yourself.

Dr. Stay recommends that you mix about ¼ teaspoon of the gel with enough baking soda to make a thick paste. Add a drop or two of clove oil and soak a little cotton in the mixture. "Wedge the paste-covered cotton right into the hole or crack and leave it there until you get to the dentist," she says.

TOOTH GRINDING

*E*ver get the impression that stress seems to be responsible for more than its fair share of maladies? Well, add another one to the list. Nervous tension, anger, frustration—name your source of stress, and it can lead to what the dental profession calls bruxism, the Bible calls the gnashing of teeth, and the rest of us call tooth grinding.

If you're a bruxer (as tooth grinders are called in medical parlance), you're probably converting your stress into dental problems by grinding your teeth, clenching your jaw, or biting down hard for no good reason. You're usually not conscious of your habit. In fact, many people grind their teeth while they're asleep. All this wasted effort can result in damaged teeth, an aching jaw, and other facial pain.

Herbs offer the advantage of not only helping with your stress relief but also easing the soreness that so often accompanies tooth grinding. Here are some home herbal remedies recommended by Flora Parsa Stay, D.D.S., a dentist in Oxnard, California, and author of *The Complete Book of Dental Remedies*.

Comfrey

Use an herbal compress on your jaw once a day. Comfrey's one of those all-around healing herbs that have been used internally for centuries. For tooth grinders, though, it has a special function. "If you soak a washcloth in warm comfrey tea and use it as a compress, it will ease tension and relieve pain in your jaw," Dr. Stay says.

That should be music to any bruxer's ears, because jaw pain is one of the more common and bothersome effects of tooth grinding. This is an herbal remedy that goes straight to the problem, since you put your comfrey-soaked cloth right on your jaw and hold it there to let the herb medicine soak in and the pain melt away.

You can buy cut or powdered root or even dried leaves loose at well-stocked health food stores. It doesn't matter which form you use, since you won't be drinking the "tea." "Make it nice and strong, with $\frac{1}{4}$ cup of herb for each cup of water," Dr. Stay says. "Simmer it for 30 minutes to get the full effect." Strain out the herb and let the liquid cool a little, but soak your washcloth in it while it's still warm. Settle back and press the cloth to the outside of whichever jaw hurts (it's usually just one side, Dr. Stay says) for at least several minutes.

Comfrey can cause liver problems in high or prolonged doses, Dr. Stay warns. Don't drink this extra-strong tea for bruxism, and limit your daily compress treatment to a few weeks at most.

Arnica

Rub ointment into your jaw once daily. The flowers of this mountain-growing plant have a circulation-stimulating effect that helps rid your aching jaw muscles of toxins accumulated from all that grinding. Arnica in tea or tincture form is sometimes used as a digestive aid or fever fighter, but the best and safest route for bruxers is to use it topically, Dr. Stay says. In other words, rub it right into your jaw.

"Arnica comes in oils, lotions, creams, and ointments," Dr. Stay says. "Those are the best forms that I recommend to relieve pain and muscle tension. Just use your fingers and rub the arnica on your jawline and face," she says. "It's very important to

Fast FACTS

Cause: Sometimes, tooth grinding is an unconscious attempt to correct a physical problem in your mouth—an ill-fitting filling, a misaligned bite, or a missing tooth. More often, it's a reaction to stress, nervous tension, or suppressed anger.

Incidence: In our stressful times, bruxism is no rarity. About one in three people suffers from it, with a higher prevalence among women. Aggressive and competitive types may be at higher risk.

When to see the doctor: Herbal remedies can ease pain while they enhance professional dental treatment for bruxism, but they shouldn't replace it. If you're waking up in the morning with jaw pain or believe that you are grinding your teeth, see your dentist.

---

massage your jaw muscles as you do it. That really helps the soothing effect."

Skullcap

Drink two cups of tea a day. Knowing that stress and nervous tension have been causing humans to grind their teeth throughout time may not make you feel any better about your own grinding. A couple of cups a day of skullcap tea just might.

"People who are bruxing are usually high-stress people," points out Dr. Stay. "Skullcap is very good for anxiety. It has a calming effect and also relieves spasms and cramps."

The dried skullcap that you find at health food stores may be the whole herb, although it's really the leaves that yield the stress relief you're looking for. Either way, make your tea with 1 tablespoon of skullcap in 1 cup of water. Dr. Stay recommends letting the water simmer over very low heat (with the herb in it, of course) for 30 minutes, so you may want to start with a tad more water to yield a drinkable tea after allowing for evaporation.

"Drink a cup in the morning and one every night at bedtime," she says. "Do this for 21 to 30 days, because it takes at least that long to break a habit."

Black Cohosh, Cayenne, and Skullcap

Drink two cups of this tea blend daily. Here's a daily tea recommended by Dr. Stay that comes at your tooth-grinding problem from three different directions. You'll be using a root (black cohosh), a leaf (skullcap), and a powder made from dried fruit (cayenne).

The skullcap, of course, is a useful herbal component of your stress-relief campaign. Helping it along is the black cohosh, a common herb for menstrual problems whose cramp-soothing properties address your jaw pain. Cayenne is a circulation stimulator, helping to rid your aching jaw muscles of toxins.

The popularity of black cohosh makes it easy to find at health food stores. Look for dried, cut root. Put 1 teaspoon of it, along with a teaspoon of dried skullcap leaves (or whole herb), into a little more than 1 cup of boiling water. Cayenne is hot stuff, so Dr. Stay suggests that you add considerably less of it than the other herbs, perhaps ¼ teaspoon. Simmer for 30 minutes and strain. Drink a cup in the morning and one in the evening. Continue at that pace for about a month. Stay within the recommended tea strength, because too much black cohosh can lead to nausea and vomiting, according to Dr. Stay.

TYPE A PERSONALITY

*Y*ou can suspect that something's amiss in a culture in which the same personality traits that make for success are also a prescription for an early death.

That's the way it is with Type A personalities. Identified and named in the 1970s by two cardiologists, Meyer Friedman and Ray Rosenman, the characteristics of the Type A personality are by now famous, or infamous: hard-driving, impatient, highly competitive, deadline-oriented people with a tendency toward hostility. According to Bill Roedel, Ph.D., chair of the psychology department at Bastyr University in Kenmore, Washington, if you combine a profile like this with a lack of attention to things such as diet, exercise, and rest, you're asking for trouble—heart trouble in particular.

It's easy to say that Type A personalities should simply stop being Type A personalities, but that's neither realistic nor necessary, says C. Leigh Broadhurst, Ph.D., an herbal researcher and nutrition consultant based in Clovery, Maryland. "People who have that kind of personality simply operate that way," she says. "What appears to be stressful to other people is not at all stressful to them. The problem is that they often don't take care of themselves. There's nothing wrong with burning the candle, but don't burn it at both ends. Type A personalities are fully capable of a higher output than other people, but they need quality input." Part of that quality input, she says, consists of daily, high-quality supplements of antioxidants and B vitamins.

Learning to meditate when you have the chance so that you can truly relax and come in contact with your quiet centers would be tops on the list of psychiatrist James Gordon, M.D., director of the Mind/Body Center in Washington, D.C., and author of *Manifesto for a New Medicine*. Physical exercise would be next. "You need to get all that energy moving in a productive way, as opposed to just sitting and steaming with it," he says.

One way to accomplish both goals is to exercise meditatively by doing yoga, suggests Thomas Kruzel, N.D., former president of the American Association of Naturopathic Physicians, who practices in Portland, Oregon. That's a step toward addressing what he sees as the real underlying problem that often leads Type A personalities to the brink of breakdown: a lack of physical, psychic, and spiritual balance.

Restoring that balance requires a holistic treatment program that addresses all three of those areas. Herbs can't do it all, but they can definitely help.

Asian Ginseng

Take 75 to 150 milligrams of extract twice a day with meals. If restoring balance is the issue, ginseng is the herb, says Timothy Birdsall, N.D., director of naturopathic medicine at Midwestern Regional Medical Center in Zion, Illinois. Herbalists call it an adaptogen because it helps the body adapt to a wide variety of stresses in the environment. Type A personalities are typically immersed in stress.

Dr. Birdsall recommends buying an extract of Asian ginseng (also called panax, Chinese, or Korean ginseng) extract with 10 to 30 percent ginsenosides. Siberian ginseng is also an effective adaptogen, he says. Look for capsules that contain 0.8 percent eleutherosides; the dosage is the same as for the Asian type. He suggests starting with the lower dosage, then increasing it after 3 to 4 weeks if necessary and continuing for about 6 to 12 months to see the best results.

Schisandra

Take 400 to 600 milligrams of extract three or four times a day. Schisandra is another adaptogenic herb from China, but it's somewhat more aggressive than ginseng, according to Dr. Broadhurst, who recommends it often to her athlete clients. It helps the body deal with stress by enhancing its use of glucose, she says, and it helps the liver flush toxins from the bloodstream. It also improves the efficiency of respiration and is an antioxidant.

The dosage above is recommended to help carry you through times of high stress. If you prefer a more concentrated extract, look for one that has 200 to 300 milligrams of standardized extract. Once you're back to a more routine schedule, you can cut back to two doses a day on an ongoing basis, Dr. Broadhurst says. Tincture forms of schisandra are widely available, she adds, as are combination formulations that contain schisandra. Either option is fine, she feels. Follow the instructions on the label.

Garlic

Eat two cloves a day or take a 500-milligram capsule three times a day. Besides being an excellent tonic for the immune system, says Dr. Broadhurst, garlic can help protect Type A personalities from one of their principal enemies: heart attack. Type A personalities tend to have high levels of epinephrine (adrenaline) in their systems, she

Fast FACTS

Cause: Why some people develop Type A personalities is unknown, but some combination of genetic predisposition, learned behaviors, and environment is considered likely.

Incidence: Once considered primarily a male phenomenon, recent research has shown that women are as likely as men to be Type A's. Ages generally range from the twenties to the forties. Type A behaviors are more likely to emerge in high-pressure work situations that reward competitiveness and quick results.

When to see the doctor: If you're having trouble controlling your emotions, particularly rage, see a therapist or psychologist.

says, which increases the thickness of the blood. That makes heart attacks more likely. Garlic helps keep the blood thin, thereby lowering blood pressure and reducing the likelihood of abnormal blood clots.

Romaine Lettuce and Nutmeg

Brew a soothing broth of romaine lettuce seasoned with ¼ teaspoon of nutmeg. "This is an old gypsy remedy," says Dr. Gordon. "Take a head of romaine, chop it finely, and boil it in 3 pints of water until it's reduced to 1½ pints. Drink one cup three times a day when needed. It's calming; you should feel the effects within 30 minutes or so. It's a smooth-muscle relaxant. Also, just the act of making the broth takes time, and that slows you down more. Make the broth meditatively."

Adding the dash of nutmeg provides an additional mellowing effect, he says. "Nutmeg in small doses is a tranquilizer. In very large doses, it causes psychic disturbances, including hallucinations, so don't overdo it."

Valerian

Take 300 milligrams in capsule form at bedtime. Type A personalities often don't get enough sleep, Dr. Birdsall says, because they're too wound up to relax. Valerian can help. "Valerian has a calming effect on the receptors that stimulate action in the central nervous system," he says.

Combinations of relaxation-inducing herbs actually work best, he has found, and health food stores sell many of them. Look for capsules that have about 100 milligrams of hops and 100 milligrams of passionflower added to the valerian. "You can go back for a couple of hundred years and find herbalists recommending combinations very similar to this," he says.

Skullcap

Drink a cup of tea at bedtime, or take two to four 250-milligram capsules twice a day with meals. Another herb that's long been known for its sedative qualities is skullcap. To make the tea, simply pour hot water over a wire tea ball filled with 1 to 2 teaspoons of dried herb and steep for 5 minutes. Add lemon and honey if you prefer. You should see results within 7 to 10 days. While skullcap can be used safely for a considerable period of time, Dr. Kruzel says that it's always best to take a rest period of 1 to 2 weeks when you use an herb long-term.

ULCERS

*F*or actor Lorne Greene, ulcers were no bonanza. Indirectly, the disease killed him.

Greene, perhaps best-known for his role as the widower Ben Cartwright on the television show *Bonanza*, was hospitalized in 1987 for surgery on a perforated ulcer. He developed pneumonia and never recovered. Sadly for fans of the popular actor, doctors didn't know then what they know now.

In the year Greene died, no one had ever heard of *Helicobacter pylori*. It wasn't until several years later that Australian doctors found the bacteria in the stomach lining of many people with peptic ulcers and were able to identify it as the cause of the ulcers. Until then, it was believed that ulcers were caused by stress and poor diet.

Antibiotics that target *H. pylori* have changed the way doctors tackle ulcers and in the process, have saved lives and allowed many more people to go through their days without the burning, stabbing pain that marks this disorder.

Nevertheless, says Mark J. S. Miller, Ph.D., professor of pediatrics and physiology at Albany Medical College in New York, as helpful as antibiotics have been in the fight against ulcers, they aren't a cure-all. *H. pylori* is becoming increasingly resistant to some of the antibiotics used to treat it. And, even if antibiotics do work, you can still be reinfected.

What's more, for 30 percent of the people with peptic ulcers, the bacteria aren't the cause. For them, ulcers are more likely to be associated with chronic use of caustic nonsteroidal anti-inflammatory drugs, such as aspirin, that they take for other conditions such as headaches, says Dr. Miller.

That's where herbs can help. There is a goodly number of plants that battle ulcers on multiple fronts. Some are antibacterial, going after *H. pylori* itself. Others are anti-inflammatory, calming the ravaged tissues in your stomach. Still others are soothing, helping your damaged stomach lining heal itself. Here's where to start.

Cat's Claw

Take 300 milligrams in capsule form twice a day with meals. Also known as *uña de gato*, cat's claw has been at the center of some highly promising laboratory research, says Dr. Miller. He should know, since he and a colleague are conducting it at Albany Medical College.

A climbing vine from South America, cat's claw has been used for hundreds, if not thousands, of years in the Peruvian Amazon to treat a wide variety of ailments. But you don't have to voyage to the steamy tropics to get the benefits. They're as close as a well-stocked health food store.

Anti-Ulcer Fruit Cocktail

In his book The Green Pharmacy, *James A. Duke, Ph.D., an herbalist and ethnobotanist in Fulton, Maryland, gives a delicious home remedy for ulcer disease. Every ingredient in this fruit/herb cocktail contains large amounts of soothing, anti-ulcer compounds. (Try to be especially generous with the ginger, since it has 11 anti-ulcer compounds concentrated in one humble spice.) If only all medicine tasted like this!*

Bananas
Pineapple
Blueberries
Ground cinnamon
Ground ginger
Ground cloves
Honey (optional)

Cut up the bananas and pineapple; the amounts and proportions will vary according to the number of servings and which fruits you like best. Put them in a serving bowl and add the blueberries. Season to taste with the spices and sweeten with the honey (if using).

Cat's claw works in a number of ways against ulcers. First, it is a powerful anti-inflammatory that calms the ulcerated tissue itself by preventing the immune system's attack on the stomach lining. Its second action relates to the development of stomach cancer down the road. Although it's not well-known, stomach cancer is one of the top cancer killers in the world. Research suggests that cat's claw actually inhibits the toxic effects of compounds that are thought to be involved in gene mutations in the stomach that can lead to cancer.

To get the benefits of cat's claw, you need to know how it's manufactured. The dosage above is for cat's claw that's been atomized, or ground exceptionally fine. If the herb has only been pulverized, a less-refined form, you'll need to increase the dosage to 1,500 milligrams twice daily with meals. The reason for this is that fewer of the active compounds are digested with the cruder form, says Dr. Miller. The best form is freeze-dried, in which 3,000 milligrams of micropulverized cat's claw is concentrated into a single 90-milligram tablet, he says.

To tell which form you have, check the label or break open a capsule and pour the powdered herb into a glass of water. If most of it settles to the bottom without dissolving, it was pulverized, and you should take the higher dose, says Dr. Miller.

Garlic

Eat two cloves a day. Garlic has strong antibiotic properties, says James S. Sensenig, N.D., distinguished visiting professor at the University of Bridgeport College of Naturopathic Medicine in Connecticut and founding president of the American Association of Naturopathic Physicians. Research bears this out.

Scientists at the Fred Hutchinson Cancer Research Center in Seattle exposed *H. pylori* to garlic and found that the herb consistently knocked the bug dead. And unlike its reaction to antibiotics, the bacteria showed no ability to become resistant to garlic.

Now for the taste. Eating raw garlic isn't a pleasant experience for most people. It's hot and it's strong. No problem; mash or crush the cloves as smoothly as you can, then spread the paste on dry toast or crackers. "That masks the strong taste. It's actually pretty good," says Dr. Sensenig.

German Chamomile

Slowly drink one cup of tea three or four times daily. German chamomile is one of the best-known and most versatile medicinal plants, says Varro E. Tyler, Ph.D., Sc.D., distinguished professor emeritus of pharmacognosy at Purdue University in West Lafayette, Indiana, and co-author of *Tyler's Honest Herbal*. And so it is for ulcer disease.

It's believed that chamomile's healing properties come from three sources—volatile oils, which are anti-inflammatory; flavonoids, which are antispasmodic; and mucilages, which soothe irritation of the mucous membrane in the stomach.

Fast FACTS

Cause: Peptic ulcers have two main causes. The first, and most common, is infection with *Helicobacter pylori* bacteria. This infection can result in an open sore, or ulcer, developing on the stomach wall or in the duodenum (the first part of the small intestine that's connected to the stomach).

The other cause is long-term use of nonsteroidal anti-inflammatory drugs such as aspirin. Over time, these caustic drugs can lay waste to the stomach lining.

Incidence: *H. pylori* infects a lot of people. In developing countries, about 80 percent of the population harbors the bug. In countries like the United States, it's about 30 percent. Still, not everyone who's infected develops ulcers, and doctors don't know why. Stress, smoking, and food allergies may play a role.

When to see the doctor: If home remedies don't work within 2 weeks, and you have sustained abdominal pain and burning, have a doctor check you out. Ulcers can turn into stomach cancer in some cases. If you experience abdominal pain or chronic indigestion during or after meals, see your doctor immediately.

To make a tea from chamomile flowers, buy some of the dried herb. Cover 1 teaspoon with 1 cup of hot water and steep for 5 to 10 minutes, then let it cool slightly.

Licorice

Chew one or two DGL lozenges four to six times daily, or take one or two 400-milligram capsules before each meal. Licorice contains flavonoids that can reduce the inflammation of an ulcer, says Dr. Sensenig. Deglycyrrhizinated licorice, or DGL, is a modified form of licorice root that contains no glycyrrhizic acid, a compound that can raise blood pressure and deplete potassium stores in the body.

DGL lozenges have no such side effects, and they're a relatively pleasant way to get the medicine to go down. Buy the chewable kind and chew them slowly, holding the compound in your mouth for at least a minute to absorb more of the active ingredients and reap all of its benefits.

Slippery Elm

Take ¼ teaspoon of powder three or four times a day. If you're having a flare-up of symptoms, slippery elm can help you out, says Dr. Sensenig. Consider it nature's antacid.

"It doesn't do much to get at the root of the problem," he explains, "but it can help you out in a pinch." Speaking of pinches, if you weigh more than 150 pounds and the dosage above isn't working, you can add a pinch more slippery elm, up to a total of ½ teaspoon. In either case, mix the powder with a small amount of water or your favorite beverage until it's the consistency of paste. Then slide the slippery elm down the hatch.

UNDERWEIGHT

*O*urs is a culture in which beauty is often a question of thinness. But if you're thin enough to be considered underweight, the main question that needs to be asked is whether your weight is affecting your health.

To be considered underweight, you would have to weigh 10 percent less than the standard weight ranges for your height and frame. Some people are thinner than average and are perfectly healthy that way. For others, underweight may be associated with health problems and put them at risk for illness or malnutrition. If you weigh less than you should, your doctor may advise you to gain a few pounds. If you have a constitution that burns calories like a blast furnace, however, that may be easier said than done.

Generally, healthy weight gain requires a combination of nutrient-rich, energy-dense foods combined with gentle exercise to build lean tissue, says Robert Rountree, M.D., a holistic physician at the Helios Health Center in Boulder, Colorado.

You can reasonably expect to gain about 1 pound a week, which means eating 500 more calories a day than you burn, says Dr. Rountree. To do this, pick the highest-calorie items from each food group. Have a milk shake instead of skim milk or a whole-wheat muffin instead of a slice of whole-wheat bread. Make sure that you eat at least three meals a day, with snacks in between.

Most people who are underweight eat small portions, so you need to force yourself to eat larger ones, advises Dr. Rountree. The herbs discussed here can help stimulate your appetite and aid digestion so that you can achieve a healthy weight.

Bromelain

Take two 500-milligram capsules between meals two or three times a day. Bromelain, an enzyme derived from the pineapple plant, helps your body digest protein, so you absorb calories and nutrients more readily, says Alan Tillotson, a professional member of the American Herbalists Guild and a medical herbalist at the Chrysalis Natural Medicine Clinic in Wilmington, Delaware.

Sold in health food stores, bromelain is standardized by a measurement called milk-clotting units (mcu), which simply indicates how much of the enzyme is needed to curdle milk. Look for capsules with a strength of at least 600 mcu, advises Tillotson. Bromelain can be used for as long as needed to aid weight gain.

Ashwaganda

Drink ½ teaspoon of powdered leaves mixed with ¼ cup of milk four times a day. Called Indian ginseng because it is used in Ayurvedic medicine in the same vitality-boosting way that Asian ginseng is used in Chinese medicine, ashwaganda works as an overall tonic. "It will help restore a sense of calm," Tillotson notes. "It's a very nourishing and nutrifying herb, so you also tend to gain weight when you take it." You can take it for as long as necessary to gain weight. If you are

Fast FACTS

Cause: Unexplained weight loss can result from digestive problems, particularly as you age, or from intestinal disorders such as Crohn's disease, ulcerative colitis, or diverticulitis. Chronic illnesses, including type 1 (non-insulin-dependent) diabetes, or hyperthyroidism can lead to underweight. So can surgery, stress, or emotional trauma. Underweight can also be caused by treatments such as chemotherapy and radiation therapy, whose side effects include nausea, vomiting, and loss of appetite.

Incidence: No more than 10 percent of adults in the United States are underweight.

When to see the doctor: Sudden weight loss that cannot be explained by a change in diet or physical activity should be evaluated by your physician.

---

chronically underweight due to stress and overwork, he recommends incorporating ashwaganda root into your daily diet.

Cardamom

Mix ¼ teaspoon into applesauce for flavor. One of the world's oldest spices, cardamom has been used throughout history to relieve digestive problems. Eaten daily, this aromatic, tasty spice works as a warming digestive stimulant to improve a poor appetite.

"This is a good herb for someone who has weak digestion and is averse to food," says Tillotson. You can pick up a jar of cardamom in the spice aisle of the grocery store and take it for as long as needed.

Gentian

Take 2 to 5 drops of tincture in water 20 to 30 minutes before meals until appetite is restored. Gentian contains possibly the most bitter substance on the planet—amarogentin, which can still be tasted even when diluted at 1 part per 50,000. The bitter constituents stimulate saliva and gastric juice secretion, says Dr. Rountree. This in turn improves appetite and digestive function, which can help you absorb more nutrients from your food. "This herb is more likely to be effective in older people, who tend to have a decrease in gastric secretions," says Dr. Rountree. Gentian can be taken safely for a month.

Flaxseed

Take 1 to 2 tablespoons of oil every day. With 115 calories per tablespoon, flaxseed oil provides a healthy concentration of calories that won't be converted into fat, says Dr. Rountree. Contrary to popular belief, the body does need fat, especially the bodies of people who are underweight. Rich in essential fatty acids, flaxseed oil promotes strong bones, nails, and teeth as well as healthy skin. Every living cell in the body needs essential fatty acids for rebuilding and producing new cells.

Fresh, high-quality flaxseed oil has a pleasant, nutty flavor. Stir it into a glass of orange juice in the morning, add it to yogurt, or drizzle it over vegetables. Dr. Rountree also recommends eating freshly ground flaxseed, which some people find more palatable.

URINARY TRACT INFECTIONS

*W*hen it comes to measurements, men always seem to get hung up on issues of length. But where urinary tract infections (UTIs) are concerned, women should be a little worried about length, too.

Thanks to a cruel twist of anatomy, women get UTIs 25 percent more often than men do. That's because the male urethra is several inches long, while the female urethra is barely an inch, giving infection-causing bacteria a short, easy trip to the bladder.

Who says size doesn't matter?

As they wend their short way up the urinary tract, those bacteria multiply in the moist, dark environment. By the time they make their presence known, you already have the classic symptoms of a full-blown UTI—burning, pain, and urgency.

That's why drinking eight 8-ounce glasses of water every day is the best medicine to prevent UTIs, says Connie Catellani, M.D., medical director of the Miro Center for Integrative Medicine in Evanston, Illinois. Those regular trips to the bathroom help flush the bad guys out before they have a chance to reach their destination. Also, once you have an infection, a steady flow of fluids will help wash it away sooner, she says.

Infections generally occur in the lower urinary tract, which means the bladder and urethra. To prevent the bacteria from traveling farther up the tract to the kidneys, your doctor may prescribe an antibiotic. The herbs listed here can complement conventional treatment by soothing spasms, easing burning, and helping to get the bacteria and debris cleaned out of your urinary tract more quickly.

Goldenrod

Drink three to four cups a day of gentle, stimulating diuretic tea to help relieve pain and burning. "Goldenrod is the number one urinary herb in Europe," says Ed Smith, a professional member of the American Herbalists Guild (AHG) and founder of Herb Pharm in Williams, Oregon. A tea made from the yellow flowering tops of this perennial herb is an ultra-safe, mildly astringent antiseptic to promote healing of inflammation in the urinary tract. Steep 1 well-rounded teaspoon in 1 cup of hot water for 5 to 10 minutes, then strain. Drink the tea until your symptoms are gone.

Pipsissewa

To wash away bacteria and relieve pain and itching, drink this tea three times a day. By increasing urine flow, pipsissewa stimulates the removal of waste products from the body. The herb contains substances called hydroquinones, which have a disinfectant effect on the urinary tract.

"If you wanted to dye a white tablecloth, you'd wash it first so that the color is absorbed evenly," says Smith. This herb works in a similar way to clean debris from the kidneys and urinary tract so that other healing agents can be absorbed more effectively.

Pipsissewa is gentler than uva-ursi, its sister plant that is often used to treat inflammation of the urinary tract, and almost never causes adverse reactions. Steep 1 teaspoon of dried leaves in 1 cup of hot water for 10 to 15 minutes, then strain. Drink the tea until your infection is gone.

Marshmallow

One to three times a day, drink a solution of 1 teaspoon of root powder soaked in 1 cup of cold water overnight. Marshmallow makes a thick, rather slimy tea that works as a demulcent to soothe irritation in the urinary tract, says Lynn Newman, a professional member of the AHG and a medical herbalist in Glen Head, New York.

Both the leaves and root contain mucilagen, the substance in the plant that makes it slimy. The root, which contains about 35 percent mucilagen, is generally available in the United States. Marshmallow is particularly useful for older adults who have chronic inflammation of the urinary tract. Take this remedy for as long as you have the infection.

Corn Silk

Take 3 to 6 milligrams of tincture three times daily, or drink a tea made from 2 teaspoons of the dried herb. A soothing diuretic, corn silk is helpful for any irritation of the urinary system, says Newman. The more trips you make to the bathroom, the more quickly the bacteria are flushed from your system.

Because it must be collected before the seeds begin to form, it is difficult to find good-quality corn silk, Smith explains. Smell is a good way to tell if you're getting a quality product. Corn silk tincture should have the nice aroma of fresh corn on the cob, he says.

- **Cause:** Urinary tract infections are caused by bacteria that enter the bladder by traveling up the urethra. In most cases, the culprits are *Escherichia coli* bacteria. Generally, this passageway from the bladder is protected, but if the opening becomes irritated, bacteria can grow there. Bubble baths and shampoos are common irritants, as is careless wiping after a bowel movement. A rare cause is obstruction of the urinary tract that results in incomplete emptying of the bladder.
- **Incidence:** By the time they're 30, nearly 50 percent of American women have had a urinary tract infection. One in five of them will have recurring infections. For both men and women, the chances of having a UTI increase with age.
- **When to see the doctor:** If you have more than two urinary tract infections (or what you think are urinary tract infections) within 6 months or more than three episodes a year, see a doctor. And always consult a physician if you experience blood in your urine, chills, nausea, vomiting, or back pain with a UTI.

To make tea, steep 2 teaspoons of dried herb in 1 cup of hot water for 10 to 15 minutes in order to get the full benefit. You can take corn silk until the infection is gone.

Cleavers

To help relieve burning in the bladder and urethra, drink a cup of tea three times a day. "Cleavers is *the* urinary herb for fever and infections," says Smith. Tea made from this herb, which is sometimes called goose grass, works as a weak, soothing diuretic. "It's not a super-strong medicine," he says.

If you've ever had to pick burrs off your clothing after a walk in a field, you've come across cleavers. Since the straggling, square-stemmed annual grows prolifically in gardens and along roadsides, it isn't usually cultivated. To capture the healing properties of the plant, the whole flowering herb must be picked when it is just about to flower in the late spring. Smith recommends buying it from a reputable wildcrafter. Use 1 teaspoon of dried cleavers per cup of hot water and steep for 10 to 15 minutes. Drink this tea until your symptoms are gone.

Cranberry or Blueberry

Stop infection before it starts with a daily dose of berries. If you're prone to UTIs, your doctor may have told you to drink at least 10 ounces of cranberry juice cocktail every day to help prevent bacteria from adhering to the walls of the urinary tract. Tired of tart, red juice? Research shows that you can get the same anti-infection protection from a handful of blueberries, a serving of cranberry sauce, or a slice of blueberry pie, says Amy Howell, Ph.D., a researcher for the Blueberry and Cranberry Research Center of Rutgers University in Chatsworth, New Jersey.

Scientists there have identified the healing compounds in the native North American berries. These compounds, which have eluded researchers since the nineteenth century, are proanthocyanidins, condensed tannins that help keep the bacteria from sticking. The bacteria are flushed from the system in the normal urine flow, says Dr. Howell.

VAGINITIS

*I*n healthy women, a certain amount of odorless, clear or white vaginal discharge is considered normal. The actual amount and type (sticky or slippery) depends on where a woman is in her lifetime and her menstrual cycle, as well as whether she's pregnant or on birth control pills.

Fast FACTS

Cause: Inflammation of the vagina can happen for many reasons. Sexually transmitted diseases, bacterial or yeast infections, microscopic tears in delicate vaginal tissue, and the use of spermicides, bubble bath, deodorant sprays, and douches are all among the factors that can lead to the itching and discharge common with vaginitis.

Incidence: Three-quarters of all women will have at least one vaginal infection during their lifetimes. Many, unfortunately, will have repeated infections.

When to see the doctor: If you are experiencing unusual (bloody or foul-smelling) discharge, itching, pain in the lower abdomen, or pain during sex, you should see your doctor for an accurate diagnosis. Proper treatment of vaginitis varies depending on what's causing the irritation.

Vaginitis is the general term for inflammation that causes discharge that is odorous, plentiful, and off-color. It's also the label that's applied any time the vagina and vulva (the outer part of the genitals) begin to burn, itch, and swell.

Relieving the uncomfortable effects of vaginitis begins with a doctor's diagnosis. That's because correct treatment depends on what's causing the problem, says Mercedes Cameron, M.D., family practitioner at The Woman's Place at St. Mary's Hospital in Grand Junction, Colorado. Some common inflammation instigators include yeast or bacterial infections, physical irritation from a diaphragm or tampon, hormone imbalances, and certain sexually transmitted diseases.

After discovering the reason behind the rawness, your doctor may prescribe antibiotic or antimicrobial medication or special douches or baths. While you follow the treatment your doctor recommends, a certain herb can help make the wait for complete relief less worrisome.

Comfrey

Make a batch of double-strength tea and use it topically as needed for 3 to 5 days. An active bout of vaginitis—no matter what the cause—brings burning and stinging. This is especially apparent during trips to the bathroom, when urine makes contact with raw skin. While you are using other treatments or medications to directly address the cause of the problem, the herb called comfrey can be a symptom-relieving comfort, says Virginia Frazer, N.D., a naturopathic physician and licensed midwife in Kennewick, Washington.

Comfrey leaf has anti-inflammatory properties. While it won't cure an infection, rinsing your vaginal area with a tea made from comfrey will soothe inflamed tissues.

Make a double-strength tea using 2 heaping tablespoons of dried comfrey leaf to 1 cup of boiling water. Steep, covered, for 10 minutes, then strain the cooled tea into a plastic spray bottle.

Keep the bottle handy when you visit the bathroom, recommends Dr. Frazer. Spray your nether parts liberally as needed to ease the burning.

VARICOSE VEINS

*A*h, summertime. The flowers are in bloom, the skies are blue, and the beach beckons. Meanwhile, you're rifling through your closet, desperately trying to find something to wear that will keep your legs covered and hide those unsightly blue veins that you'd rather not share with the world at large.

If this tactic sounds familiar, you're one of the millions of Americans who are bothered by varicose veins. More than twice as common in women as in men, varicose veins can be brought on by pregnancy, obesity, prolonged standing, or unlucky genes. Whatever the catalyst, the root cause is the same: misbehaving veins and the valves in them.

A varicose vein happens when valves in a leg vein malfunction or the vein wall becomes weak and can't support the blood as it's pumped back to the heart. When the valves don't close as they should, some of the blood pools in the veins and flows backward due to gravity. Pressure builds up, and the veins begin to stretch and twist. The result? Those knotted, purple veins that make summer—with its almost compulsory uniform of shorts and swimsuits—the least favorite season for many women.

Varicose veins rarely indicate a serious problem, says Howard C. Baron, M.D., associate professor of surgery at the New York University School of Medicine, chief of vascular surgery at the Cabrini Medical Center, both in New York City, and author of *Varicose Veins: A Guide to Prevention and Treatment*. Although your legs may ache by the end of the day, symptoms are often mild or even nonexistent. The veins do tend to become more prominent over time, though, so the sooner you start taking steps to hinder their progress, the better.

The "three E's"—elevation, elastic stockings, and exercise—should be the core of your anti-varicosity program, says Dr. Baron. Whenever you can, sit or lie down with your feet elevated above heart level. Wear fitted elastic stockings. For these, you'll need to see your doctor, who will give you a prescription for the correct size and degree of compression, then you can buy them at a surgical supply store.

Don't ignore exercise such as walking, biking, or swimming, says Dr. Baron. It gets the calf muscles pumping and your blood moving toward your heart. If you are overweight, exercise helps you reduce.

"A lot of people who have jobs where they stand all day don't want to do exercise when they get home," says Sally LaMont, N.D., a naturopathic doctor and licensed acupuncturist in Marin County, California. "They don't do the kind of movement that would allow the muscles in the leg to massage the blood back up."

Diet also plays a key role, says Dr. Baron. Cut down on saturated fats and cholesterol, which can constrict blood vessels and impede blood flow. Also, make sure that you get plenty of fiber in your diet. The more you get, the less likely that you'll have to strain when you move your bowels. Believe it or not, such straining raises pressure in the body, which in turn obstructs the flow of blood up the legs. Eat plenty of vegetables, fruits, legumes, and whole grains, he suggests. And try these herbal remedies to thwart those bothersome veins.

Horse Chestnut

Take 45 drops of tincture three times a day. Mix the tincture with 2 tablespoons of hot water to help it taste better, says Mark Stengler, N.D., a naturopathic doctor in Oceanside, California, and author of *The Natural Physician: Your Health Guide for Common Ailments*. "Let it stand for a couple of minutes so the alcohol evaporates out. Then you can add more water or juice to it." If your veins are inflamed, take this until the swelling goes away. If you have chronic varicose veins, take this dose for 3 months. You can cut the dose in half and take it indefinitely.

Horse chestnut is a varicose vein's worst nightmare. Germany's Commission E, which evaluates herbs for safety and effectiveness, confirms that its principal ingredient, aescin, tightens the veins. "We call it a venotonic," says Dr. Stengler. "That's an herbal substance that increases the contraction of the elastic fibers in the vein wall. Usually, varicose veins have lost their elasticity and are sagging, so it tones them up." It also tones and strengthens the valves, he adds.

One study found that horse chestnut seed extract was as effective as elastic stockings in reducing swelling in the legs of 240 people with vein problems.

Witch Hazel

Dab on this astringent herb with a cotton swab twice a day. Available in liquid form in almost any supermarket or drugstore, witch hazel is one of the most widely available and inexpensive herbs you can buy. Soak a cotton swab in witch hazel water and rub it over varicose veins twice a day, says Dr. Stengler. It acts as an astringent to help tighten vein walls. It's fine to use this remedy for as long as needed.

Butcher's Broom

Take 300 milligrams of extract standardized to 10 percent ruscogenin with breakfast, lunch, and dinner. This shrubby relative of asparagus got its name because the branches were once bound

Fast FACTS

Cause: Experts don't really know why some people get varicose veins and others don't, but obesity, pregnancy, and even tight clothing can aggravate a preexisting tendency for varicose veins. Heredity is the only obvious culprit.

Incidence: Affecting about 15 to 20 percent of Americans, varicose veins occur most often in women over 50. In fact, women are two-and-a-half times more likely than men to have the problem. One study showed that while varicose veins in men seemed to be unrelated to obesity, being overweight was a big risk factor for women.

When to see the doctor: If you have varicose veins and experience shortness of breath or chest pain, see your doctor at once. In severe cases, blood clots form in the vein and can end up lodged in the lung. If your leg is painful, red, swollen, or warm, you should see a doctor; these are symptoms of inflammation in a vein. Also, consult your doctor if the skin around a varicose vein, especially on your ankle, is turning purplish brown and is itchy or flaky; these symptoms could indicate that a varicose ulcer is developing. And if you accidentally cut the skin over a varicose vein, see a physician.

---

into bundles and sold to butchers for sweeping their blocks. The herb is used extensively in Europe for varicose veins and hemorrhoids.

The active ingredient in butcher's broom is ruscogenin, which, says Dr. Stengler, has an anti-inflammatory, vasoconstricting (vein-tightening) effect. You can take this dosage for about 3 months or indefinitely, if you wish.

Bilberry

Take an 80-milligram capsule of extract standardized to 25 percent anthocyanosides three times a day. Also known as huckleberries, these cousins of the blueberry grow on the heaths and moors of Europe and in the western United States. "They help to stabilize the connective tissue around a vein so it's not so lax," says Dr. Stengler. That may help prevent blood from pooling in the vein. Bilberry is safe to take long-term.

Ginger

Brew a tea and drink it three times a day. One of the problems with varicose veins, says Christopher Robbins, a member of Britain's National Institute of Medical Herbalists who practices herbal medicine in Ross-on-Wye, Herefordshire, England, and has written several books, including *The Natural Pharmacy*, is that you tend to get a slowdown in circulation, which can lead to venous ulcers.

His advice: Take herbs such as ginger that stimulate the peripheral circulation. You need a substantial amount, so it's easier to take as a tea rather than just using it in cooking, he says.

To make the tea, grate 1 inch of fresh, unpeeled ginger, pour 1 cup of boiling water over it, and steep for 10 minutes. It's not necessary to strain the tea, since the fiber in the ginger helps maintain regularity. You can also make tea with 1 teaspoon of dried ginger per cup of boiling water.

VERTIGO

*H*itchcock fans everywhere, take note, vertigo is *not* a fear of heights. What Jimmy Stewart experienced as he climbed to the top of that bell tower in one of the suspense master's most riveting movies was, technically speaking, acrophobia. But what kind of movie title would that have made?

Vertigo, which comes from the Latin verb meaning "to turn," is a specific kind of dizziness in which you or everything around you seems to be turning or spinning. Plus, it's more likely to happen when you sit up in bed than when you're perched on a ledge 50 feet above the ground.

Even if it's not the stuff of Hollywood thrillers, it's unnerving when your world starts spinning out of control. It's also extremely common. But it's not a disease, it's a symptom, frequently tipping you off to a problem in the inner ear, the control center of your body's balance system, says Connie Catellani, M.D., medical director of the Miro Center for Integrative Medicine in Evanston, Illinois.

You need to find out what's causing your vertigo before you can determine whether herbs can help alleviate it, says Anne McIntyre, a member of Britain's National Institute of Medical Herbalists and co-owner of the Midsummer Cottage Clinic in Oxfordshire, England.

Once you know what's causing the room to spin, herbs can help by clearing up congestion, increasing blood flow, fighting viral infections, and soothing the inflammation that may be affecting your balance. And they can do it without the side effects of the antihistamines, anti-nausea drugs, or sedatives that doctors often prescribe, says Dr. Catellani.

Herbal remedies for vertigo work best in tandem with diet and lifestyle changes. "I would restrict salt, because it encourages fluid retention," says Andrew Lucking, N.D., a naturopathic doctor in Minneapolis. "And I'd want to check the person's cholesterol and fat intake."

Your doctor may also recommend cutting out nicotine and caffeine, both of which decrease blood flow to the head. Depending on what kind of vertigo you have, you'll also want to try the following herbs.

Ginkgo, Rosemary, Wood Betony, and Cramp Bark

Take 5 milliliters of this tincture blend in 20 milliliters of water three times a day after meals. If you're experiencing vertigo because of impeded blood flow, herbs that stimulate the circulation can be helpful. Germany's Commission E, which evaluates herbs for safety and effectiveness, has endorsed ginkgo as a treatment for vertigo and dizziness, and it's a popular choice with European herbalists. Rosemary and wood betony also stimulate blood flow to the head, says McIntyre, and cramp bark relaxes the arteries, therefore aiding blood flow as well.

Using a child's medicine dropper, measure 25 milliliters of each tincture into an amber bottle, says McIntyre. You can continue taking this for as long as the problem persists.

Ginger and Rosemary

Massage your neck twice a day with a soothing oil. If muscle tension in your neck is impeding blood flow to your head, McIntyre suggests massaging the area with a combination of ginger and rosemary essential oils. Both help loosen tight muscles and speed blood flow. Look for them in your health food store and make your massage oil using 2 drops of each essential oil per 5 milliliters of vegetable oil.

Elder, Peppermint, and Yarrow

Drink this tea frequently throughout the day. If mucus buildup caused by a simple cold is the culprit, it makes sense to use decongestant herbs, says McIntyre. She recommends this traditional English infusion for clearing up congestion. Make it by mixing equal quantities of dried elder flowers, peppermint, and yarrow, then using 1 teaspoon of the mixed herbs for each cup of boiling water. Let stand to infuse in a teapot for 10 to 15 minutes and drink the tea while it's comfortably warm.

Mullein or Garlic

Place 3 drops of either oil in the affected ear (or ears) at bedtime. If there's a buildup of fluid in the inner ear, these eardrops can help draw it out, says Barbara Silbert, N.D., D.C., a naturopathic doctor and chiropractor who is president of the Massachusetts Society of Naturopathic Physicians and has a family practice in Boston and Newbury, Massachusetts.

Cause: The spinning dizziness of vertigo can be a symptom of a number of very different conditions. What they have in common is that they all affect the fragile mechanism of the inner ear, the key to your sense of balance. Specific ailments that can cause vertigo include labyrinthitis (a viral inflammation of the inner ear) and Meniére's disease, a problem in the fluid-filled canals of the inner ear. High blood pressure, high cholesterol, atherosclerosis (hardening of the arteries), and anemia can all result in poor circulation that impedes blood flow to the inner ear, resulting in vertigo. Often, however, it's impossible to determine the cause.

Incidence: It seems the world just won't stay still for a lot of us. Dizziness is the third most frequent reason that people visit their doctors.

When to see the doctor: Play it safe and check with your doctor if you have repeated, severe, or prolonged episodes of vertigo. Special diagnostic tests can pinpoint the cause of your dizziness.

Garlic has antibacterial and anti-inflammatory properties, and mullein is well-known for its soothing action. The eardrops are readily available at health food stores, but try to find drops in a base of glycerin rather than olive oil, says Dr. Silbert, because the osmotic property of the glycerin will help pull the fluid out of your ear.

To administer the drops, warm the bottle by immersing it in hot water, then lie on your side and have a friend or your mate drop the oil into the ear canal. Place a cotton ball in your ear and stay put for at least 5 to 10 minutes to give the drops a chance to find their target. Continue with this treatment until the condition improves.

Eucalyptus and Lemon

Make a steamy mixture with these essential oils and inhale the vapors for 5 minutes twice a day. If congestion is the problem, McIntyre suggests this hot inhalation of eucalyptus and lemon oils. Buy the pure essential oils at a health food store and put 20 drops of each in a large bowl of steaming hot water. Put a towel over your head, lower your face over the bowl, and breathe in the vapors. Be careful not to burn your face by getting too close to the water. Do this until your congestion clears up.

Black Cohosh

Take 3 milliliters of tincture in 4 ounces of water three times daily until the condition improves. If inflammation of the inner or middle ear is the cause of your dizziness, this anti-inflammatory herb can be helpful. "It has a reputation for all sorts of things to do with ears and dizziness," says McIntyre. She also recommends it if your vertigo is the result of high blood pressure or tension in the muscles of your neck. It's an excellent muscle relaxant, and it also has painkilling properties, she says.

Echinacea

Take ¼ teaspoon of tincture every 2 hours. If your vertigo is associated with an acute viral infection like a cold or the flu, Dr. Catellani recommends taking a proactive approach with frequent doses of that antiviral champ, echinacea. Continue taking it for about a week, along with your physician's recommended treatment.

Ginger

Sip tea throughout the day. Fresh ginger makes a sweet and spicy tea that can ease mild vertigo associated with a cold, says Dr. Catellani. Simply grate a ½-inch slice of fresh ginger into 1 to 2 cups of steaming water. Steep for 5 to 10 minutes, strain, and drink. You can drink this tea as often as needed.

People on the go may want to try this trick: Place 1 inch of sliced fresh ginger in a 4-cup thermos, fill it with near-boiling water, seal it, and take it with you to wherever you may be going. The tea is ready in an hour or so, says Dr. Catellani, and you can add more hot water to the same ginger to top off your tea later in the day.

VOMITING

$\mathcal{W}$hen you've eaten a bad clam, contracted a stomach virus, or taken a car trip that seems like an eternal ride on the Roller Coaster of Death, it's usually not a matter of *if* you'll throw up. It's a matter of *when*. And "when" is determined not by your stomach or your prayers but by your brain.

That's right: Your brain makes you vomit. Not your whole brain, just a tiny sliver called, appropriately enough, the vomiting center. A variety of things activate Vomit Central, most often stomach ailments such as infection or food poisoning or middle ear disturbances, which cause motion sickness or dizziness.

What happens next is out of your control. Your windpipe closes. The muscles of your abdominal wall and diaphragm tighten suddenly and forcefully. These sudden spasms make the limp little bag of your stomach eject its contents up and out of your esophagus.

Along with herbal remedies, try the time-honored treatments for nausea and vomiting. For nausea, try clear liquids such as flat soda, nonacidic fruit juices, or ice pops, suggests Bruce Luxon, M.D., associate professor of gastroenterology at St. Louis University Medical Center in Missouri. They may calm your stomach.

If you've passed nausea and progressed to vomiting, stick to clear liquids such as cranberry, grape, or apple juice; fruit-flavored "snack drinks"; gelatin; ice pops; or bullion or clear broth.

When you haven't vomited for 24 hours, you can start eating solid food again, says Dr. Luxon. He suggests small amounts of starchy food, such as crackers, bread, or pasta. If that goes well for 24 hours, you can resume your normal diet, he says. Avoid spicy, fatty, or fried foods, which may start your stomach a-churnin' once again.

Certain herbs can help quell queasiness or treat vomiting. Some are known as anti-emetics, which means that they reduce nausea and help relieve or prevent vomiting, says Ellen Kamhi, R.N., Ph.D., a professional member of the American Herbalists Guild (AHG), an herbalist in Oyster Bay, New York, and author of *The Natural Medicine Chest*. Others are antispasmodic herbs—that is, they ease or prevent spasms of the smooth muscles lining the gastrointestinal tract.

German Chamomile

Drink one cup of tea as needed. "The species name for German chamomile, *Matricaria recutita*, means 'mother of the stomach.' It's a powerful antispasmodic and one of the main herbs for digestive complaints," says Dr. Kamhi. To make the tea, pour 1 cup of boiling water over 2 teaspoons of dried herb and steep for 5 to 10 minutes.

Cinnamon

Drink one to three cups of tea a day as needed. Cinnamon is wonderful for relieving nausea and vomiting, says Mary Bove, N.D., a naturopathic physician at the Brattleboro Naturopathic Clinic in Vermont and a member of Britain's National Institute of Medical Herbalists. Indeed, this common, pleasantly spicy herb is a traditional remedy for stomach upset. To make the tea, break up one stick of cinnamon in a cup and cover with boiling water. Steep for 10 minutes, remove the cinnamon, and drink.

Ginger

Chew on a small piece of fresh ginger, take 250 milligrams in capsule form four times a day, or drink tea as needed. In Europe, this gnarled and knobby root is commonly used to calm churning stomachs. Ginger contains oils that increase digestive fluids and neutralize toxins and stomach acid, thereby reducing nausea and vomiting, says Dr. Kamhi.

There are several ways to take ginger medicinally, she says. If you happen to have fresh ginger on hand, cut off a small piece, about 1

Fast FACTS

Cause: Food poisoning, overeating, infection (such as a viral stomach flu), or other illnesses, especially those that cause a high fever.

Incidence: At some time, everyone has had nausea or lost their breakfast, lunch, or dinner to a bug, bacteria, or nerves.

When to see the doctor: In both adults and children, prolonged vomiting can signal a serious illness or cause severe dehydration. See your doctor if vomiting continues for more than 2 days or you experience significant diarrhea along with the vomiting. You should also seek medical attention if you see blood in the vomit or if vomiting is accompanied by dizziness when standing, a fever higher than 104°F, a stiff neck, or a severe headache.

---

inch by ½ inch, peel it, and chew on it for about 30 minutes. (You can either swallow it or spit it out.)

You can also take ginger capsules, or, if you're up to it, you can drink ginger tea. To make the tea, cut a 2-inch piece of root and slice it into a saucepan. Add 3 to 4 cups of water and simmer for 10 minutes. You can also use 1 to 2 teaspoons of dried ginger in 3 to 4 cups of water.

Goldenseal

Take ½ teaspoon of tincture every 2 to 3 hours as needed until you feel better. Vomiting caused by food poisoning responds well to goldenseal, says Dr. Kamhi. "I give it to people who are traveling to foreign countries, where they may pick up any number of parasites," she says. You may wish to dilute the tincture in some water, she suggests, since it has a very bitter taste.

Meadowsweet

Drink one cup of tea three times a day as needed. Meadowsweet is one of the best digestive remedies available, says Dr. Bove. This herb protects and soothes the mucous membranes of the digestive tract, thereby helping to reduce excess stomach acid and relieve queasiness. Pour 1 cup of boiling water over 1 teaspoon of dried herb, steep for 3 to 5 minutes, and strain before drinking. You can mix in a little spearmint if you wish.

Peppermint, Meadowsweet, and Slippery Elm

Drink one cup of tea every 1 to 2 hours as needed. "Peppermint is great for nausea," says Barry Sherr, a professional member of the AHG who practices in Danbury, Connecticut. Indeed, this spicy herb has been called upon by countless people to calm sick stomachs for centuries.

This tea protects and soothes the gastric lining and relieves nausea and stomach spasms, says Sherr. To make it, pour 1 cup of boiling water over 1 heaping tablespoon of dried peppermint leaves and ½ teaspoon each of dried meadowsweet and slippery elm bark. Steep for 10 minutes, strain, and drink.

Slippery Elm

Drink ½ cup of tea three times a day until you feel better. Slippery elm bark is a traditional remedy for inflammatory conditions of the digestive system, such as gastritis, colitis, and ulcers. Today, herbalists still recommend it for all of those ailments as well as for vomiting. Dr. Kamhi, for example, suggests slippery elm tea to soothe nausea and vomiting caused by chemotherapy, and Dr. Bove recommends it as an all-around safe, effective treatment for vomiting.

Slippery elm is loaded with mucilage, a gelatinous substance made of proteins and sugars, which has a soothing effect on irritated or inflamed digestive tissue. To make the tea, mix 1 teaspoon of powder with 1 cup of boiling water. If you like, add a teaspoon of honey and a sprinkle of cinnamon. This tea can be a little thick, so Dr. Bove often suggests taking it by the spoonful.

WARTS

*T*hink of something vulgar, and it has probably been used to treat warts—saliva, brackish rainwater, fish heads, tobacco juice, even dog dung. Compared to these remedies, herbs seem downright conventional. The strange thing is, sometimes these revolting folk remedies work almost as well as more appealing wart removers.

There's a psychological factor at play with warts. Many doctors think that just believing in the cure seems to marshal the body's defenses. The power of suggestion aside, there may be another scientific explanation of sorts. Whether the remedy is spit, tobacco juice, or a fragrant herb, all that daily dabbing is a signal for your immune system to wake up and notice that there's a virus afoot.

With their bumpy, fleshy presence, warts seem to scream "Look at me!" To your body's immune system, however, the virus that causes warts is like the wallflower at the dance. Since it lives on the outskirts of the top layer of skin—the epidermis—it sometimes simply goes unnoticed.

Warts often heal on their own, but if you want to rid yourself of these pesky protuberances, you might try at-home treatments. One common remedy is low-strength salicylic acid that you paint on every day for several weeks or months until the wart goes away, says Mary Ruth Buchness, M.D., chief of dermatology at St. Vincent's Hospital and Medical Center in New York City. For stubborn warts, doctors may try freezing or burning, both of which can involve pain, bleeding, and potential scarring. While these treatments are usually successful, the virus often spreads, and another wart crops up right next door, says Dr. Buchness.

The herbs discussed below can help kick your immune system into gear so that your body can heal the wart by itself. Healing times can vary widely, though, from a few weeks to a few months. Because topical remedies for warts tend to be caustic, Claudia Wingo, R.N., a medical herbalist in College Park, Maryland, and a member of the National Herbalists Association of Australia, tells her patients to protect the surrounding skin with zinc oxide ointment. These remedies are intended for ordinary warts that appear on the hands and for plantar warts on the soles of your feet. It's not a good idea to use any of these remedies on your face.

Arbor Vitae and Bloodroot

Apply an oil or salve made from these antiviral herbs twice a day. Before arbor vitae became a landscaping ornamental, Native Americans used it as a medicine for fever, headache, and coughs. Because it has established antiviral activity, herbalists today often prescribe it topically for warts.

To make your own wart-be-gone oil, put a handful of fresh arbor vitae greens in a slow cooker. Add two 1-inch pieces of bloodroot. Cover the herbs with 2 cups of olive oil and simmer on low heat overnight. "This takes all the essential oils out," says Wingo. Let it cool completely, then strain it into a container. You can use the oil directly on the wart, she explains, or mix it with coconut oil or beeswax to make a salve.

Salves last longer and keep better, says Gayle Eversole, Ph.D., a certified nurse practitioner and a professional member of the American Herbalists Guild in Everett, Washington.

Astragalus, Calendula, Nettle, and Cleavers

Drink one to two cups of this immune-boosting tea daily for 2 to 6 months. "People tend to get warts when they are run down," explains Wingo. "You can't just work topically." After a month of drinking this tea blend, you should find that your skin is starting to clear, and you may feel less tired, she says.

As one of the important tonic herbs in Traditional Chinese Medicine, astragalus has been extensively researched by Asian scientists. Numerous studies confirm its ability to stimulate the immune system and fight viruses. In the Chinese tradition, the dried sliced root, which looks like a tongue depressor, is simmered for several hours to make a thick, strong tea.

Cause: Warts can be caused by any one of the more than 60 types of human papillomavirus (HPV). The virus enters the skin through tiny breaks and can be transmitted by direct contact with another person or with a piece of skin shed from a wart. Nongenital warts are only mildly contagious. Just as some people are more likely than others to catch a cold virus, some people contract HPV more easily than others. People with weakened immune systems have a higher risk for developing persistent warts. And, contrary to traditional belief, you cannot get them from handling frogs or toads.

Incidence: Warts are more common among children and adolescents. Adults often develop immunity to them. Commonly appearing on the hands, elbows, face, and soles of the feet, warts can also grow on the genitals, where the infection is more serious.

When to see the doctor: Many warts disappear on their own within 1 to 2 years. If you are over 45 and develop warts, call your doctor. New or unusual skin growth should be evaluated to rule out skin cancer. Warts on the genitals are associated with an increased risk of cancer and need to be treated by a physician.

You're more likely to find the powdered herb in health food stores, however. Mix it with equal parts of calendula, nettle, and cleavers, which all gently support the immune system, says Wingo. Use 1 heaping teaspoon of the blend for each cup of tea. Although this combination makes a pleasant-tasting tea, you can add some peppermint or lemon balm for flavor. Fresh herbs are best, but dried will also work, says Wingo.

Calendula

Dab on some herbal cream twice a day. In Europe, calendula cream is used to promote healing of topical wounds. Although a wart isn't a wound, studies of calendula extracts have confirmed that the herb has antiviral properties and an ability to stimulate the immune system.

To heal a wart, mix a few drops of essential oil of lemon into the cream, says Wingo. Lemon balm in oil or cream form is another antiviral wart treatment favored by herbalists, she says.

Dandelion

Rub sap from a fresh root on the wart twice a day until it goes away. Here's one way to control the scourge of weeds in your yard and get rid of a wart at the same time. Traditionally, dandelion tea has been used internally to treat skin conditions, but the milky sap from the fresh root can also be directly applied to a wart, says Dr. Eversole. (Make sure that the dandelion you harvest hasn't been treated with chemical herbicides for at least 3 years.)

Be patient. It may take weeks or months to erase the fleshy evidence of the virus. Of course, if you're snowed in for the winter, you may have to wait until spring to try this remedy. This same technique also works with sap from milkweed, says Dr. Eversole.

Fenugreek

Apply a paste made from seeds once a day until the wart goes away. Since they're used as a spice and a flavoring agent, you may have a jar of these sweet-tasting seeds in your kitchen. You can also use them to make a paste to treat warts, says Dr. Eversole. Put 1 tablespoon of seeds in a small jar and add enough water to cover them completely. Soak the seeds for about 2 days in the refrigerator until they form a thick solution similar to ointment. Apply it to the wart once a day and let it dry, she says.

Lemon

Before you go to bed, tape a piece of lemon peel to the wart. The pith, or white flesh of the peel, and the fragrant yellow outer part of the fruit contain volatile oil that has antiseptic properties. Regular overnight application of the inside of the peel can help soften and heal a wart or callus, says Dr. Eversole.

WINDBURN

*I*f you're impelled to brave the great outdoors on days that make mailmen reconsider their career choice, the ruddy complexion that you come home with may be more than just a healthy glow. It may be windburn.

Something of a misnomer, windburn isn't actually a burn, although the redness and swelling it brings about can make it look and feel like one. It's more accurate to describe windburn as a skin irritation. What happens to your skin when it's exposed to severe winds, especially when it's cold out, is that it loses moisture rapidly and becomes dry and chafed. The physical friction of the wind whipping past your tender epidermis further aggravates the situation.

Petroleum jelly is a big favorite of M.D.'s when it comes to treating windburn, which makes sense because it provides a soothing, protective layer that prevents further moisture loss. Herbalists and naturopaths have their own favored remedies for windburned skin. Here are some to try.

Calendula and St. John's Wort

Mix these herbal oils with a basic skin lotion and use as needed. Whitney Miller, N.D., a naturopathic doctor who has a family practice in New London and Colchester, Connecticut, likes combining the soothing, anti-inflammatory properties of calendula and St. John's wort with a simple face lotion such as Eucerin.

Fill a 4-ounce screw-top jar almost to the brim with lotion and squirt in approximately 1 teaspoon of each of the herbal oils. "The exact amount isn't important," says Dr. Miller. Just be sure to mix the lotion well, as the oils have a tendency to separate out.

Jojoba

Apply this gentle oil directly to your face. You have to be careful about applying oils directly to your skin, because they can

Fast FACTS

Cause: Windburn happens when skin is exposed to severe winds, particularly when the temperature is low. Rapid moisture loss causes the skin to become dry and chafed.

Incidence: Skiers and yachtsmen suffer from windburn, but so do joggers, dog walkers, and just about anyone else who takes on the elements without adequate protection.

When to see the doctor: Consult a doctor if your skin is still red and inflamed after 4 to 5 days of home treatment.

make it break out. But, says Dr. Miller, "I've never met anyone who reacted badly to jojoba oil." That may be because jojoba isn't technically an oil; it's a substance known as a liquid wax ester that has excellent emollient properties but also allows the skin to breathe.

Jojoba oil is extracted from the seeds of a woody, evergreen shrub indigenous to two places on opposite sides of the globe: the American Sonoran Desert and Israel. Historically, the oil was used by Apaches and other Native Americans.

Calendula and Aloe

Mix 2 parts calendula succus and 1 part aloe gel in a spritzer bottle and spray on your skin as often as needed. Aloe and calendula top many herbalists' lists as the best all-around skin-care herbs. Sharol Tilgner, N.D., a naturopathic physician, professional member of the American Herbalists Guild (AHG), and president of Wise Woman Herbals in Eugene, Oregon, likes to combine them in a handy spray for irritated skin.

Calendula succus is a low-alcohol tincture. If you can't find it in a health food store, try a mail-order company. Be sure to use at least twice as much calendula as aloe, says Dr. Tilgner, so that the mixture has enough alcohol in it to preserve it.

Chamomile, Frankincense, and Lavender

Add 2 drops of each essential oil to 1 ounce of skin lotion and smooth it onto your skin. Both the German and Roman varieties of chamomile are good anti-inflammatory herbs, says Mindy Green, a founder and professional member of the American Herbalists Guild, director of educational services at the Herb Research Foundation in Boulder, Colorado, and co-author of *Aromatherapy: A Complete Guide to the Healing Art*. "Frankincense is very moisturizing and wonderful for cracked, dry skin," says Green. An unscented skin lotion that doesn't contain mineral oil would be best for this mixture.

WORKAHOLISM

*I*t's considered quite fashionable by the fast-paced crowd to call yourself a workaholic. True to the prevailing attitude of more pain, more gain, the problem has even been referred to as "the best-dressed addiction." But workaholism isn't just working late hours or having a tough job. It's actually a compulsive disorder.

Hard work is almost universally praised as a sign of dedication, intensity, and ambition. Contrary to this idea, though, workaholics—people who are addicted to their jobs—actually don't make better employees. They can be irritable and controlling, with narrow points of view that stifle creativity.

In spite of the fact that many people don't take it seriously, workaholism is a potentially serious problem that can destroy relationships, reduce productivity on the job, and eventually cause mental and physical breakdown.

If you think that you're a workaholic or are worried that you have some tendencies toward the problem, there are some herbal remedies

ADVENTURES IN HERBALISM

HOW TO MAKE A KAVA COCKTAIL—
THE TRADITIONAL WAY

*H*erbs are often covered in boiling water for a time, then strained and taken as a tea. Sometimes, herbalists more fully extract the active properties of a plant by steeping it in alcohol for weeks, then filtering out the solids to create what's called a tincture. In some cases, as with culinary herbs, the herbs need no blending and can be taken—eaten—as they are.

The medicinal plant kava, however, has traditionally been prepared in an altogether unique way. In its native land of Polynesia, kava "mixologists" have a very intimate involvement in their herbal creation. In order to make the kava drink, they first chew the fresh root, combining it thoroughly with saliva to help break it down. Then they collect the mush in a vat of coconut milk. The resulting kava "cocktail" is then strained and drunk at public ceremonies and social gatherings.

Now, of course, kava is available in tincture, tea, and capsule form, but it's said that the traditional, hands-on, fresh root concoction is much more potent.

that can soften the harmful effects of being too devoted to your job. Try the following to help you slow down the pace of your outside world by bringing some focus to the internal one.

Kava Kava

Take 100 milligrams of standardized root extract two or three times a day for up to 3 months. If you'd like to be as mellow as a Pacific islander—or at least a little less uptight—do what the natives

Fast FACTS

Cause: While workaholism is primarily related to personality, certain situations can make work addiction more likely. Financial responsibilities or debts that are greater than income can create an urgent need to earn overtime wages. A high-pressure work environment can make an employee feel that more "face time" is required for job stability or a promotion. Domestic problems may make staying late at the office seem a better choice than calling it a day. In addition, cultural beliefs that value labor as a godly antidote to evil only reinforce the misconception that there's no such thing as too much work.

Incidence: No one really knows how many people are addicted to their work. It's estimated that the average American clocks 52 work hours per week, and a good portion of those people would be willing to push it to 62 hours in exchange for overtime pay. In Japan, 10,000 workers a year succumb to *karoshi*—fatal heart attack or stroke brought on by steadily laboring 60 to 70 hours a week.

When to see the doctor: Most workaholics are entrenched in denial; they don't know or can't admit that they need help. People who are addicted to work may only learn about their problems from their spouses or children. Symptoms of forgetfulness, chronic fatigue, grouchiness, mood swings, and stress-related physical illnesses (such as high blood pressure and temporomandibular joint problems) are all signs that the body is breaking down. At this point, a visit to a physician—as well as an appointment with a counselor or therapist—is crucial to good physical and mental health.

---

who live there do. Try some kava, a tropical plant with a history of reverential ceremonial use.

The anxiety-relieving effects of kava have been compared to those of potent benzodiazepine drugs like diazepam (Valium), alprazolam (Xanax), and chlordiazepoxide (Librium). The advantage of kava is that it can positively alter brain activity without the same sedative effect or potential for addiction as anti-anxiety drugs.

Rather than feeling "knocked out," people who take kava report less nervousness and a better sense of general well-being. Anxiety-ridden workaholics can use kava as part of an overall program that includes relaxation techniques and counseling to help ease tension, says William Page-Echols, D.O., an osteopathic physician at Full Spectrum Family Medicine in East Lansing, Michigan. He recommends looking for a product standardized for 55 percent kavalactones, the active ingredients in kava.

Lavender

Combine 5 drops of this essential oil with 2 ounces of carrier oil, then add to warm bathwater and soak for 20 minutes each night. Taking the time to soak in the tub is something a workaholic would never do, right? Well, that's just the point of this tip. Breaking set with a bath is a time-honored way to signal the end of a stressful, too-long workday.

Adding essential oil of lavender to the tub will compound the soothing effects of the warm water. Its sweet floral fragrance is known in the practice of aromatherapy (the therapeutic use of scent) for its calming and quieting properties. Scientifically, it has been proven to positively affect the central nervous system. "It may just help do the trick," says Nancy Welliver, N.D., director of the Institute for Medical Herbalism in Calistoga, California.

Buy a bottle of pure lavender essential oil, which is the most highly concentrated form of the herb. Since it won't disperse easily in water and may irritate your skin, Dr. Welliver recommends combining lavender oil with a carrier oil such as almond or olive oil in a glass bottle and shaking them together.

You can also mix the essential oil with 2 tablespoons of milk or 1 tablespoon of baking soda, according to Kal Kotecha, an aromatherapist and director of the Kal Kotecha Academy of Aromatherapy and Massage in Ontario. Add the mixture to the bath just before you are ready to step in, then swish the water with your hand to mix it in. This ensures that the fragrance will be at its most potent when you take the plunge.

WRINKLES

*I*n truth, we're all "thin-skinned." The body's largest organ, skin ranges from only $\frac{1}{25}$ to $\frac{1}{8}$ inch deep, and what you do with it makes a lasting impression. After decades of smiling and frowning, furrowing and squinting, a few of your favorite expressions are bound to end up etched in the tapestry of your visage.

Three factors influence how soon those fine lines will turn into full-fledged wrinkles—genetics, exposure to sunlight, and smoking, which damages the skin internally, making it less elastic. There's nothing you can do about your DNA, but you can take the smart path and avoid the things that promote wrinkles. Sun damage is responsible for most wrinkles, but the good news is that by using sunscreen regularly, beginning in childhood, you can prevent this type. A face-shielding, wide-brimmed hat also helps.

Look for sunscreen products that contain antioxidants like vitamin C or vitamin E as well as vitamin A, says David Edelberg, M.D., founder of American WholeHealth in Chicago. To stay healthy and supple, your skin depends in part on antioxidant vitamins, minerals, herbs, and enzymes. Although we get many of these cell protectors from foods and supplements, research shows that your skin can also benefit from using them externally to counteract the damage caused by sun exposure and environmental factors. Regularly slathering on an antioxidant-rich sunscreen will not only prevent any further damage, it will also allow the skin to heal and repair itself.

Changes in your skin's elastic layer start long before the fine lines and crinkles start to show. Collagen—the glue that holds your skin together—decreases by about 1 percent a year during adulthood. To combat this natural process, Alan M. Dattner, M.D., a holistic dermatologist in New Rochelle, New York, recommends a daily supplement of vitamin C to help your body produce more of the connective tissue. He suggests slowly working up to 1,000 milligrams of vitamin C daily by taking 250 milligrams to start, then 500 milligrams, then

1,000. Try to include natural sources of vitamin C, such as oranges and red peppers, in your diet, says Dr. Dattner.

For the most part, herbal treatments for skin focus on keeping it healthy and vibrant rather than on reversing the signs of aging. Herbalists tend to accept wrinkles and the gray hair and wisdom that go along with them. That's not bad advice.

Flaxseed

Each day, mix 1 tablespoon of oil into something you eat. Flaxseed oil has compounds that will help keep your skin moist, says Dr. Edelberg. Cooking destroys its healing properties, so use it straight from the bottle. You can add it to cereal, stir it into juice, or drizzle it over pasta or vegetables.

Buy fresh, cold-pressed, refrigerated flaxseed oil packaged in a dark, opaque bottle. The oil turns rancid quickly when exposed to light or high temperatures. Good-quality oil has a pleasant, nutty flavor.

Apple, Strawberry, and Grape

Strip away wrinkle-emphasizing skin with a natural fruit acid mask three times a week. A natural fruit acid peel can reduce the harshness of heavy wrinkles and sometimes eliminate fine lines by gently exfoliating the skin, says Dina Falconi, a medical herbalist, author of *Earthly Bodies and Heavenly Hair*, and founder of Falcon Formulations in New York state.

"Fruit acids are extremely effective at removing the loose layer of dead skin," says Falconi. Citrus fruits, berries, apples, tomatoes, kiwifuit, peaches, and grapes have the same active ingredients available in cosmetic products that contain alpha hydroxy acids.

To make your own version and avoid paying cosmetic counter prices, mix 1 tablespoon of mashed fruit with the same amount of whole-wheat flour and water, ½ tablespoon of cornmeal, and a few drops of oil (such as jojoba or peanut oil), says Falconi. If the mixture seems either too runny or too thick, adjust it by adding a bit more

Fast FACTS

Cause: Wrinkles are caused by the breakdown of collagen, the intertwined cell layer that forms an elastic, spongy base under the second layer of your skin. When you're young, collagen easily absorbs moisture and swells to keep your skin plump, smooth, and resilient. As you age, though, your body makes less collagen, and the existing collagen loses some of its ability to soak up water. Crevices in the collagen eventually cause the skin to collapse and fold on the surface.

Incidence: Your skin's tendency to wrinkle is determined largely by genetics, sun exposure, and whether you smoke.

When to see the doctor: The appearance of severely wrinkled skin can be improved with surgery, laser treatments, or chemical peels. Before you undertake any type of treatment, discuss your options with a dermatologist.

flour or water to get the desired consistency. Apply it to just-washed skin and leave it on for about 20 minutes. Rinse with cool water.

Papaya

To remove fine lines, use this peel twice a month. Dermatologists use chemicals to remove wrinkles by stripping away the outer layers of skin. You can try a milder, do-it-yourself version of the same procedure with papaya, says Claudia Wingo, R.N., a medical herbalist in College Park, Maryland, and a member of the National Herbalists Association of Australia.

Papaya contains proteolytic enzymes, compounds that help break down protein. That's why this tropical fruit is typically used as a digestive agent. Those same protein-eating enzymes can help shine up your complexion by dissolving the first layer of skin.

Here's how to make your own papaya peel. In a small food processor, grind 2 tablespoons of washed and peeled papaya. Mix it with 1 tablespoon of dry oatmeal, pat it onto clean skin, and let it set for 10 minutes. Gently scrub it off with a washcloth in an outward, circular motion. The oatmeal helps to remove debris from the skin.

Witch Hazel and Lavender

Try this herbal toner anytime you want a refreshing lift. Falconi recommends blotting your skin with lavender-infused witch hazel to temporarily tighten small wrinkles. This inexpensive astringent is distilled from the leaves and young twigs of the witch hazel tree. It contains large quantities of tannins, which have a drying, astringent effect that tightens the proteins of the skin surface.

To make a scented skin toner, add 6 drops of lavender essential oil to 4 ounces of witch hazel and apply it with your fingers. "I don't like using cotton pads. They absorb many of the essential components of the herbs," says Falconi.

Lavender, Coriander, and Anise

Invigorate your skin with a facial steam one to three times a week. "As we age, our skin tends to become dry, thin, and dull. An herbal steam treatment stimulates and increases circulation to the skin," says Falconi. "Steaming encourages vibrancy and sparkle without causing mechanical or chemical irritation." She developed this sweet, refreshing recipe specifically for mature skin. Combine two handfuls of lavender flowers, two palmfuls of crushed coriander seeds, and two palmfuls of crushed aniseed, then follow this basic facial steam technique.

Cleanse any makeup or surface dirt from your face. Put one palmful of the herbal mix into a heatproof quart bowl and pour in 1 pint of boiling water. Slowly lower your face over the bowl and place a bath towel over both your head and the bowl to create a tent that captures the steam. Be careful not to lower your face too close to the steaming liquid, cautions Falconi. Remain in the steam tent for about 20 minutes. In general, it's best to let your skin air-dry following any skin treatment, she says.

YEAST INFECTIONS

*I*f you are a woman who's ever had a yeast infection, you know that you never want to have another one.

Infection with an overgrowth of the yeast organism known as *Candida albicans* causes vaginal itching and burning, plus a thick-textured, bready-smelling discharge. Not a pretty picture for that most private of places.

Unfortunately, yeast infections are fairly common occurrences. On the brighter side, though, while the situation may feel absolutely unbearable, life and limb aren't actually in danger. This makes self-treatment an option, with either over-the counter medications, which have been found to work only a little more than half the time, or natural remedies.

Two nonherbal but natural treatments to try for beating a yeast infection include sea salt and yogurt. Sea salt actually has the ability to kill candida, says Virginia Frazer, N.D., a naturopathic physician and licensed midwife in Kennewick, Washington. Once a day, dissolve 1 cup of sea salt in warm bathwater, swish it around, then ease yourself in for a soak. Repeat until symptoms subside.

Yogurt also has a reputation for getting a yeast overgrowth under control naturally. Let a few tablespoons of plain, organic, live-culture yogurt come to room temperature, then use clean fingers to cover the outside and inside of your vagina with it. Do this for 15 minutes several times a day for up to a week. Rinse off the yogurt with warm water, then use a blow-dryer on the warm setting to make sure that you are totally dry, says Dr. Frazer.

If you've been diagnosed with the yeast beast before and can reliably recognize the symptoms, it's okay to proceed with the following home remedies for their specified duration.

White Grape Vinegar

Douche with white vinegar and water twice a day for 2 days. This plant-based home remedy for yeast infections involves vinegar, which

Fast FACTS

Cause: Yeast infections are caused by an overgrowth in the vagina of the candida fungus, usually the strain named *Candida albicans*. In healthy women, the number of normally harmless candida organisms remains stable. Certain factors, however, such as using antibiotics, wearing tight clothing, being pregnant, or having diabetes or a compromised immune system, can allow yeast to grow out of control, leading to symptoms of infection.

Incidence: More than one million American women are diagnosed with yeast infections each year.

When to see the doctor: If you've never been diagnosed with a yeast infection before, if you're pregnant, or if you have diabetes, you should see your doctor to determine the exact cause of your symptoms. You could have another type of infection that requires different treatment. You should also turn to your doctor if you see no improvement after using home remedies for a maximum of 2 weeks.

is really just the fermented juice of white grapes. Douching is never recommended for healthy women because it can throw a perfectly normal vaginal environment off-balance. During a yeast infection, though, the vagina's pH balance is already off-kilter. That's when an internal cleansing with the mild acidity of a vinegar solution can really help, says Mercedes Cameron, M.D., a family practitioner at The Woman's Place at St. Mary's Hospital in Grand Junction, Colorado.

Twice a day for 2 days, use a standard douche bag to douche with 2 tablespoons of white vinegar added to 1 quart of water. If you are clearly getting better, continue douching until symptoms subside, but for no longer than 1 week. If you don't see any improvement in 2 days, you may have a problem other than a yeast infection, so it's time to visit your doctor, says Dr. Cameron.

Echinacea

Take one dropper of tincture in ½ cup of water up to four times daily for up to 2 weeks. Echinacea is known in herbal circles for its cold-curing ability. But the same immunity-stimulating effect that can send sniffles scrambling can stem a yeast infection as well, says Larry Kincheloe, M.D., chairman of the department of obstetrics and gynecology at the Central Oklahoma Medical Group in Oklahoma City.

During a yeast infection, your immune system is involved in a battle against the candida fungus. Studies show that echinacea encourages immunity by boosting levels of white blood cells, which are the body's first line of defense against infection.

A good-quality echinacea tincture will cause a tingling sensation on your tongue.

Since echinacea becomes less effective the longer you take it, you should discontinue this herbal treatment after 2 weeks. If you're still experiencing symptoms after that time, you should seek advice and treatment from your doctor.

YOUR GUIDE TO SAFE
USE OF HERBS

*W*hile herbal home remedies are generally safe and cause few, if any, side effects, herbalists are quick to caution that botanical medicines should be used cautiously—and knowledgeably.

First, if you are under a doctor's care for any health condition or are taking medication, do not take any herb or alter your medication regimen without your doctor's knowledge. Do not give herbs to children without consulting a physician. Also, if you are pregnant, do not self-treat with any natural remedy without the consent of your obstetrician or midwife. The same advice applies to nursing mothers and women who are trying to conceive.

Some remedies may cause adverse reactions if you are allergy-prone, have a major health condition, take prescription medication, take an herb for too long, take too much, or use the herb improperly. The guidelines in this chart are intended for adults only and usually refer to internal use.

Since some herbs can cause a skin reaction when used topically, it's always wise to do a patch test before applying an herb for the first time. Apply a small amount to your skin and observe it for 24 hours to be sure that you aren't sensitive. If redness or a rash occurs, discontinue use.

Before you try the remedies in this book, check the following safety guidelines, based on the American Herbal Products Association's *Botanical Safety Handbook*, a recognized source of herb safety information, and on the advice of experienced herbal healers. Then you can enjoy the world of herbal healing with confidence.

Herb	Cautions and Safety Guidelines
Agrimony (*Agrimonia eupatoria*)	None; generally regarded as safe.
Alfalfa (*Medicago sativa*)	None; generally regarded as safe.
Aloe (*Aloe barbadensis*)	Do not use gel topically on any surgical incision; may delay wound healing. Do not ingest dried leaf; it is a habit-forming laxative.
Alpha hydroxy acids (AHAs)	Discontinue use if stinging, redness, itching, or any other symptoms of skin irritation occur.
American ginseng (*Panax quinquefolium*)	May cause irritability if taken with caffeine or other stimulants. Do not use if you have high blood pressure.
Arbor vitae (*Thuja occidentalis*)	Not recommended for long-term use. Do not exceed the recommended dose.
Arnica (*Arnica montana*)	Do not use on broken skin.
Ashwaganda (*Withania somnifera*)	Do not use with barbiturates; it may intensify their effects.
Asian ginseng (*Panax ginseng*)	May cause irritability if taken with caffeine or other stimulants. Do not use if you have high blood pressure.
Astragalus (*Astragalus membranaceous*)	None; generally regarded as safe.
Basil (*Ocimum basilicum*)	Generally regarded as safe when used as a spice. Do not take large amounts (several cups a day) for extended periods.
Bayberry (*Berberis vulgaris*)	None; generally regarded as safe.
Bilberry (*Vaccinium myrtillus*)	None; generally regarded as safe.
Bitter melon (*Momordica charantia*)	None; generally regarded as safe.

Herb	Cautions and Safety Guidelines
Black cherry (*Prunus serotina*)	Not recommended for long-term use. Do not exceed the recommended dose.
Black cohosh (*Actea racemosa*)	Do not use for more than 6 months.
Black haw (*Viburnum prunifolium*)	Do not use without medical supervision if you have a history of kidney stones; it contains oxalates, which may cause kidney stones.
Black horehound (*Ballota nigra*)	None; generally regarded as safe.
Bladderwrack (*Fucus vesiculosus*)	Do not use for more than 6 weeks; may reduce gastrointestinal absorption of iron, sodium, and potassium. Not recommended if you have hyperthyroidism. May aggravate existing acne.
Bloodroot (*Sanguinaria canadensis*)	Safe when used in commercial dental products or under the supervision of a qualified health-care practitioner. May cause nausea and vomiting in doses higher than 5 to 10 drops of regular-strength tincture if taken more than twice a day.
Blueberry (*Vaccinium angustifolium*; *V. corymbosum*; *V. pallidum*)	None; generally regarded as safe.
Blue cohosh (*Caulophyllum thalictroides*)	None; generally regarded as safe.
Blue-green algae (*Aphanizomeon flos-aquae*)	Discontinue use if you experience diarrhea or nausea.
Boneset (*Eupatorium perfoliatum*)	May cause an allergic reaction in those with allergies or sensitivities, especially to chamomile, feverfew, ragweed, or other members of the daisy family. May cause vomiting and severe diarrhea in large doses.

Herb	Cautions and Safety Guidelines
Boswellia (*Boswellia serrata*)	None; generally regarded as safe.
Brahmi (*Bacopa monniera*)	None; generally regarded as safe.
Brewer's yeast (*Saccharomyces cerevisiae*)	Do not use without medical supervision if you have diabetes or hypoglycemia. Do not use if you have candidiasis, gout, or high blood levels of uric acid. Use with caution if you have a known allergy to molds. Take on an empty stomach unless indigestion occurs; then take with food.
Bromelain	May cause nausea, vomiting, diarrhea, skin rash, and heavy menstrual bleeding. May increase the risk of bleeding in people taking aspirin or anticoagulants (blood thinners). Do not use if you are allergic to pineapple.
Burdock (*Arctium lappa*)	None; generally regarded as safe.
Cabbage (*Brassica oleracea*)	None; generally regarded as safe.
Calendula (*Calendula officinalis*)	None; generally regarded as safe.
California poppy (*Eschscholzia californica*)	Do not use with antidepressant MAO inhibitor drugs such as phenelzine sulfate (Nardil) and tranylcypromine (Parnate) without medical supervision.
Cardamom (*Elettaria cardamomum*)	None; generally regarded as safe.
Cascara (*Rhamnus purshianus*)	Do not use if you have any inflammatory condition of the intestines, intestinal obstruction, or abdominal pain. May cause laxative dependency and diarrhea. Do not use for more than 14 days.
Castor (*Ricinus communis*)	Do not use oil internally if you have an intestinal obstruction or abdominal pain. Do not use for more than 8 to 10 days.

Herb	Cautions and Safety Guidelines
Cat's claw (*Uncaria tomentosa*)	Do not use if you have hemophilia. May cause headache, abdominal pain, or difficult breathing. Also has contraceptive properties.
Catnip (*Nepeta cataria*)	None; generally regarded as safe.
Cayenne (*Capsicum annuum; C. frutescens*)	May cause gastrointestinal irritation if taken on an empty stomach. Do not use topically near eyes or on injured skin.
Celandine (*Chelidonium majus*)	Generally regarded as safe for topical use. Do not use internally without the supervision of a qualified health-care practitioner.
Celery seed (*Apium graveolens*)	Use therapeutic doses with caution if you have a kidney disorder. Avoid overexposure to direct sunlight; may cause photosensitivity.
Chamomile (*Matricaria recutita*)	Very rarely, may cause an allergic reaction when ingested. Drink tea with caution if you are allergic to closely related plants such as ragweed, asters, and chrysanthemums.
Chasteberry (*Vitex agnus-castus*)	May counteract the effectiveness of birth control pills.
Chickweed (*Stellaria media*)	None; generally regarded as safe.
Chinese honeysuckle (*Lonicera japonica*)	None; generally regarded as safe.
Cinnamon (*Cinnamomum zeylanicum*)	None; generally regarded as safe.
Cleavers (*Galium aparine*)	None; generally regarded as safe.
Clove (*Syzygium aromaticum*)	None; generally regarded as safe.
Collinsonia (*Collinsonia canadensis*)	None; generally regarded as safe.

Herb	Cautions and Safety Guidelines
Comfrey (*Symphytum officinale*)	For external use only. Do not use on deep or infected wounds; may promote surface healing too quickly and not allow healing of underlying tissue.
Coriander (*Coriandrum sativum*)	None; generally regarded as safe.
Corn silk (*Zea mays*)	None; generally regarded as safe.
Cottonwood (*Populus deltoides*)	None; generally regarded as safe.
Couch grass (*Agropyron repens*)	None; generally regarded as safe.
Cramp bark (*Viburnum opulus*)	None; generally regarded as safe.
Cranberry (*Vaccinium macrocarpon*)	None; generally regarded as safe.
Damiana (*Turnera diffusa; T. aphrodisiaca*)	None; generally regarded as safe.
Dandelion (*Taraxacum officinale*)	Do not use root preparations without medical supervision if you have gallbladder disease.
Dang gui (*Angelica sinensis*)	None; generally regarded as safe.
Devil's claw (*Harpagophytum procumbens*)	Do not use if you have gastric or duodenal ulcers. Consult your physician before using if you have gallstones.
Echinacea (*Echinacea angustifolia; E. purpurea; E. pallida*)	Do not use if you are allergic to closely related plants such ragweed, asters, and chrysanthemums. Do not use if you have tuberculosis or an autoimmune condition such as lupus or multiple sclerosis; it stimulates the immune system.
Elder (*Sambucus canadensis; S. nigra*)	Seeds, bark, leaves, and unripe fruit may cause vomiting or severe diarrhea.
Elecampane (*Inula helenium*)	None; generally regarded as safe.

Herb	Cautions and Safety Guidelines
Ephedra (*Ephedra sinica*)	Use only under the supervision of a qualified health-care practitioner.
Evening primrose (*Oenothera biennis*)	None; generally regarded as safe.
Eyebright (*Euphrasia officinalis*)	None; generally regarded as safe.
Fennel (*Foeniculum vulgare*)	Do not use seeds medicinally for more than 6 weeks without the supervision of a qualified health-care practitioner.
Fenugreek (*Trigonella foenum-graecum*)	None; generally regarded as safe.
Feverfew (*Tanacetum parthenium*)	Chewing fresh leaves may cause mouth sores in some people.
Figwort (*Scrophularia marilandica*)	Do not use if you have rapid heartbeat.
Flax (*Linum usitatissimum*)	Do not use seeds if you have a bowel obstruction. Take with at least 8 ounces of water.
Garlic (*Allium sativum*)	Do not use supplements if you are taking anticoagulants (blood thinners) or before undergoing surgery; it thins the blood and may increase bleeding. Do not use if you are taking hypoglycemic drugs.
Gentian (*Gentiana lutea*)	May cause nausea and vomiting in large doses. Do not use if you have high blood pressure, gastric or duodenal ulcers, or gastric irritation and inflammation.
Ginger (*Zingiber officinale*)	Do not use therapeutic amounts of dried root or powder without medical supervision if you have gallstones; it may increase bile secretions.

Herb	Cautions and Safety Guidelines
Ginkgo (*Ginkgo biloba*)	Do not use with antidepressant MAO inhibitor drugs such as phenelzine sulfate (Nardil) or tranylcypromine (Parnate), aspirin or other nonsteroidal anti-inflammatory drugs, or anti-coagulant (blood-thinning) medications such as warfarin (Coumadin). May cause dermatitis, diarrhea, and vomiting in doses higher than 240 milligrams of concentrated extract.
Goldenrod (*Solidago virgaurea*)	Do not use if you have a chronic kidney disorder.
Goldenseal (*Hydrastis canadensis*)	Do not use if you have high blood pressure.
Gotu kola (*Centella asiatica*)	Rarely, may cause rash or headache. Do not use for extended periods without the supervision of a qualified health-care practitioner.
Grape seed (*Vitus vinifera*)	None; generally regarded as safe.
Gravel root (*Eupatorium purpureum*)	For external use only. Do not use on broken skin.
Grindelia (*Grindelia camporum*)	None; generally regarded as safe.
Ground ivy (*Glechoma hederacea*)	None; generally regarded as safe.
Guaiacum (*Guaiacum officinale*)	May cause gastrointestinal irritation.
Guarana (*Paullina cupana*)	Not recommended for long-term use in high amounts; it contains twice the amount of caffeine found in coffee and stimulates the nervous system. May cause gastrointestinal irritation.
Guggul (*Commiphora mukul*)	Rarely, may cause diarrhea, restlessness, apprehension, or hiccups.
Gymnema sylvestre	May influence blood sugar levels. Do not use without medical supervision if you have diabetes.

Herb	Cautions and Safety Guidelines
Hawthorn (*Crataegus oxycantha*; *C. laevigata* ; *C. monogyna*)	Do not use regularly for more than a few weeks without medical supervision if you have a cardiovascular condition; you may require lower doses of other medications such as high blood pressure drugs. Do not use without medical supervision if you have low blood pressure caused by heart valve problems.
Hibiscus (*Hibiscus sabdariffa*)	None; generally regarded as safe.
Horse chestnut (*Aesculus hippocastanum*)	May interfere with the action of other drugs, especially anticoagulants (blood thinners) such as warfarin (Coumadin). May cause gastrointestinal irritation.
Horsetail (*Equisetum* spp.)	Do not use tincture if you have heart or kidney problems. May cause thiamin deficiency. Do not take more than 2 grams a day of powdered extract or use for prolonged periods.
Hyssop (*Hyssopus officinalis*)	None; generally regarded as safe.
Jewelweed (*Impatiens capensis*; *I. biflora*; *I. pallida*)	Generally regarded as safe for topical use. Do not use internally without the supervision of a qualified health-care practitioner.
Jojoba (*Simmondsia chinensis*)	None; generally regarded as safe for topical use.
Johnny jump-up (*Viola tricolor*)	None; generally regarded as safe.
Juniper (*Juniper* spp.)	None; generally regarded as safe.
Kava kava (*Piper methysticum*)	Do not use with alcohol or barbiturates. Do not exceed the recommended dose. Use caution when driving or operating equipment; it is a muscle relaxant.
Kudzu (*Pueraria lobata*)	None; generally regarded as safe.

Herb	Cautions and Safety Guidelines
Lavender (*Lavandula officinalis*; *L. angustifolia*; *L. vera*)	None; generally regarded as safe.
Lemon (*Citrus limon*)	None; generally regarded as safe.
Lemon balm (*Melissa officinalis*)	None; generally regarded as safe.
Licorice (*Glycyrrhiza glabra*)	Do not use if you have diabetes, high blood pressure, liver or kidney disorders, or low potassium levels. Do not use daily for more than 4 to 6 weeks; overuse may lead to water retention, high blood pressure due to potassium loss, or impaired heart and kidney function.
Linden (*Tilia* × *europaea*)	None; generally regarded as safe.
Lobelia (*Lobelia inflata*)	None; generally regarded as safe.
Lomatium (*Lomatium dissectum*)	May cause low-grade fever or rashes when used internally.
Maitake (*Grifola frondosa*)	None; generally regarded as safe.
Marshmallow (*Althaea officinalis*)	May slow the absorption of medications taken at the same time.
Meadowsweet (*Filipendula* spp.)	Do not use if you need to avoid aspirin for any reason; its active ingredient, salicin, is related to aspirin.
Milk thistle (*Silybum marianum*)	None; generally regarded as safe.
Motherwort (*Leonurus cardiaca*)	None; generally regarded as safe.
Muira puama (*Ptychopetalum olacoides*)	None; generally regarded as safe.
Mullein (*Verbascum thapsus*)	None; generally regarded as safe.
Myrrh (*Commiphora myrrha*)	May cause diarrhea and irritation of the kidneys. Do not use if you have uterine bleeding for any reason.

Herb	Cautions and Safety Guidelines
Nettle (*Urtica dioica*)	May aggravate allergy symptoms; take only one dose a day for the first few days.
Nutmeg (*Myristica fragrans*)	Generally regarded as safe when used as a spice. Do not use therapeutic amounts without the supervision of a qualified health-care practitioner.
Oak (*Quercus* spp.)	Do not use topically if you have extensive skin damage.
Oats (*Avena sativa*)	Do not use if you have celiac disease (gluten intolerance); it contains gluten, a grain protein.
Olive (*Olea europaea*)	None; generally regarded as safe.
Orange (*Citrus sinensis*)	None; generally regarded as safe.
Oregano (*Origanum heracleoticum*)	None; generally regarded as safe.
Oregon grape (*Mahonia aquifolium*)	None; generally regarded as safe.
Osha (*Ligusticum poteri*)	None; generally regarded as safe.
Papaya enzymes (*Carica papaya*)	May influence blood sugar levels. Do not use without medical supervision if you have diabetes.
Parsley (*Petroselinum crispum*)	Generally regarded as safe when used as a garnish or ingredient in food. Do not use large amounts (several cups a day) if you have kidney disease; may increase urine flow.
Partridgeberry (*Mitchella repens*)	None; generally regarded as safe.
Passionflower (*Passiflora incarnata*)	None; generally regarded as safe.
Pau d'arco (*Tabebuia impetiginosa*)	None; generally regarded as safe.

Herb	Cautions and Safety Guidelines
Pennyroyal (*Mentha pulegium; Hedeoma pulegioides*)	None; generally regarded as safe.
Peppermint (*Mentha piperita*)	None; generally regarded as safe.
Pine (*Pinus strobus*)	None; generally regarded as safe.
Pipsissewa (*Chimaphila umbellata*)	None; generally regarded as safe.
Plantain (*Plantago lanceolata; P. major ; P. media*)	None; generally regarded as safe.
Poplar (*Populus tremuloides*)	None; generally regarded as safe.
Propolis	Do not use if you have asthma; it contains allergens that may aggravate the condition. May cause a rash when handled.
Psyllium (*Plantago ovata*)	Do not use if you have a bowel obstruction. Take 1 hour after other drugs, and take with at least 8 ounces of water.
Pygeum (*Prunus africana*)	May cause nausea and stomach pain.
Quercetin	None; generally regarded as safe.
Red clover (*Trifolium pratense*)	None; generally regarded as safe.
Red raspberry (*Rubus idaeus*)	None; generally regarded as safe.
Reishi (*Ganoderma lucidum*)	May cause dry mouth or stomach upset when used for more than 3 months.
Rhubarb (*Rheum officinale*)	Do not use if you have a known intestinal obstruction, abdominal pain of unknown origin, or any inflammatory condition of the intestines, such as appendicitis, colitis, or irritable bowel syndrome. Use with caution if you have a history of kidney stones. Do not use continuously for more than 8 to 10 days.
Rose (*Rosa* spp.)	None; generally regarded as safe.

Herb	Cautions and Safety Guidelines
Rose hips (*Rosa canina*)	None; generally regarded as safe.
Rosemary (*Rosmarinus officinalis*)	Generally regarded as safe when used as a spice. In therapeutic amounts, may cause excessive menstrual bleeding.
Sage (*Salvia officinalis*)	Generally regarded as safe when used as a spice. In therapeutic amounts, may increase sedative side effects of drugs. Do not use if you are hypoglycemic or undergoing anticonvulsant therapy.
St. John's wort (*Hypericum perforatum*)	Do not use with antidepressants without medical supervision. Avoid overexposure to direct sunlight; may cause photosensitivity.
Saw palmetto (*Serenoa repens*)	Consult your doctor before using to treat enlarged prostate.
Schisandra (*Schisandra chinensis*)	None; generally regarded as safe.
Senna (*Cassia senna*)	Do not use if you have a bowel obstruction. Take 1 hour after other drugs, and take with at least 8 ounces of water.
Shepherd's purse (*Capsella bursa-pastoris*)	Do not use if you have a history of kidney stones.
Shiitake (*Lentinus edodes*)	None; generally regarded as safe.
Siberian ginseng (*Eleutherococcus senticosus*)	None; generally regarded as safe.
Skullcap (*Scutellaria laterifolia*)	None; generally regarded as safe.
Slippery elm (*Ulmus rubra*)	None; generally regarded as safe.
Spearmint (*Mentha spicata*)	None; generally regarded as safe.
Stevia (*Stevia rebaudiana*)	None; generally regarded as safe.
Tea (*Camellia sinensis*)	Green tea is generally regarded as safe. Fermented black tea is not recommended for excessive or long-term use because it can stimulate the nervous system.

Herb	Cautions and Safety Guidelines
Thyme (*Thymus vulgaris*)	None; generally regarded as safe.
Tribulus (*Tribulus terrestris*)	None; generally regarded as safe.
Turmeric (*Curcuma domestica*)	Generally regarded as safe when used as a spice. Do not use in therapeutic amounts as a home remedy if you have high levels of stomach acid, ulcers, gallstones, or bile duct obstruction.
Usnea (*Usnea barbata*)	None; generally regarded as safe.
Uva-ursi (*Arctostaphylos uva-ursi*)	Do not use for more than 2 weeks without the supervision of a qualified health-care practitioner. Do not use if you have kidney disease; it contains tannins, which may cause further damage. May cause stomach irritation.
Valerian (*Valeriana officinalis*)	Do not use with sleep-enhancing or mood-regulating medications; it may intensify their effects. May cause heart palpitations and nervousness in sensitive individuals. If such stimulant action occurs, discontinue use.
Vervain (*Verbena officinalis*)	None; generally regarded as safe.
Wheat grass (*Triticum aestivum*)	None; generally regarded as safe.
White oak (*Quercus alba*)	Do not use topically if you have extensive skin damage. Do not use internally for more than several days at a time.
White willow (*Salix alba*)	Do not use if you need to avoid aspirin, especially if you are taking anticoagulant (blood-thinning) medication such as warfarin (Coumadin); its active ingredient is related to aspirin. May interact with barbiturates or sedatives such as aprobarbital (Amytal) or alprazolam (Xanax). May cause stomach irritation when consumed with alcohol.

Herb	Cautions and Safety Guidelines
Wild cherry (*Prunus serotina*)	Not recommended for long-term use. Do not exceed the recommended dose.
Wild indigo (*Baptisia tinctoria*)	Not recommended for long-term use, except under the supervision of a qualified health-care practitioner. May cause vomiting and diarrhea in doses larger than 10 drops of tincture taken three times daily.
Wild yam (*Dioscorea villosa*)	None; generally regarded as safe.
Witch hazel (*Hamamelis virginiana*)	None; generally regarded as safe.
Wood betony (*Stachys officinalis*)	None; generally regarded as safe.
Yarrow (*Achillea millefolium*)	Generally regarded as safe. Rarely, handling the flowers may cause a skin rash.
Yellow dock (*Rumex crispus*)	Do not use without medical supervision if you have a history of kidney stones; it contains oxalates and tannins that may aggravate this condition.
Yucca (*Yucca* spp.)	None; generally regarded as safe.

SAFE USE OF ESSENTIAL OILS IN THIS BOOK

*U*sing essential oils is a common and highly effective way to tap the healing power of herbs, but if you've never used oils before, it pays to follow some commonsense guidelines.

Essential oils are inhaled or placed on the skin but are never taken internally because they are so concentrated that they can be toxic.

You should never apply essential oils undiluted unless instructed otherwise. Dilute them in a neutral base, which can be an oil (such as almond), a cream, or a gel, before application. Many essential oils may cause skin irritation or allergic reactions in people with sensitive skin.

Always do a patch test before applying any new oil to your skin. Put a few drops of diluted oil on the back of your wrist and wait for an hour or more. If irritation or redness occurs, bathe the area with cold water. For future use, prepare a dilution with half the amount of essential oil or avoid it altogether.

As with herbs, if you are pregnant or nursing, do not use essential oils without first consulting your doctor. Store your oils in dark bottles, away from light and heat and out of the reach of children and pets. By familiarizing yourself with the list that follows, you can use the remedies in this book with confidence.

Essential Oil	Cautions and Safety Guidelines
Basil (*Ocimum basilicum*)	Do not use for more than 2 weeks without the guidance of a qualified health-care practitioner.
Bay laurel (*Laurus nobilis*)	Do not use for more than 2 weeks without the guidance of a qualified health-care practitioner. May cause lethargy and unconsciousness.

Essential Oil	Cautions and Safety Guidelines
Bergamot (*Citrus bergamia*)	Avoid direct sunlight after topical application; may cause photosensitivity (except with bergapten-free types).
Clove (*Syzygium aromaticum*)	Do not use for more than 2 weeks without the guidance of a qualified health-care practitioner. May be used undiluted for tooth pain.
Eucalyptus (*Eucalyptus* spp.)	Do not use for more than 2 weeks without the guidance of a qualified health-care practitioner.
Ginger (*Zingiber officinale*)	Avoid direct sunlight after topical application; may cause photosensitivity.
Juniper (*Juniperus communis*)	Do not use for more than 2 weeks without the guidance of a qualified health-care practitioner. Do not use if you have kidney disease.
Lavender (*Lavandula* spp.)	May be used undiluted, but do not get it near your eyes.
Lemon (*Citrus limon*)	Avoid direct sunlight after topical application; may cause photosensitivity.
Orange (*Citrus* spp.)	Avoid direct sunlight after topical application; may cause photosensitivity.
Peppermint (*Mentha piperita*)	Do not use more than 3 drops in bathwater. May be used internally, but ingestion may lead to stomach upset in sensitive individuals. Do not use without medical supervision if you have gallbladder or liver disease.
Rosemary (*Rosmarinus officinalis*)	Do not use if you have high blood pressure or epilepsy.
Tagetes (*Tagetes minuta*)	Do not use for more than 2 weeks without the guidance of a qualified health-care practitioner.
Tea tree (*Melaleuca alternifolia*)	May be applied undiluted to the skin.
Thyme (*Thymus vulgaris*)	Do not use red thyme. Do not use white and common thyme if you have high blood pressure.
Ylang ylang (*Cananga odorata*)	Use in moderation; its strong smell may cause nausea or headaches.

WHERE TO FIND THE BEST HERBS

*Y*ou may find all the herbs and herbal products you need in your local health food store, herb specialty store, or aromatherapy shop. These days, herbs are even crowding the shelves of supermarkets, drugstores, and large discount chain stores. Still, there may be times when you cannot find exactly what you need. A product may be out of stock, or an unusual herb may not be available.

Luckily, there is a wealth of mail-order suppliers that carry everything from bulk herbs (including Chinese and Ayurvedic herbs) to herb capsules and exotic essential oils. This resource guide represents just a sampling of the many companies that carry herbal products and supplies.

The fact that a company is listed does not imply an endorsement. Also, this list is not all-inclusive: If a company has been omitted, that doesn't mean that it's not reputable. Rather, this directory is provided to point you in the right direction and give you an idea of the types of products available. The descriptions included here are just an overview; many of these companies carry additional items.

To request catalogs, write to the addresses below or call directory assistance for phone numbers. Some companies may charge a small fee for their catalogs. Many companies also have Web sites on the Internet.

Aroma Vera
5901 Rodeo Road
Los Angeles, CA 90016-4312
Essential oils and spa products.

Avena Botanicals
219 Mill Street
Rockport, ME 04856
Tinctures (extracts), infused oils, bulk herbs, and books.

Ayurveda Holistic Center
82-A Bayville Avenue
Bayville, NY 11709
Ayurvedic dried herbs and herbal blends.

Black Kat Herbals
P.O. Box 271
Smithville, TN 37166
Tinctures, capsules, salves, teas, herbal soaps, and massage oils.

Blessed Herbs
109 Barre Plains Road
Oakham, MA 01068
Bulk herbs, liquid extracts, and skin-care products.

Catskill Mountain Herbals
P.O. Box 1426
Olive Bridge, NY 12461
Tinctures, infused oils, salves, and some dried herbs.

Cheryl's Herbs
836 Hanley Industrial Court
St. Louis, MO 63144
Essential oils, aromatherapy products, and dried herbs.

The Chopra Center for Well-Being
7630 Fay Avenue
La Jolla, CA 92037
Books, audio and video tapes, Ayurvedic herbal formulas as tablets and jam, massage oils, teas, and skin-care products.

Dancing Willow Herbs
960 Main Avenue
Durango, CO 81301
Full-strength tinctures.

Devonshire Apothecary
2105 Ashby Avenue
Austin, TX 78704
Tinctures, teas, salves, and books.

Dragon River Herbals
P.O. Box 28
El Rito, NM 87530
Tinctures.

Dry Creek Herb Farm and Learning Center
13935 Dry Creek Road
Auburn, CA 95602
Bulk herbs, tea blends, books, tapes, tinctures, essential oils, and skin-care products.

Earth Essentials
6349 Filbert Avenue
Orangevale, CA 95662
Essential oils and skin blends.

East Earth Herb, Inc.
P.O. Box 2802
Eugene, OR 97402
Tablets and tinctures.

East Earth Trade Winds
P.O. Box 493151
Redding, CA 96049-3151
Chinese herbal products, dried herbs, essential oils and books, tea, and teapots.

Eclectic Institute, Inc.
14385 Southeast Lusted Road
Sandy, OR 97055-9549
Tinctures, freeze-dried herbs in capsules and chewable herb tablets, and medicinal mushrooms.

Fragrant Earth
c/o Samarkand Trading Company
4925 6th Avenue, NW
Maysville, WA 98271
Essential oils.

The Fragrant Garden
P.O. Box 281
Port Perry, ON L9L 1A3
Canada
Essential oils, dried herbs, and body-care products.

Frontier Natural Products Co-op
P.O. Box 299
Norway, IA 52318
Dried herbs, tinctures, herb capsules, salves, essential oils, Chinese herb teas, and skin- and hair-care products.

The Gaia Garden Herbal Dispensary
2672 West Broadway
Vancouver, BC V6K 2G3
Canada
Tinctures, dried herbs, supplements, capsules, vitamins, essential oils, salves, skin- and hair-care products, and books.

Gaia Herbs
108 Island Ford Road
Brevard, NC 28712
Tinctures, including Ayurvedic, Chinese, and rain forest liquid herbal extracts; solid extracts; salves and infused oils; and phytocaps.

Ginseng Select Products, Inc.
611 Druid Road East, Suite 711
Clearwater, FL 33756
Ginseng in many forms; no laboratory products used.

Green Terrestrial Herbs
Warm Brooke Road
Arlington, VT 05250
Infused oils, salves, herbal tea blends, and dried herbs.

Healing Spirits Organically Grown and Wildcrafted Medicinal Herbs
9198 State Route 415
Avoca, NY 14809
Dried and fresh herbs by special order.

Herbalist and Alchemist
51 South Wandling Avenue
Washington, NJ 07882
Tinctures, including Chinese, Ayurvedic, and mushroom extracts; dried Chinese herbs and tea blends; infused oils and ointments; and books.

Herbally Yours, Inc.
P.O. Box 26
Changewater, NJ 07831
Skin- and hair-care products, essential oils, cosmetics ingredients, dried herbs, tea blends, tinctures, and books.

The Herb Cupboard
113 Pittsburg Street
Scottsdale, PA 15683
Tinctures, capsules, salves, teas, body-care products, and books.

The Herb Farm
13 Wayne Court
Quispamsis, NB E2G 1E0
Canada
Dried herbs and tea blends.

The Herb Garden
P.O. Box 773-RD
Pilot Mountain, NC 27041
Herb plants.

Herb Hill
71 Ferris Lane
Poughkeepsie, NY 12601
Herbal salves and skin-care products.

Herb Pharm
P.O. Box 116
Williams, OR 97544
Liquid extracts, herbal oils, and books.

The Herb Shoppe
4372 Chris Greene Lake Road
Charlottesville, VA 22911
Dried herbs, including Chinese herbs and custom-order combinations; special-order Ayurvedic herbs and formulas; herbal oils; liniments; and Ayurvedic beauty products.

HomeHealth
1233 Montauk Highway
P.O. Box 9007
Oakdale, NY 11769-9007
Herb supplements, skin- and hair-care products, vitamins, and minerals.

Indiana Botanic Gardens, Inc.
3401 West 37th Avenue
Hobart, IN 46342
Dried herbs, teas, essential oils, and books.

Indian River Herb Farm
RD #4, Box 268A
Riverdale Park
Millsboro, DE 19966
Teas, tinctures, dried herbs, capsules, and aromatherapy products.

Lin Sister Herb Shop, Inc.
4 Bowery
New York, NY 10013
Chinese herbal remedies.

Materia Medica, LLC
4940 Pan American Freeway, NE
Albuquerque, NM 87109
Tinctures, creams, capsules, tablets, essential oils, and vegetable oils.

Mountain Herbals
7 Langdon Street
Montpelier, VT 05602-2908
Dried herbs and tinctures.

Mountain Rose Herbs
20818 High Street
North San Juan, CA 95960
Infused oils, tinctures, essential oils, vegetable oils, and dried herbs.

Mountain Spirit
P.O. Box 368
Port Townsend, WA 98368
Tinctures, teas, bulk herbs, bath herbs, and massage oils.

National College of Naturopathic Medicine
Natural Health Centers
11231 Southeast Market Street
Portland, OR 97216
Tinctures, capsules, dried herbs, and essential oils.

Nature's Meadow
P.O. Box 510
Gainesville, MO 65655
Tinctures.

Original Swiss Aromatics
P.O. Box 6842
San Rafael, CA 94903
Essential oils and facial and massage oils.

Pacific Botanicals
4350 Fish Hatchery Road
Grants Pass, OR 97527
Certified organic fresh and dried herbs, spices, and sea vegetables.

Puritan's Pride
1233 Montauk Highway
P.O. Box 9001
Oakdale, NY 11769-9001
Herb supplements, skin- and hair-care products, vitamins, and minerals.

Raven's Nest Herbals
P.O. Box 370
Duluth, GA 30096
Custom-blended dried herbs and oils.

Sage Mountain Herbs
P.O. Box 420
East Barre, VT 05649
Tinctures, herbal formulas in capsules, and beauty products. (Also an herbal education center.)

Sage Woman Herbs
206-B South 8th Street
Colorado Springs, CO 80905
Herbal formulas in capsules, tea blends, dried herbs, tinctures, vegetable oils, salves, and skin- and hair-care products.

San Francisco Herb Company
250 14th Street
San Francisco, CA 94103
Dried herbs.

Ten Ren Tea and Ginseng Company
5817 8th Avenue
Brooklyn, NY 11220
135-18 Roosevelt Avenue
Flushing, NY 11354
825-G Rockville Pike
Rockview, MD 20852
Ginseng and Chinese teas.

Turtle Island Herbs
2825 Wilderness Place, Suite 350
Boulder, CO 80301
Tinctures, syrups, and salves.

The Ultimate Herb and Spice Shoppe
Box 395
Duenweg, MO 64841
Dried herbs and massage oils.

Unitea Herbs
1705 14th Street, Suite 318
Boulder, CO 80302
Tea blends.

The Vitamin Shoppe
4700 Westside Avenue
North Bergen, NJ 07047
Tinctures and herb capsules.

Western Botanicals
7122 Almond Avenue
Orangevale, CA 95662
Herbal formulas in capsules, teas, tinctures, and massage oils; also some dried herbs.

Wild Weeds
1302 Camp Weott Road
Ferndale, CA 95536
Tea blends, herbal salves and oils, skin- and hair-care products, tinctures, dried herbs, essential oils, books, and packaging for herbs.

Wise Woman Herbals
P.O. Box 279
Creswell, OR 97426
Tinctures, salves, solid extracts, capsules, suppositories, herbal oils, and essential oils.

INDEX

Underscored page references indicate boxed text and tables.

D

Damiana
    safety guidelines for, 552
    for treating
        erection problems, 212
        low sex drive, 338–39
Dandelion
    Dandy De-Itching Dandelion Coffee,
        435
    for preventing osteoporosis, 389
    safety guidelines for, 552
    for treating
        carpal tunnel syndrome, 140
        fibrocystic breasts, 220–21
        fibroids, 222–23
        hangover, 259
        high cholesterol, 278
        kidney stones, 326
        premenstrual syndrome, 426
        tick bites, 490
        urinary tract infections, in pets,
            413–14
        warts, 533
Dandruff, 186–88
    Fast Facts, 187
    treating, with
        nettle, horsetail, Johnny jump-up, and
            lavender, 187–88
        tea tree, 186–87
Dang gui
    safety guidelines for, 552
    for treating
        low sex drive, 339
        menstrual cramps, 353–54
        menstrual irregularities, 356–57
Deodorant, herbal, 103
Depression, mild. See Blues, the
Dermatitis. See Eczema and dermatitis
Devil's claw
    for premenstrual syndrome, 425–26
    safety guidelines for, 552
Diabetes, 188–95
    Fast Facts, 194
    treating, with
        Asian ginseng, 191–92
        bilberry, 194–95
        bitter melon, 191
        cinnamon, 192–93
        flaxseed, 193
        ginkgo, 195
        Gymnema sylvestre, 192
        prickly pear, 193

Diarrhea, 195–98
    Fast Facts, 197
    treating, with
        black tea, 197–98
        carrot, 198
        cinnamon, 197
        cinquefoil, 196
        green tea, 197–98
        slippery elm, 198
Dizziness. See Vertigo
Doctrine of Signatures, in herbal medicine,
    113
Douche, for yeast infections, 544–45
Dry hair, 199–201
    Fast Facts, 200
    treating, with
        jojoba, 199–200
        lavender, 200–201
        rosemary, 200–201
        sandalwood, 200–201
        sweet almond, 199–200
Dry hands. See Chapped or dry hands
Dry skin, 201–5
    Fast Facts, 204
    treating, with
        calendula, 203–4
        chamomile, 205
        flaxseed, 202
        glycerin and rosewater, 202–3
        Happy Hands Oil, 203
        lemon balm, 205
        olive oil, 204–5
        peppermint, 205

E

Eardrops, for swimmer's ear, 485–86
Echinacea
    Cold-Sore-No-More Herbal Helper, 151
    Home Run Allergy Relief, 53
    safety guidelines for, 552
    for herbal starter kit, 22
    Superstar Flu Decoctail, 231
    for treating
        boils, 105
        bronchitis, 109–11
        canker sores, 135, 136
        colds, 154, 156–57
        cold sores, 150
        cough, 180
        flu, 230–32
        gingivitis, 250
        laryngitis, 330

G

Garcinia cambogia, avoiding, in weight-loss
    formulas, <u>393</u>

Garlic
  Ginger-Garlic Super Soup, <u>155</u>
  safety guidelines for, <u>553</u>
  for herbal starter kit, <u>22</u>
  for treating
    angina, 59
    athlete's foot, 78–79
    bronchitis, 111
    flu, 232–33
    food poisoning, 237–38
    foot odor, 242–43
    high blood pressure, 271
    high cholesterol, 275–76
    insect bites and stings, 298–99
    intermittent claudication, 308–9
    low immunity, 337
    nail fungus, 369
    shingles, 448
    sinusitis, 451
    sties and chalazia, 460
    swimmer's ear, 485–86
    Type A personality, 501–2
    ulcers, 506
    vertigo, 523–24
    worms, in pets, 415

Gas. *See* Flatulence

Gastroesophageal reflux disease (GERD).
    See Heartburn

Gentian
  Bitters-to-Burn Beverage, <u>395</u>
  safety guidelines for, <u>553</u>
  for treating
    eczema and dermatitis, 208–9
    heartburn, 266
    underweight, 510

Geranium
  Burnout Blend, <u>119</u>
  for treating
    burnout, 119
    menstrual cramps, 354
    premenstrual syndrome, 427

GERD. *See* Heartburn

German chamomile, for treating
  ulcers, 506–7
  vomiting, 527

Ginger
  Anti-Ulcer Fruit Cocktail, <u>505</u>
  Bitters-to-Burn Beverage, <u>395</u>
  Distress Express Fizz, <u>364</u>
  Ginger-Garlic Super Soup, <u>155</u>
  Herbal Sprain Soother, <u>464</u>
  for preventing osteoporosis, 390
  safety guidelines for, <u>553</u>, <u>563</u>
  for herbal starter kit, <u>23</u>
  Superstar Flu Decoctail, <u>231</u>
  Take-Five Cramp Relief, <u>352</u>
  for treating
    aches and pains, 40
    angina, 60–61
    arthritis, 68
    boils, 106–7
    burping, 125–26
    cold hands and feet, 147–48
    fatigue, 217
    food poisoning, 240
    forgetfulness, <u>246</u>, 247–48
    gout, 253–54
    hangover, 258
    heartburn, 264
    infertility in men, 288
    inflammatory bowel disease, 296
    irritable bowel syndrome, 314
    jet lag, 319–20
    menstrual cramps, 351, 354
    motion sickness, 364
    nausea, 370–71
    sore throat, 458
    stomachaches, 461
    varicose veins, 521
    vertigo, 523, 525
    vomiting, 527–28

Gingivitis, 248–52
  Fast Facts, <u>251</u>
  treating, with
    echinacea, 250
    goldenseal, 250–51
    goldenseal, myrrh, and aloe, 251–52
    In-the-Pink Gum Swab, <u>249</u>
    myrrh, 251
    propolis, 252
    rosemary, thyme, peppermint, and
      myrrh, 252

Ginkgo
  safety guidelines for, <u>554</u>
  for herbal starter kit, <u>23</u>
  for treating
    angina, 59–60
    anxiety, 64
    asthma, 73–74
    the blues, 101
    cold hands and feet, 148–49
    diabetes, 194–95

Partridgeberry
  for infertility in women, 292
  Perimenopausal Relief Tincture Tonic, 346
  safety guidelines for, 557
Passionflower
  safety guidelines for, 557
  for treating
    anxiety, 64
    burnout, 118–19
    carpal tunnel syndrome, 139–40
    insomnia, 304
    jet lag, 318–19
    poison plant rashes, 422–23
    stress, 470–71
Pau d'arco
  safety guidelines for, 557
  for treating
    nail fungus, 368
    rectal itch, 440–41
Peanut oil, for dry skin, 203
Pear juice
  Slippery Elm Soother, 455
Pennyroyal
  Aromatic Flea Repellent, 404
  safety guidelines for, 558
Peppermint
  Aromatic Flea Repellent, 404
  Five-Herb Gas-Blasting Tea, 225
  Herbal Sprain Soother, 464
  Pain-Pacifying Compress, 82
  safety guidelines for, 558, 563
  for treating
    aches and pains, 40–41
    back pain, 84
    bad breath, 86–87
    burping, 124–25
    colds, 157–58
    commuter fatigue, 159–60
    dry skin, 205
    flatulence, 224–25
    flu, 229–30, 233
    forgetfulness, 246
    gingivitis, 249, 252
    headaches, 260–61, 262–63
    insect bites and stings, 299–300
    irritable bowel syndrome, 314
    jet lag, 20
    motion sickness, 363
    nausea, 372
    poison plant rashes, 421–22
    sinusitis, 449–50
    sore throat, 456
    stomachaches, 461–62

strains and sprains, 467–68
sunburn, 477–78
toothache, 494
vertigo, 523
vomiting, 529
Pet problems, 397–415
  anxiety, 398–99
  arthritis, 400–402
  bad breath, 402–3
  dosage recommendations for, 410
  fleas, 403–5
  hairballs, 405–6
  hot spots, 406–8
  itching, 408–9
  overweight, 409, 411–12
  urinary tract infections, 412–14
  when to see the vet about, 401
  worms, 414–15
Phlebitis, 415–19
  Fast Facts, 418
  treating, with
    arnica, 417
    bromelain, 418–19
    calendula, yarrow, and echinacea, 417–18
    horse chestnut and calendula, 416–17
    white oak, 418
Pine
  safety guidelines for, 558
  for treating
    bursitis and tendinitis, 130
    macular degeneration, 342–43
Pineapple
  Anti-Ulcer Fruit Cocktail, 505
Pipsissewa
  safety guidelines for, 558
  for urinary tract infections, 512–13
Plantain
  Chanchal's Tonic Tea for the Lungs, 109
  safety guidelines for, 558
  for treating
    blisters, 92
    hot spots, in dogs, 407
    itching, in pets, 408
    tick bites, 488
PMS. See Premenstrual syndrome
Poison plant rashes, 419–23
  Fast Facts, 422
  treating, with
    jewelweed, 420–21
    oats, 421
    passionflower, oats, skullcap, and St.
      John's wort, 422–23
    peppermint, 421–22

Reishi
   safety guidelines for, <u>558</u>
   for treating
      hangover, 259
      high blood pressure, 272
      low immunity, 336–37
Rhubarb, safety guidelines for, <u>558</u>
Rice, for oily skin, 383–84
Robert's Formula, for inflammatory bowel
      disease, 295–96
Rocky Mountain spotted fever, from tick
      bites, 487, <u>489</u>
Romaine lettuce, for treating
   irritability, 312–13
   Type A personality, 502
Roman chamomile
   Victoria's Anti-Ballistic Formula, <u>310</u>
Rose
   Herbal Sleepytime Pillow, <u>303</u>
   safety guidelines for, <u>558</u>
   for treating
      dry skin, 202–3
      oily skin, 386–87
Rose hips
   for bruises, 115
   safety guidelines for, <u>559</u>
Rosemary
   safety guidelines for, <u>559</u>, <u>563</u>
   for treating
      aches and pains, 40–41
      back pain, 84
      bursitis and tendinitis, 127–28
      concentration problems, 167
      cuts and scrapes, 183–84
      dry hair, 200–201
      forgetfulness, 246
      gingivitis, 252
      jet lag, 320
      laryngitis, 331–32
      migraine, 361
      oily hair, 381–82
      sinusitis, 449–50
      strains and sprains, 467–68
      stuffy nose, 473–74
      vertigo, 522–23
   Victoria's Aromatic Foot Powder, <u>77</u>

S

Safety guidelines
   for essential oils, 562, <u>562–63</u>
   for herbs, 547, <u>548–61</u>

Sage
   safety guidelines for, <u>559</u>
   for treating
      acne, 44–45
      body odor, 103
      canker sores, 136
      colds, 156
      laryngitis, 331–32
      menopausal problems,
         345–46
      oily skin, 385
      sore throat, 456–57
      stuffy nose, 473–74
Salves, herbal, 20
Sandalwood, for treating
   arthritis, <u>67</u>
   dry hair, 200–201
San qi ginseng, for promoting surgery
      recovery, 480–81
Saw palmetto
   safety guidelines for, <u>559</u>
   for treating
      erection problems, 212–13
      kidney stones, 328
      prostate problems, 430–31
Scars, 441–44
   Fast Facts, <u>443</u>
   treating, with
      bromelain, 444
      calendula, 442–43
      calendula and cottonwood,
         444
      gotu kola, 443
Schisandra
   safety guidelines for, <u>559</u>
   for treating
      burnout, 117
      Type A personality, 501
Scrapes. *See* Cuts and scrapes
Senna
   for constipation, 169–70
   safety guidelines for, <u>559</u>
Sex drive, low. *See* Low sex
      drive
Shepherd's purse
   safety guidelines for, <u>559</u>
   for treating
      cuts and scrapes, 181
      nosebleeds, 378
Shiitake
   for low immunity, 335–36
   safety guidelines for, <u>559</u>